Physical Activity and Public Health Practice

Physical Activity and Public Health Practice

Edited by
Barbara E. Ainsworth and Caroline A. Macera

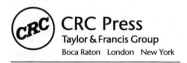

CRC Press
Taylor & Francis Group
Boca Raton   London   New York

CRC Press is an imprint of the
Taylor & Francis Group, an **informa** business

CRC Press
Taylor & Francis Group
6000 Broken Sound Parkway NW, Suite 300
Boca Raton, FL 33487-2742

Printed in the United States of America on acid-free paper
Version Date: 20120123

International Standard Book Number: 978-1-4398-4951-4 (Hardback)

**Visit the Taylor & Francis Web site at
http://www.taylorandfrancis.com**

**and the CRC Press Web site at
http://www.crcpress.com**

Contents

Preface

PHYSICAL INACTIVITY AS A PUBLIC HEALTH PROBLEM: CHALLENGES AND OPPORTUNITIES

INTRODUCTION

Physical inactivity is an emerging public health concern worldwide. Many adults and children are not active at health-enhancing levels. This situation provides a great opportunity to improve population health by increasing levels of physical activity. Health is a dynamic state influenced by multiple influences including personal, social, cultural, institutional, and environmental factors. Although this poses a challenge in understanding how these factors influence physical activity in ways that constrain individuals' choices to become and remain active, the opportunities of an active society are seen in reduced morbidity and mortality due to physical inactivity.

The World Health Organization (WHO) defines health as "a state of complete physical, mental, and social well-being, not merely the absence of disease or infirmity" (World Health Organization 2011). As the world's leading public health agency, WHO sets the agenda for activities to prevent diseases, prolong life, and promote health and efficiency through organized community action. As such, public health has the charge to address threats to health among people in developing countries and in developed countries. The scope of public health is broad; it aims to modify the social conditions resulting in disease and injury and promote activities to assure community conditions that are conducive to well-being. Many of the conveniences taken for granted in developed countries, such as clean water, sanitation services, and control of communicable diseases, can be attributed to organized public health efforts. Public health practice focuses on two levels to assure the community's health. Activities that require no action are termed "passive protection" and include water treatment, legislative smoking bans, and preservation of food quality. Activities designed to ensure health that require action by an individual are termed "active protection." These include laws requiring motorcyclists and bicyclists to wear helmets and people in cars to wear seat belts. Engaging in regular physical activity is a form of active protection in that it requires effort by an individual to ensure health benefits.

PHYSICAL ACTIVITY AND PUBLIC HEALTH

Over the past century, many advances in public health have been documented, and during the last half of the twentieth century, physical activity became recognized as a major health-enhancing behavior. Surveillance to identify physical activity levels in populations began in the 1970s and 1980s and continue to the present day. During this time, physical inactivity was identified as a major risk factor for coronary heart disease with equal strength as previously recognized risk factors of cigarette smoking, hypertension, and hypercholesterolemia (Fletcher et al. 1992). In 1995, the U.S. Centers for Disease Control and Prevention and the American College of Sports Medicine issued a consensus statement on the value of regular, moderate intensity physical activity as a health-enhancing behavior for the prevention of many chronic diseases (Pate et al. 1995), which led to the first U.S. Surgeon General's Report on Physical Activity and Health, released in 1996 (U.S. Department of Health and Human Services 1996). In 2008, the U.S. government updated the physical activity guidelines for children, adults, and older adults (U.S. Department of Health and Human Services 2011). Since the turn of the twenty-first century, recognition of the health promoting benefits of physical activity has occurred globally.

PHYSICAL INACTIVITY AS A PUBLIC HEALTH PROBLEM

Criteria have been used to identify the breadth of physical inactivity as a public health problem instead of merely a social or popular cultural issue. Four criteria will be discussed to answer the question: "Is physical inactivity a public health problem?"

1. Physical inactivity crosses geographic, political, and other boundaries. Differences in physical activity by race and ethnicity, cultural traditions, economic and educational strata, and geographic boundaries suggest a widespread condition not limited to a single population group or geographic location. Data are consistent that physical inactivity is higher in women than men, graded by educational attainment and social class, and influenced by cultures and traditions.

2. Physical inactivity affects the health, function, and well-being of a large number of people. Physical inactivity is causally associated with many types of chronic diseases, including coronary heart disease, type 2 diabetes, colon cancer, breast cancer, and potentially disabling conditions of overweight and obesity, depression, osteoporosis, and frailty among older adults (U.S. Department of Health and Human Services 2011). Globally, 1.9 million deaths are attributed to physical inactivity, a number which could be eliminated if all persons received at least 150 minutes per week of moderate and vigorous intensity physical activity (Lopez et al. 2006).

3. The causal mechanisms of physical inactivity, which involves a large number of people, are unknown. While a great deal is known about the causal mechanisms for the effects of physical activity on health and disease conditions, little is known about the many possible factors that contribute to sedentary lifestyles. How do age, sex, body mass, and self-efficacy influence decisions to be active or sedentary? Can social support, cultural traditions, and family dynamics help people to be more active? Or do they inhibit physical activity for selected individuals? Are worksite policies and access to recreational areas effective in promoting decisions to be physically active? And how do the urban form, transportation choices, and legislative mandates affect how people make choices to live active or sedentary lives? These are difficult questions, but it is essential to know the answers for effective promotion of physical activity at the community level.

4. Physical inactivity will get worse if it is not addressed as a community responsibility. A hallmark of the public health approach to preventing disease and ensuring good health is that a public health problem must be addressed at the community level and as a community responsibility. Community efforts reflect the sum of individuals, groups, institutions, organizations, and governments within cities, towns, and villages to act in coordination for optimal results. Physical activity surveillance in England shows a steady increase in the proportion of adults who meet their physical activity recommendations, increasing from 20% to 25% in women and 33% to 40% in men from 1997 to 2006 (Craig and Mindell 2008). This reflects a tremendous effort from government and volunteer groups to intentionally increase opportunities for physical activity. While a 5% increase in the prevalence of physically activity may not seem very large, every 1% decrease in sedentary behaviors can translate into thousands of lives saved from a chronic disease diagnosis or early mortality.

COMMUNITY PHYSICAL ACTIVITY PROGRAMS

Public health problems are best solved with coordinated, community approaches. An example of a community physical activity promotion project that has had a global influence on the promotion of physical activity is called Agita São Paulo (Agita São Paulo 2011). Led by Dr. Victor Matsudo, Agita São Paulo was launched in 1996 to encourage physical activity as a way of life in Brazil. At the start of the program, nearly 70% to 80% of residents in São Paulo, a city of 34.7 million people, did not meet the state's recommendation for 30 minutes per day and 5 days per week of moderate intensity physical activity. The program was so successful that it was exported to other states in Brazil, other countries in South America, and ultimately adopted by WHO as a network. The Agita Mundo Network (Move for Health for All) includes 59 countries and 263 member institutions.

From research performed in the past 50 years, we have learned a great deal about the health benefits of regular physical activity and of enhanced physical fitness (U.S. Department of Health and Human Services 2011). Almost all disease risks can be reduced by living a lifestyle with regular periods of moderate and/or vigorous physical activity. However, we remain challenged with identifying the best approaches to encouraging people to initiate and maintain active lifestyles on a regular basis.

SUMMARY

The philosophy of public health is that preventable death and disability ought to be minimized; that activities are conducted as an ethical enterprise as an agent for social change; and that change is made in the face of superstition, ignorance, public apathy, political interference, and with inadequate resources. We act as public health professionals to increase physical activity for community citizens because it is the right thing to do, not because it is the popular thing to do. As such, it is a goal of all physical activity health promotion advocates to increase the opportunity for citizens of any city and state to live active, healthy lives.

This book is a summary of the latest scientific research in the area of physical activity and health and is designed to guide public health practitioners and public health researchers. The 18 chapters in this book provide a comprehensive review of the field of physical activity starting with a historical approach and the latest information on physiological adaptation to physical activity and the unique contribution of sedentary behavior to overall health. This book also includes chapters describing the role of physical activity in the prevention and treatment of chronic disease as well as its role in relation to growth and development, among healthy adults and older adults, and in relation to obesity. Also covered are practical aspects such as measurement, national recommendations, and surveillance. The final chapters focus on promoting physical activity among hard to reach populations, worksites, and schools, as well as the contribution of the built environment and policy decisions in promoting physical activity.

Barbara E. Ainsworth
Caroline A. Macera

REFERENCES

Agita São Paulo. Promoting Physical Activity in São Paulo, Brazil. http://www.agitasp.org.br/ (accessed on June 23, 2011).

Craig, R., and J. Mindell. 2008. *Health Survey for England—2006. Volume 1—Cardiovascular Disease and Risk Factors in Adults*. Leeds, UK: The Information Center.

Fletcher, G. F., S. N. Blair, J. Blumenthal et al. 1992. Statement on exercise. Benefits and recommendations for physical activity programs for all Americans. A statement for health professionals by the Committee on Exercise and Cardiac Rehabilitation of the Council on Clinical Cardiology, American Heart Association. *Circulation* 86: 340–344.

Lopez, A. D., C. D. Mathers, M. Ezzati et al., eds. 2006. *Global Burden of Disease and Risk Factors*. New York: Oxford University Press.

Pate, R. R., M. Pratt, S. N. Blair et al. 1995. Physical activity and public health: A recommendation from the Centers for Disease Control and Prevention and the American College of Sports Medicine. *JAMA* 273: 402–427.

U.S. Department of Health and Human Services. 1996. Surgeon General's Report on Physical Activity and Health. Washington, DC: US Government Printing Office, 1996.

U.S. Department of Health and Human Services. 2008 Physical Activity Guidelines for Americans. Available at http://health.gov/PAGuidelines/ (accessed June 23, 2011).

World Health Organization. Definition of health. Available at: http://www.who.int/governance/eb/who_constitution_en.pdf (accessed June 23, 2011).

Editors

Barbara E. Ainsworth, PhD, MPH, FACSM, FNAK, is a professor in the Exercise and Wellness Program within the School of Nutrition and Health Promotion at Arizona State University (ASU). Dr. Ainsworth received her graduate degrees in exercise physiology and epidemiology from the University of Minnesota. Her research relates to physical activity and public health with focuses on the assessment of physical activity in populations, the evaluation of physical activity questionnaires, and physical activity in women. Dr. Ainsworth is best known as the lead author for the Compendium of Physical Activities, an exhaustive list of the energy cost of human physical activities. With more than 200 publications, Dr. Ainsworth is a fellow in the American College of Sports Medicine (ACSM); the Research Consortium of American Alliance for Health, Physical Education, Recreation and Dance; the National Academy of Kinesiology; and the North American Society of Health, Physical Education, Recreation and Dance Professionals. She serves on the editorial board of several journals and has lectured in many countries. Dr. Ainsworth holds honorary academic appointments at the Karolinska Institute in Stockholm, Sweden, and the Akershaus University College in Oslo, Norway. She has served as president for the ACSM and was a 2006 ACSM Citation Award recipient. Her teaching assignment at ASU includes graduate courses on research methods, physical activity and public health, and physical activity epidemiology.

Caroline A. Macera, PhD, is a professor of epidemiology and associate director at the Graduate School of Public Health at San Diego State University. Dr. Macera received her training in epidemiology from the University of California at Berkeley and taught at the University of South Carolina for 17 years before joining the Centers for Disease Control and Prevention as a team leader for surveillance and epidemiology in the Physical Activity and Health Branch. During this time, she was involved in developing the Healthy People 2010 physical activity and fitness objectives. Dr. Macera has more than 30 years' experience as an epidemiologist and is a fellow of the ACSM. She is also a member of the American Public Health Association, the Society for Epidemiology Research, and the American College of Epidemiology, and serves on the editorial board of the *Journal of Physical Activity and Health*. She has more than 200 publications (peer-reviewed manuscripts, commentaries, and book chapters) in the fields of epidemiology and public health, most with a focus on the role of physical activity and health. Dr. Macera is a coauthor of an undergraduate text entitled *Basics of Epidemiology: The Distribution and Determinants of Disease in Humans* and teaches courses in epidemiology and chronic disease prevention.

Contributor List

Semra A. Aytur, PhD, MPH
Department of Health Management and
  Policy
University of New Hampshire
Durham, New Hampshire

Fátima Baptista, PhD
Exercise and Health Laboratory
Faculty of Human Movement
Technical University of Lisbon
Lisbon, Portugal

Jack W. Berryman, PhD, FACSM
Department of Bioethics and
  Humanities
School of Medicine
University of Washington
Seattle, Washington

Steven N. Blair, PED, FACSM
Department of Exercise Science and
  Department of Epidemiology and
  Biostatistics
Arnold School of Public Health
University of South Carolina
Columbia, South Carolina

Scott Brown, MS
Laboratory of Physiological Hygiene
  and Exercise Science
School of Kinesiology
University of Minnesota
Minneapolis, Minnesota

David M. Buchner, MD, MPH
Department of Kinesiology and
  Community Health
University of Illinois
Urbana–Champaign, Illinois

Keith Burns, MS
Department of Exercise Science
Arnold School of Public Health
University of South Carolina
Columbia, South Carolina

Susan A. Carlson, MPH
Physical Activity and Health Branch
Division of Nutrition, Physical Activity
  and Obesity
Centers for Disease Control and
  Prevention
Atlanta, Georgia

Ryan Cheek, MS
Department of Exercise Science
Arnold School of Public Health
University of South Carolina
Columbia, South Carolina

Joan Dorn, PhD
Departments of Exercise and Nutrition
  Sciences and Social and Preventive
  Medicine
School of Public Health and Health
  Professions
University of Buffalo
Buffalo, New York

and

Physical Activity and Health Branch
Division of Nutrition, Physical Activity
  and Obesity
Centers for Disease Control and
  Prevention
Atlanta, Georgia

J. Larry Durstine, PhD, FACSM, FAACVPR
Department of Exercise Science
Arnold School of Public Health
University of South Carolina
Columbia, South Carolina

Kelly R. Evenson, MS, PhD, FACSM
Department of Epidemiology
Gillings School of Global Public Health
University of North Carolina
Chapel Hill, North Carolina

Christopher Ford, MPH
Department of Nutrition
Gillings School of Global Public Health
University of North Carolina
Chapel Hill, North Carolina

Sarah Foster, PhD
Center for the Built Environment and
    Health
School of Population Health
University of Western Australia
Perth, Australia

Janet E. Fulton, PhD, FACSM
Physical Activity and Health Branch
Division of Nutrition, Physical Activity
    and Obesity
Centers for Disease Control and
    Prevention
Atlanta, Georgia

Kelley K. Pettee Gabriel, PhD
Division of Epidemiology, Human
    Genetics and Environmental
    Sciences
School of Public Health
University of Texas Health Science
    Center at Houston–Austin Regional
    Campus
Austin, Texas

Jennifer L. Gay, PhD
Department of Health Promotion and
    Behavior
College of Public Health
University of Georgia
Athens, Georgia

Bethany Barone Gibbs, PhD
Department of Health and Physical
    Activity
University of Pittsburgh
Pittsburgh, Pennsylvania

Billie Giles-Corti, PhD
Center for the Built Environment and
    Health
School of Population Health
University of Western Australia
Perth, Australia

Genevieve N. Healy, PhD
School of Population Health
University of Queensland
Brisbane, Australia

and

Baker IDI Heart and Diabetes Institute
Melbourne, Australia

Stephen D. Herrmann, PhD, ATC
Department of Internal Medicine
Cardiovascular Research Institute
Center for Physical Activity and Weight
    Management
University of Kansas Medical Center
Kansas City, Kansas

Cassandra Hoebbel, PhD
Departments of Exercise and Nutrition
    Sciences and Social and Preventive
    Medicine
School of Public Health and Health
    Professions
University at Buffalo
Buffalo, New York

Paula Hooper, BSc (Hons), MS
Center for the Built Environment and
    Health
School of Population Health
University of Western Australia
Perth, Australia

Kathleen F. Janz, EdD, FACSM
Department of Health and Human
    Physiology
University of Iowa
Iowa City, Iowa

Arthur S. Leon, MD, MS, FACSM
Laboratory of Physiological Hygiene
    and Exercise Science
School of Kinesiology
University of Minnesota
Minneapolis, Minnesota

Andrea Nathan, BHlthSc (Hons)
Center for the Built Environment and
    Health
School of Population Health
University of Western Australia
Perth, Australia

Amanda E. Paluch
Department of Exercise Science
Arnold School of Public Health
University of South Carolina
Columbia, South Carolina

Deborah Parra-Medina, PhD, MPH
Institute for Health Promotion Research
University of Texas Health Science
    Center at San Antonio
San Antonio, Texas

**Kenneth E. Powell, MD, MPH,
    FACSM**
Public Health and Epidemiologic
    Consultant
Atlanta, Georgia

Jared P. Reis, PhD
Division of Cardiovascular Sciences
National Heart, Lung, and Blood Institute
National Institutes of Health
Bethesda, Maryland

**Charles M. Tipton, MD, MPH,
    FACSM**
Department of Physiology
University of Arizona
Tucson, Arizona

Richard P. Troiano, PhD
Division of Cancer Control and
    Population Sciences
Risk Factor Monitoring and Methods
    Branch Applied Research Program
National Cancer Institute
Bethesda, Maryland

Catrine Tudor-Locke, PhD, FACSM
Walking Behavior Laboratory
Pennington Biomedical Research
    Center
Baton Rouge, Louisiana

Ilkka Vuori, MD, PhD, FACSM
Finnish Bone and Joint Association
Helsinki, Finland

Dianne Stanton Ward, EdD, FACSM
Department of Nutrition
Gillings School of Global Public Health
University of North Carolina
Chapel Hill, North Carolina

Zenong Yin, PhD
Department of Health and Kinesiology
College of Education and Human
    Development
University of Texas at San Antonio
San Antonio, Texas

1 History of Physical Activity Contributions to Public Health

Amanda E. Paluch, Jack W. Berryman,
Kenneth E. Powell, Ilkka Vuori,
Charles M. Tipton, and Steven N. Blair

CONTENTS

INTRODUCTION

Surveys show that a large majority of adults believe that regular physical activity is good for health, although this does not necessarily translate into them getting sufficient activity. This concept of the importance of regular activity has a long history. In this chapter, we review some of the early comments on this topic, and trace the development of this theme throughout the twentieth century and up to the present. Space limitations prevent an exhaustive review of information on physical activity and health, and our comments are based on our own experience, a selective review, and recent events.

HEALTH, EXERCISE, AND EXERCISE PRESCRIPTION DURING ANTIQUITY

The importance of physical activity for good health and, in some instances, to cure disease, dates back to India and the river civilization in the Indus River Valley. Here, in about 1500 BC, were the 1,028 sacred hymns of the Rgveda (Rig-Veda) written in Sanskrit that included requests for benevolence and blessings from gods and goddesses and divine remedies for diseases. When health was mentioned, it was not related to disease or recovery from disease; it was viewed as a condition of the pleasure or displeasure of the gods. One hymn makes reference to the existence of three humors that influence health. Another sacred text, the Atharaveda (Atharva-Veda), also contains detailed information about medicine, health, and disease. Many of these Vedic texts were foundational elements in the development of what would later become Ayurvedic medicine (i.e., the science of life).

Between 1500 and 800 BC, the tridosa doctrine (also known as the trihautu doctrine and considered to be the Indian humoral theory) was developed. It was introduced to help explain the meaning of life, death, health, and disease while describing how the elements of water, fire, air, earth, and ether contributed to the formation of the human body. Interacting within the body were nutrient particles derived from the wind, sun, and moon that later became transformed into air, bile, and phlegm. These were regarded by the physician Susruta (ca. 600 BC) as *dosas* (humors) and were identified as *vayu*, *pitta*, and *kapha*, respectively. He added a fourth humor, blood, since he believed it was capable of influencing interactions between the other humors.

According to the tridosa doctrine, the humors controlled and regulated all functions of the body. When they were in equilibrium, health was present. But if one or more humors were displaced or out of balance with the others, health was impaired and illness or death could occur. In addition to disease, conditions that could alter the equilibrium between the humors were climate, food, fatigue, psychic changes, poisons, sedentary living, and exercise (Tipton 2008a).

Susruta's views on the importance of physical activity are contained in *The Sushruta Samhita*. He defined exercise as a "sense of weariness from bodily labor and it should be taken every day." It included walking, running, jumping, swimming, diving, riding, archery, wrestling, and javelin throwing. As a physician, Susruta prescribed exercise because it increased the growth of limbs; improved muscle mass, strength, endurance, and tone; reduced corpulence; increased resistance against fatigue; enhanced mental alertness, retentive memory, and keen intelligence; and improved appearance and complexion. In general, he believed that regular moderate exercise provided resistance to disease and "against physical decay" and stated, "Diseases fly from the presence of a person, habituated to regular physical exercise. . . ." Susruta was convinced that a sedentary lifestyle that included lack of physical activity, sleeping through the day, and excessive food or fluids, would sufficiently elevate the kapha humor to a level that would disrupt humoral equilibrium resulting in a disease state and potential death. Obesity was the likely result for which Susruta prescribed exercise (Tipton 2008b). Many of the themes in Susruta's works would be echoed centuries later in the Yoga-Sûtra of Pâtanjali. The Yoga-Sûtra, a Sanskrit manual of nearly 200 aphorisms, emphasizes that the path to enlightenment necessitated physical activity. This text forms the basis of modern Hatha Yoga.

Just as the early religious and philosophical writings of Hinduism (i.e., the Vedic texts) laid the foundation for Ayurvedic medicine, early Taoist philosophy and thought strongly influenced the development of traditional Chinese medicine. Taoism, usually translated as "the Way" or "the Path," reflected the simplicity of nature and imbued ancient Chinese culture with a reverence for the relationship between life and death, as well as man's eternal struggle with nature. The gradual accumulation of Taoist and folk knowledge during antiquity further developed during the Warring States period (475–221 BC). The *Huangdi Neijing* (*The Yellow Emperor's Inner Canon*) was the culmination of centuries of observation and medical experience. This book is rich in the philosophy of physical activity. To remain healthy and avoid disease, one must first understand the body. Dietary modifications according to the alterations of yin and yang were emphasized along with paying attention to the duration of physical postures and activity (e.g., sitting, lying, standing, and walking). In another text, the *Annals of Mr. Lü*, a historical miscellany from the point of view of the Qin Kingdom (about 239 BC), the politician Buwei Lü referred to longevity as maintaining health that includes "conforming to natural laws of life," "abstinence," "removal of harmful factors," and "movement." "Movement" refers to exercise. This book uses simple truths from the daily life of ordinary people and highlights the influence of exercise on the human body. In the third century, the Chinese physician and surgeon Hua Tuo prescribed moderate exercise as a method to increase "yang" (i.e., masculine energy) and overcome disease.

Exercise also played a central role in ancient Greek and Roman culture from the 400s BC and the time of the Greek physician Hippocrates (460–370 BC) to the death of the Roman physician Galen (129–210 AD). They both emphasized that medicine consisted of two fundamental parts—hygiene (named after the goddess Hygieia) and therapeutics, or the treatment of disease. Accordingly, the physician was involved with patients on a regular basis to advise them on how to stay healthy and how to avoid sickness, along with restoring health if they became ill. In the era of Hippocrates, this involved an understanding of the four bodily fluids, or humors (blood, phlegm, yellow bile, and black bile), because the patient's health was believed to be dependent on their balance and harmony. The humors then had to be understood as they related to the four elements (earth, air, fire, and water) and the four primary qualities (hot, cold, wet, and dry) (Berryman 2010).

For his part, Hippocrates—based on observation and analysis of a patient's physiological information—would provide advice and a prescription of regimen. The main ingredients of his regimen were food and exercise since he believed that they—independently or in combination—had the greatest potential to alter the body's humoral makeup. To this end, Hippocrates wrote at least three separate books on regimen: *Regimen in Health*, *Regimen*, and *Regimen in Acute Diseases*. In *Regimen in Health*, he noted that "eating alone will not keep a man well; he must also take exercise. For food and exercise, while possessing opposite qualities, yet work together to produce health" (Berryman 2003).

The most prominent figure in medicine, anatomy, and physiology after Hippocrates was Galen. His theories and writings dominated medicine and went unchallenged through the Middle Ages and were still widely accepted during the Renaissance. He built upon the regimen of Hippocrates and introduced his version of humoral theory, which he divided into naturals (physiology), nonnaturals (things not innate—hygiene or health), and contranaturals (against nature—pathology). The nonnaturals were factors external to the body over which a person had some control: (1) air and environment, (2) food and drink, (3) sleeping and waking, (4) motion (exercise) and rest, (5) retention and evacuation, and (6) passions of the mind (emotions). Known as the "six things nonnatural," they had to be used in moderation, balance, and order in terms of quantity, quality, and time, since too much or too little would put the body out of balance. They played a central role in hygiene, the science of health and its preservation, but their regulation also came into use as therapy (Berryman 1992).

Overall, Galen regarded exercise as one branch of hygiene and hygiene as part of the science of medicine. Accordingly, his book *On Hygiene* provides the best collection of his views on exercise and health. In this book, he discusses the need for exercise, the value of exercise, the definition of exercise, the time for exercise, the varieties of exercise, and the different qualities of exercise, among others. Galen's discussion of the nonnaturals and the important role of exercise is found in *The Pulse for Beginners*, *To Thrasyboulos: Is Healthiness a Part of Medicine or of Gymnastics?* and *The Art of Medicine*. His thorough understanding of exercise is exhibited in his treatise, *The Exercise with the Small Ball*, and he writes more extensively about exercise, health, and "condition" in *The Best Constitution of Our Bodies* and *Good Condition*. Here, Galen described a continuum of healthfulness going from illness or "impairment of function," to health described as "well-conditioned" and the "peak of good condition" (Berryman 2003).

THE BEGINNINGS OF SCIENTIFIC WORK ON PHYSICAL ACTIVITY AND HEALTH

EXERCISE PHYSIOLOGY AND HEALTH OUTCOMES

The development of research in health-related biological sciences and its significance to the field is perhaps best seen in Copenhagen, Denmark. August Krogh (1874–1949), often recognized as the father of exercise physiology in Scandinavia, performed groundbreaking studies on respiration and circulation at rest and during and after exercise. He launched the hypothesis of "central commands" in 1913, and received the Nobel Prize for research on the mechanism regulating capillaries in 1919. He found that tissues extracted more oxygen during exercise than at rest, and concurrently circulation and ventilation increased. One of the many innovative devices for research constructed by Krogh was a new cycle ergometer with magnets and weights to quantify exercise intensity. He summarizes his broad interests and great skills in a paper published in 1913: "The tracheal system of the hind limb of a grasshopper can be rapidly and extensively ventilated by the respiratory movements of the insect. About 20% of the air contained can be renewed by one breath. The oxygen percentage in the air of the hind legs is very high during rest (16%) but after exhausting muscular exertions it becomes very low (5%)" (Krogh 1913). In 1920, Krogh and his coworker, J. Lindhard, studied the relative contribution of fat and carbohydrate as sources of muscular energy, and determined the respiratory quotient with an accuracy of 0.005. Thus, Krogh's studies linked exercise physiology with metabolism and nutrition. Although not interested in sports himself, Krogh attracted researchers such as G. Liljestrand from the Karolinska Institute in Stockholm. Together, they measured the oxygen uptake of rowers, swimmers, and cross-country skiers during free performance in 1918–1920 (Liljestrand and Lindhard 1920).

Krogh continued his work with many coworkers, which included E. Asmussen, E. Howu-Christensen, and M. Nielsen. Asmussen, Christensen, and Nielsen published a number of studies on topics such as muscular strength and performance, ventilatory and cardiovascular responses to exercise of different intensities and in different postures, factors behind maximal strength, and concentric, eccentric, and isometric muscle contraction, and maximum working capacity during leg and arm exercise. Asmussen had a clear and broad view of the significance of exercise physiology. Muscular exercise, more than most other conditions, taxes the bodily functions to the limit, and indicates the extent to which the human organism can adapt itself to the stresses and strains of the environment.

Erik Hovu-Christensen, who was one of the members of the team, conducted numerous studies on cardiac output, body temperature, and blood sugar during heavy exercise, the responses of leg and arm exercise, and the effects of exercise training. One of the subjects in some of these studies was Marius Nielsen. He continued studies on temperature regulation using advanced techniques under strictly controlled conditions in a climatic chamber. Today, this branch continues successfully in Copenhagen. Christensen conducted further studies on energy metabolism during exercise, showing that the proportion of carbohydrates and fats as energy-yielding substrates depends on work rate, duration of heavy exercise, diet during the 3 days before the exercise, and the training state of the subject. These studies, which he conducted with Ove Hansen, also showed that hypoglycemia could induce fatigue. The findings of these studies were confirmed in the 1960s in Christensen's laboratory, now in Stockholm, by direct determination of changes in muscle glycogen concentration using needle biopsy (Bergström et al. 1967).

The career of Erik Hovu-Christensen demonstrates the importance of scientific exchange. In 1941, he was elected as the first professor at a new department in physiology at the College of Physical Education (Gymnastik-och Idrottshögskolan [GIH]) in Stockholm. During the initial years working conditions were poor and he considered returning to Copenhagen, but because Denmark was occupied by the Germans he stayed in Stockholm. This decision was very important, because he then had a major influence on the development of physiology of muscular activity in various environments and for different purposes, including sports, work, and leisure (Åstrand 1991).

Mentored by Christensen, Per-Olof Åstrand began his studies, together with Irma Ryhming (who would later become his wife), by assessing the physical working capacity of subjects of various ages beginning with 4-year-olds. An important instrument in these pioneering studies was the cycle ergometer developed by W. von Döbeln at GIH. The ergometer was later manufactured by the Monark Company in large numbers and used worldwide in laboratories and in the field. Another long-lasting product of the early studies on work capacity was the development of the

Åstrand–Ryhming nomogram for indirect assessment of maximal oxygen uptake based on submaximal workloads and corresponding heart rate, which was also used extensively for decades all over the world. The numerous innovative studies designed, led, and supervised by Åstrand, conducted in collaboration with a great number of students from Sweden and abroad, on ventilation, circulation, metabolism, and their regulations during exercise in various physical activities in the context of sports, work, and leisure, and under various environmental conditions including high altitude, have led to expansion of the knowledge of exercise physiology and approaches and methods in this field of research. This knowledge has led to a wide range of applications in sport, work, leisure and health, and aroused substantial interest in doing research related to this field not only in Sweden and not only in exercise physiology, but also in numerous countries and on many areas of basic and applied research.

Åstrand's contributions to the field of work-, sport-, and health-related physiology are attributed not only to the original research, but also to the wide and effective distribution of the results and ideas based on them via books, writings, and presentations for researchers and the general public. Åstrand and Kare Rodahl's *Textbook of Work Physiology*, translated in eight languages, has sold more than 100,000 copies and remains a classic for the field. On the popular front, the booklet *Health and Fitness* has been translated in 10 languages and distributed in about 20 million copies (Björn Ekblom, personal communication, August 2010). Åstrand has been a leader in advocating for health through physical activity and advising how to do it on a global scale.

In Finland, there was an enormous interest in exercise, especially sports physiology and medicine, in the 1930s when the country was preparing to host the Helsinki Olympic games planned to be held in 1940 (although this was later postponed to 1952 because of World War II). However, after World War II, the interest and resources had to be directed to other research questions. Martti J. Karvonen (1918–2009) was a leader in exercise research in Finland, and began research in the newly established Institute of Occupational Medicine by studying energy expenditure and energy intake of Finnish lumberjacks in postwar Finland (Karvonen et al. 1961). He applied the methods of work and clinical physiology as well as nutrition research, and discovered the very high rate and daily amount of energy expended. The results were widely publicized, attracted a lot of attention, and made the lumberjacks nearly national heroes—for good reasons. The work developed methods related to work physiology, and later expanded to address the emerging serious public health problem: coronary heart disease (CHD). These lines of research gradually helped to merge exercise physiology, epidemiology, and medicine. One of Karvonen's studies led to the development of the "Karvonen formula" for assessing training intensity by using heart rate (Karvonen, Kentala, and Mustala 1957). Although these remarks on the historical development of exercise physiology in Europe are by no means complete, they do give a general view of the development of the field.

Physical Activity Epidemiology

Physical activity epidemiology was initiated by a British epidemiologist, Jerry Morris (1910–2009). Morris was a leader in developing solid methods for collection and data analysis of epidemiological studies on causes of chronic diseases. In 1957, he published *Uses of Epidemiology*, the first text to use classical epidemiology on chronic, noncommunicable diseases.

Beginning in the late 1940s, Morris began following a large group of drivers and conductors on London's double-decker buses, and monitoring them for CHD (Morris et al. 1953). The drivers in this study spent 90% of their workday at the steering wheel, whereas the conductors climbed an average of 600 stairs per day collecting fares. The data showed that drivers had double the rate of heart attacks compared with conductors. Furthermore, conductors with CHD had less severe cases and they occurred later in life. Morris was ahead of his time when addressing the fitness–fatness debate, currently a topic of interest, finding that although protection from heart attacks could be explained by physical activity levels, it could not be attributed to body leanness. Using the trouser size as a measure of body composition, he found that conductors had a lower risk of CHD regardless of their waistband size (Heady et al. 1961).

To further validate his findings among the London bus transportation employees, he performed a longitudinal study in postal workers. Postmen, who walked or rode a bicycle on delivery routes, had significantly lower CHD rates when compared with individuals in sedentary occupations: office clerks and telephone operators (Morris et al. 1953). During the 1960s, he followed 18,000 men working sedentary civil service jobs for 8 years, and concluded that those who participated in regular aerobic activity decreased their risk of CHD by 50% (Morris et al. 1980). Morris' contributions ignited the modern era of physical activity epidemiology. He encouraged the continuation of research on occupational and leisure physical activity into the 1950s and 1960s.

Development of new areas in research requires new ideas, insight, understanding, and methods. Much of this has to be done by applying concepts, findings, and methods from related areas through innovative approaches. He developed and used new methods to study the physiological responses to work and working environments. He would often use simple, but always valid, designs and methods in laboratory and epidemiological studies corresponding to the available conditions and opportunities. His approach was to proceed gradually (step by step) toward the goal, content with what was available and possible at the moment without waiting for better opportunities.

As an eyewitness to the serious problem of CHD in the beginning of the 1950s, especially among Karelian men, Karvonen focused epidemiological research on cardiovascular disease (CVD) (Rautaharju, Karvonen, and Keys 1961). He initiated the first population study on cardiovascular health in Finland, the East–West Study, in the mid-1950s, and some years later, he linked it to the Seven Countries Study. Initiated in 1958, the Seven Countries Study pioneered the systemic evaluation of the relation among lifestyle, diet, and rates of CHD among middle-aged men in 16 contrasting cohorts in seven countries: United States, Japan, Italy, Greece, the Netherlands, Finland, and Yugoslavia. He was the godfather of several major investigations including the North Karelia Project (Karvonen 1995). Initiated in 1972, the North Karelia Project was a comprehensive <u>intervention</u> directed at reducing CVD rates among residents within a province of Eastern Finland. The project expanded into broader objectives covering the prevention of other noncommunicable diseases and overall lifestyle-health promotion. With its long-term success in improving health and reducing rates of disease, the project demonstrates approaches and evidence to the preventability of various health problems that can be disseminated to other public health efforts worldwide. However, because of several factors—his modest personality, institutional matters, and job changes—Karvonen's name was sometimes not included in some of the publications of epidemiological studies in which he had participated.

From early on in his career, Karvonen had an interest in the health effects of physical activity, such as cardiovascular effects on longevity of endurance sports, especially cross-country skiing. He saw leisure time physical activity as an important health-enhancing factor. However, in epidemiological studies, physical activity was Karvonen's secondary interest compared to the role of other risk factors and nutrition. Critical to methodology within studies, he was reluctant to see occupational physical activity as a protective factor against CHD. He observed that job titles may not correctly indicate the physical demands of the occupation. He also noticed that in most studies the influence of other known and unknown risk factors could not or had not been taken sufficiently into account, or their influence was dominant compared to physical activity. For instance, hardworking Finnish lumberjacks had a higher prevalence of CHD compared with persons in physically less demanding occupations; some of this likely due to the high animal fat consumption and heavy smoking among lumberjacks (Karvonen et al. 1961). However, in the extension of the Seven Countries Study in the Finnish population samples, in which physical activity was assessed by detailed interview, low physical activity clearly increased the risk of atherosclerotic diseases. Karvonen points out, however, that even in the most active groups, 20–30% of the men aged 50–69 years already had a diagnosed atherosclerotic disease (Karvonen 1982).

In another publication, Karvonen indicates that in a multivariate analysis of the 7-year follow-up in the North Karelia Project, men with low physical activity at work had a 1.5-fold risk of acute myocardial infarction. For women, the corresponding risk was 2.4-fold (Karvonen 1984). But, as a critical scientist, Karvonen asked which was the cause and which was the effect. Did physical activity protect against CVD, or was the higher incidence among the less active men caused by CVD at entry, still undiagnosed but already curtailing their physical activity? He concluded that the findings on the influence of leisure time and occupational physical activity on the risk of heart disease seemed discordant, the first being protective, the latter not. To settle this discrepancy, at least the amount, intensity, and type of occupational physical activity, association of physical activity with other risk factors, and the possible influence of unidentified risk factors should be considered. How right he was with his remark!

Latter Half of the Twentieth Century

Influenced by the developments in epidemiological methods and concepts from Morris and Karvonen, the latter half of the twentieth century featured several longitudinal studies further contributing to the important evidence for physical activity's relationship with chronic disease.

Ralph S. Paffenbarger Jr. (1922–2007) was a leading epidemiologist whose research advanced the study of physical activity and chronic disease, specifically CHD. His interest in studying chronic disease and activity developed when he began working with the Framingham Heart Study in the 1950s. Currently in its third generation of participants, the grandchildren of the original cohort, the Framingham Heart Study's objective was (and continues) to identify the major CVD risk factors by following thousands of men and women living in Framingham, Massachusetts, throughout their lifetime. Leaving the U.S. Centers for Disease Control in 1968, he served as faculty at the University of California–Berkeley, Harvard University, and Stanford University until 1993.

A main contribution to physical activity epidemiology came from Paffenbarger's San Francisco Longshoremen study. The study tracked 6300 longshoremen for two decades, beginning with multiphasic screening examinations in 1951. Results compared three occupations of varying activity expenditures (cargo handlers, foremen, and clerks) with the risk of CVD morbidity and mortality. For instance, Paffenbarger found that men with more sedentary occupations expended 925 fewer calories per workday (Paffenbarger et al. 1970). The death rate of less active men was twice as great; CHD death rate was one-third higher; and sudden cardiac death was two-thirds greater compared with men in the more active occupations (Paffenbarger et al. 1970).

Paffenbarger implemented the College Alumni Health Study in 1960 to examine the role of physical activity to health in a cohort of more 50,000 University of Pennsylvania and Harvard University alumni, a strategically chosen cohort that could be easily tracked. Paffenbarger used detailed social, psychological, and medical histories, obtained by mail-back surveys, as well as information from college days. There have been many reports from this study on the benefits of physical activity on health outcomes such as heart disease, stroke, cancer, diabetes, and overall longevity. An example of one finding is that Harvard Alumni with a composite physical activity index (derived from stair climbed, blocks walked, and strenuous sports played) below 2000 kcal/week were at a 64% greater risk of heart attack (Paffenbarger et al. 1978).

Paffenbarger's research brought attention to physical inactivity as a significant public health concern. For such contributions, Paffenberger, together with Jerry Morris, received the first International Olympic Committee Prize for sports science in 1996, considered a top honor in the field of physical activity academia.

Influenced by Morris's London transportation and postal worker studies displaying the link between occupational physical activity and CHD, Henry Taylor took this concept to the railroad industry, examining and following men from 1957 to 1977. He compared the death rates of three groups of employees, and found that the more sedentary occupation of clerical work had substantially higher death rates for arteriosclerotic heart disease than the more active occupations of switchmen and section men (i.e., railway laborers) (5.7 vs. 3.9 and 2.8 per 1000 men, respectively) (Taylor et al. 1962).

In 1987, a systematic review by Powell et al. amassed the early, influential studies examining varying levels of physical activity with CHD, and consolidated them into the conclusion that physical activity is a vital aspect of public health (Powell et al. 1987). The article addressed many of the longitudinal projects mentioned throughout this chapter, from London postal and transportation workers, to U.S. railroad workers and longshoremen, to residents of North Karelia, Finland, and Framingham, Massachusetts. When summarizing the studies, the review concluded that inactivity resulted in an average 2-fold risk for CHD. These findings were similar to that of the risk of CHD associated with hypertension, hypercholesterolemia, and smoking. For this reason, physical activity should be promoted to the same degree that blood pressure control, healthy diets to reduce cholesterol levels, and smoking cessation programs have been promoted. The authors close with a call for public policies to focus on encouraging higher levels of physical activity.

CARDIORESPIRATORY FITNESS AND HEALTH OUTCOMES

Earlier epidemiological studies mentioned above show the relation of physical activity to CVD. One hypothesis was that this relationship may be mediated through fitness levels. Taylor's Railroad Study examined physical fitness and health outcomes with a submaximal treadmill test administered in a Pullman car turned laboratory. After an average of 20 years follow-up, men with lower fitness levels, shown by a higher submaximal heart rate, had a higher risk of death from all causes, CHD, and overall CVD (Slattery and Jacobs 1988).

Taylor was influenced by the work of physiologists, A.V. Hill and Hartley Lupton in the 1920s (Hill and Lupton 1923), who described concepts of aerobic and anaerobic metabolism, and demonstrated that an upper limit exists in a human's capacity of the respiratory and cardiovascular system to transport oxygen to muscles. In 1955, Taylor outlined the criteria for measuring maximal oxygen consumption and established this measure as the gold standard for aerobic fitness. Taylor asked his subjects to come to his laboratory in three to five separate visits in order to establish the necessary workload to produce maximal oxygen intake. During each visit, grade or speed was increased until there were two treadmill tests that elicited similar oxygen intake. Taylor concludes that "there is a linear relationship between oxygen intake and work load until the maximum oxygen intake is reached. Further increases in work load beyond this point merely result in an increase in oxygen debt and a shortening of the time in which the work can be performed" (Taylor et al. 1955). He further states that these measurements can be used to study cardiovascular and respiratory function in the presence of various diseases, since maximal oxygen consumption can be substantially impaired by disease.

One of us (SB) has spent several years following women and men examined at the Cooper Clinic. These examinations included an extensive battery of laboratory tests, including a maximal exercise test on a treadmill to assess cardiorespiratory fitness. The first prospective data from this study on cardiorespiratory fitness and mortality were published in 1989, and showed substantially lower death rates in women and men who were at least moderately fit (Blair et al. 1989). Moderate fitness in this cohort was associated with ~140 min/week of walking or ~90 min/week of jogging, levels of activity that are consistent with current physical activity guidelines. The individuals who were moderately fit had death rates during follow-up that were about 50% lower than the low fit individuals. Numerous other studies on this population have been published over the years, with similar results for different outcomes such as CHD, diabetes, and cancer (Lee et al. 1999; Sui et al. 2008; Farrell et al. 2007). Low cardiorespiratory fitness in this cohort accounts for more deaths than other established risk factors such as diabetes, smoking, high blood pressure, high cholesterol, or obesity (Blair 2009).

Numerous large-scale epidemiological studies on physical activity or fitness over the past 50 years provide convincing evidence for the importance of an active lifestyle to maintain good health and function. The brief review presented above is only a small portion of the studies conducted on this topic, but they are representative of the overall body of literature (Physical Activity Guidelines Advisory Committee 2008). It is abundantly clear that physical inactivity is one of the leading causes of morbidity, mortality, and poor function, and is a major public health problem around the world.

COMBINING EPIDEMIOLOGY AND PHYSIOLOGY— MERGING OF TWO KEY SUBDISCIPLINES

As previously discussed, Henry Taylor made substantial contributions to both epidemiological research and the physiology field by the development of maximal oxygen uptake tests. His interest in both realms made him a leader in merging these two key disciplines. Taylor had an interest in the biologically plausible mechanisms that relate fitness to cardiovascular health. As an example, in his Railroad Study, he found that the greater risk of disease associated with low fitness levels can be largely attributed to higher blood pressure. Martti Karvonen also studied both the physiology and epidemiology of physical activity.

In 1977, Arthur Leon and Henry Blackburn published a summary of the findings of earlier studies on physical activity and its association with positive health outcomes (Leon and Blackburn 1977). In this publication, they clearly recognized that endurance exercise results in improvements in cardiovascular health and life expectancy, which come from the positive physiological adaptations due to exercise. The report states that endurance exercise results in physiological improvements, such as blood lipid changes, increased insulin sensitivity, increased myocardial vascularity, enhanced cardiovascular efficiency, and reduced blood pressure and heart rate, which all can help prevent the development of CHD.

PHYSICAL ACTIVITY AND THE PUBLIC HEALTH ESTABLISHMENT

In the middle of the twentieth century, atherosclerotic heart disease was epidemic. The proportion of deaths in the United States caused by CHD had risen from around 10% in the early 1900s to 30–35% at mid-century. Efforts to understand the causes and to develop treatments and preventions were intense. The gradual recognition during the latter half of the century that physical activity plays a key role for health produced a series of projects and organizational changes within public health agencies.

Highlights in the development of physical activity-related surveillance, etiologic research, health promotion, and policy development programs within federal health agencies are described briefly in the following paragraphs. A similar but longer list of notable events is available elsewhere (National Center for Health Statistics 2010).

The President's Council on Fitness, Sports, and Nutrition (PCFSN) was created in 1953. Originally named the President's Council on Youth Fitness, it was established in response to a survey showing European children to be more physically fit than American children. Its origins, therefore, lie more in concerns about wartime readiness than public health and its focus, especially in its early years, was fitness and performance, not health. It is, however, to our knowledge, the first federal agency with a specific interest in physical fitness, and by extension, physical activity. PCFSN has been a helpful partner in a number of more recent developments, such as the Objectives for the Nation and the development of the *2008 Physical Activity Guidelines for Americans*.

As research findings from exercise science and epidemiology combined to suggest that regular physical activity may reduce the incidence of atherosclerotic heart disease, the public health community took notice. In the early 1960s, the National Center for Chronic Disease Control (NCCDC) was established at the National Institutes of Health (NIH) to develop applications for the prevention and control of chronic diseases, especially heart disease. The NCCDC encouraged cooperation between exercise science and public health science by assigning NIH physicians to exercise science laboratories around the country and bringing exercise scientists to NIH. Discussions about how to study the relationship between activity and heart disease were held, a summary of scientific evidence was published (Fox and Skinner 1964), and pilot studies were conducted. In 1968, only 4 years after the establishment of NCCDC, the cost of the Vietnam War required the federal government to cut back on domestic programs, NIH eliminated NCCDC in favor of more clinically oriented research.

As familiar as "lifestyle" sounds today, in the 1970s the word and its concepts were new. Chronic diseases, especially heart disease, had emerged as the leading causes of death and disability, and certain behaviors—primarily tobacco use, poor dietary habits, inactivity, and alcohol abuse—had been implicated as causes. The word lifestyle came to mean the bundle of behaviors and environmental exposures with health implications. The effort to address the burden of chronic diseases was openly called the second public health revolution (the first revolution being the development of vaccines and antibiotics to prevent and control infectious diseases). In spite of the pioneering work by Krogh, Christensen, Åstrand, Taylor, and other exercise scientists and the emerging epidemiologic evidence from Morris, Paffenbarger, and others, medical practitioner groups remained reluctant to endorse the health benefits of regular physical activity throughout the 1970s. The public health community, however, with its emphasis on lifestyle was more supportive. The Lalonde Report in 1974 from Canada (Lalonde 1974), Healthy People in 1979 from the United States (Public Health Service 1979), several World Health Organization (WHO) reports in the early 1980s (WHO 1985), and probably reports from other countries as well, called for lifestyle changes including physical activity—as the key to curtailing the epidemic of coronary artery disease and other chronic diseases. In the United States, the publication of Healthy People led directly to the nation's first set of national health objectives with a target date of 1990, and physical activity was included

(Public Health Service 1980). Increasing the prevalence of beneficial physical activity has held a prominent place in all subsequent sets of national objectives: Healthy People 2000, 2010, and, just recently, 2020.

These key public health documents and national objectives produced programmatic and organizational changes. The National Center for Health Statistics (NCHS), using the ongoing National Health Interview Survey, began surveillance of self-reported physical activity behaviors in 1975. Major community-wide intervention trials in Finland (North Karelia), California, Minnesota, and Rhode Island were undertaken to explore methods to improve chronic disease control and modify health behaviors, including physical activity.

In 1983, in response to the Healthy People document declaring a second public health revolution to be driven by behavioral change to prevent chronic diseases, the Centers for Disease Control and Prevention (CDC) established the Behavioral Epidemiology and Evaluation Branch (BEEB). It focused first on physical activity. In 1984, BEEB convened a workshop to summarize the current status of the scientific evidence relating physical activity and health outcomes and to identify priority topics for future research (Powell and Paffenbarger 1985). To complement NCHS's ongoing surveillance of physical activity at the national level, the CDC included physical activity in its newly developed state-specific surveillance systems for adults (i.e., Behavioral Risk Factor Surveillance System) and youth (i.e., Youth Risk Behavior Surveillance System).

By the early 1990s, the evidence was incontestable. A series of statements and recommendations from various organizations and governmental agencies followed (see below, this chapter). Just as importantly, commitments and organizational changes solidified and broadened the array of federal activities. In 1996, CDC established the Physical Activity and Health Branch (PAHB). PAHB has taken a leading role in the provision of technical assistance to state and local health departments for the development and implementation of physical activity programs; in identifying evidence-based physical activity promotion programs for communities; in supporting training courses in physical activity epidemiology and program implementation; and in examining the cost-effectiveness of physical activity interventions (Pratt et al. 2009). Elsewhere at CDC, tests of cardiorespiratory fitness and muscular strength, and the use of accelerometers for the objective measurement of physical activity have been added to the National Health and Nutrition Examination Survey to further strengthen the national surveillance of physical fitness and activity.

Other federal agencies, especially those within the Department of Health and Human Services such as the National Cancer Institute and the NIH, have similarly expanded their physical activity-related programs. Just as importantly, nearly all state and many local health departments have programs and personnel dedicated to physical activity-related public health functions.

PHYSICAL ACTIVITY RECOMMENDATIONS

As decades of evidence accumulated regarding the link between chronic disease and low levels of physical activity, public health directed attention toward increasing physical activity among the entire U.S. population. The need for physical activity recommendations developed from the need to promote exercise while allaying the apprehension that promoting exercise, if not controlled, could cause an increase in sudden cardiac deaths due to individuals taking on too much too quickly. Therefore, the history of recommendations derived from the attempt to find the activity range that will "reduce risk while maximizing benefit" (Physical Activity Guidelines Advisory Committee 2008).

The American College of Sports Medicine (ACSM) was a leader in the initial development of guidelines for physical activity. The first recommendations for the general population came from ACSM's Position Statement on "The Recommended Quantity and Quality of Exercise for Developing and Maintaining Fitness in Healthy Adults" published in 1978 (ACSM 1978). The research to support this recommendation came solely from the exercise physiology spectrum, with Michael Pollock's review on endurance exercise and cardiorespiratory fitness titled "The Quantification of Exercise Training Programs" as the backbone for much of the evidence (Pollock 1973). The recommendations focused on "developing and maintaining cardiorespiratory fitness and body composition in healthy adults" and suggested 15 min to 60 min of rhythmical and aerobic activities at 60% to 90% of heart rate reserve ($HRR = HR_{max} - HR_{rest}$), 3 to 5 days per week (ACSM 1978).

The ACSM revised the Position Stand in 1990, with slight changes to the dose of aerobic activity (20–60 min of moderate to vigorous physical activity (MVPA), 50–85% HRR) (ACSM Position Stand 1990). Significant additions included a recommendation for muscular strength activities for 2 days/week and the recognition that health benefits can be derived from lower intensity exercise performed more frequently for longer durations. The 1990 recommendations made an important distinction that moderate activity can derive benefits beyond cardiorespiratory endurance, and significant health benefits (such as preventing chronic diseases) can occur. These recommendations began the shift of the paradigm of physical activity recommendations, moving away from the focus on exercise for optimizing performance-based fitness to a much broader emphasis on physical activity for its health-related benefits.

The ACSM began to consider feasibility and efficacy when developing recommendations. Because approximately half the population was not sufficiently active, and a quarter of the population could be categorized as sedentary, the recommendations had to target this large group. Thus, the ACSM focused on moderate rather than the past high-intensity levels and recommended the lowest, yet still effective, level of physical activity to offer health benefits (ACSM 2006).

A significant step in this health-promotion direction occurred in 1992 when the American Heart Association (AHA) declared physical inactivity the fourth leading modifiable risk factor for CHD, accompanying smoking, hypertension, and hypercholesterolemia. Additionally, the AHA recognized that moderate doses of physical activity, lower than what had currently been recognized, can have substantial health benefits (Fletcher et al. 1992).

The AHA's statement caused a heightened awareness to the importance of a physically active lifestyle. In response, the CDC and ACSM began collaborating on developing the first public health guidelines on physical activity. The report, published in 1995, selected a dose of physical activity that was manageable for the target sedentary population. These guidelines contained significant differences from the past recommendations. The key recommendation focused on moderate intensity (defined as 3–6 METs, or a high enough intensity to expend about 200 kcal in 30 min, i.e., walk 2 miles briskly) rather than vigorous, although they recognized in the report that additional benefits could accrue with higher levels of activity. Moreover, frequency was increased from 3–5 to 5–7 days/week. Additionally, these guidelines introduced the concept of accumulating activity throughout the day in 8- to 10-min bouts, rather than one continuous session (Pate et al. 1995). It is interesting to note that in past recommendations the supported research generally derived from the exercise physiology field, and in the 1995 report evidence mostly came from epidemiological studies finding significant reductions in chronic disease with increased levels of physical activity. As an indication of the influence of this report, a citation analysis on the Web of Science shows that by the end of 2010 it had been cited >5000 times. This is an astonishing number of citations, which most likely makes it the most highly cited report in the history of exercise science research. Indeed, few reports in any field have accumulated so many citations.

Shortly thereafter, the NIH gathered for a 3-day consensus conference on "Physical Activity and Cardiovascular Health." Representing many health fields from psychology to cardiology to public health, the panel closely examined and discussed the link between activity and cardiovascular health with the intention to advise both physicians and the general public (NIH 1996). The recommendations that resulted from this conference were very much similar to the 1995 public health guidelines. At the same time, the WHO (1995) published a report on physical activity and its health benefits, making the same conclusions; it emphasized 30 min of moderate-intensity activity most days of the week, which can be accumulated in bouts, and any activity beyond this can have additional benefits.

Not long after these three reports by the CDC/ACSM, NIH, and WHO, "Physical Activity and Health: A Report of the Surgeon General" was published in 1996 (U.S. Dept. of Health and Human Services 1996). Commissioned by the Secretary of Health and Human Services and a collaboration of multiple federal and nongovernment organizations such as the CDC, ACSM, NIH, AHA, and the President's Council on Physical Fitness and Sports, this large group pulled out the existing literature to summarize the high prevalence of sedentary behavior, how this sedentary behavior results in negative health outcomes, and how physical activity can counteract this issue. The Surgeon General's report suggests a regimen of 30–45 min of activity most days of the week to reduce the risk of chronic disease. The report emphasized the amount, rather than intensity, to allow a large variety of options to achieve the recommendations, such as a 30-min brisk walk, 30 min of lawn mowing or leaf raking, or 45 min of volleyball. The report created the recommendation with the idea that the "flexibility to vary activities according to preference and life circumstances, will encourage more people to make physical activity a regular and sustainable part of their lives" (U.S. Dept. of Health and Human Services 1996).

The most recent recommendations by the ACSM and the AHA came out in 2007, which sought to make improvements on the 1995 CDC/ACSM recommendations. Although fundamentally unchanged, slight clarifications were made, such as making strength training a concrete part of the recommendation, and clarifying 10 min of aerobic moderate-vigorous physical activity as the minimum duration counted toward the recommendation. Furthermore, the ACSM clarified intensity as 5 days/ week rather than "most, preferably all days." Although vigorous activity was ambiguously implied before, now it is explicitly recommended in an effort to acknowledge the preference of adults for higher intensity activities. These recommendations explain that moderate and vigorous activity can be combined, and the total volume calculated through MET values suggests a minimum goal between 450 and 750 MET min week^{-1} (Haskell et al. 2007).

Following the 2007 ACSM–AHA recommendations, the U.S. Department of Health and Human Services created a document designed to provide guidance on physical activity for Americans. The 2008 Physical Activity Guidelines provided recommendations covering all age groups, both healthy and with disabilities. Much of the recommendations remain similar to the 2007 ACSM–AHA recommendations, such as the same total volume of physical activity, utilizing the concept of accumulating 10-min bouts, 2 days of strength training, and acknowledging that additional benefits can occur if more activity is performed. However, the Physical Activity Guidelines take a slightly different approach by suggesting a total volume for the week rather than providing a specific frequency and duration (i.e., 30 min/day, 5 days/week). For instance, the Guidelines state that adults should perform 150 min of moderate intensity or 75 min of vigorous intensity activity per week, or an equivalent combination of moderate and vigorous intensity. In combining intensities, 1 min of vigorous intensity is equivalent to 2 min of moderate intensity. Additionally, rather than specific recommendations for only the minimum amount of activity required, the Guidelines suggest a volume of 300 min of moderate activity or 150 min of vigorous activity per week (or an equivalent of both) for additional health benefits (U.S. Dept. of Health and Human Services 2008). These recommendations create a more flexible way to achieve adequate levels of physical activity, thus appealing to a larger audience.

In recent years, the obesity epidemic has caused various groups to also focus their recommendations on the volume of physical activity necessary for weight loss and maintenance. In 2001, the ACSM stated that in order to have weight loss and prevent additional weight gain, overweight individuals should increase their activity to 200–300 min/week (40–60 min, 5 days/week) (Jakicic, Clarke, and Coleman 2001). In 2002, the Institute of Medicine recommended 60 min/day of moderate PA to prevent weight gain (IOM 2002). And a year later, the International Association for the Study of Obesity declared 45 min to 60 min of moderate activity per day necessary to prevent overweight adults from becoming obese, and preventing weight regain may require 60 min to 90 min (Saris et al. 2003). The 2005 Dietary Guidelines had similar recommendations of 60 min most days of the week to prevent weight gain and 60 min to 90 min to help with weight loss and to sustain this loss (U.S. Dept. of Health and Human Services 2005).

These guidelines for weight loss/maintenance led to some confusion among the public regarding what is the adequate volume of physical activity. To summarize, in order to prevent obesity, to have weight loss, and to prevent weight regain, physical activity levels most likely need to exceed 30 min/day. It is important to note, however, that these reports also acknowledge the health benefits that can derive from 30 min of activity, even among the overweight and obese population.

Despite the many efforts by the leading health authorities' recommendations, no significant increases in physical activity have occurred in the United States. Therefore, the most recent action to take place has been the development of the National Physical Activity Plan, introduced in 2010. The Plan does not provide specific recommendations; rather it provides "a comprehensive set of policies, programs, and initiatives that aim to increase physical activity in all segments of the American population" (National Physical Activity Plan 2010). The plan is a collaboration of eight societal sectors, one of them being public health. This is an example of another direction public health is taking in an attempt to increase physical activity levels. Rather than issuing recommendations, the plan provides avenues to take action to develop a heightened public awareness of the importance of physical activity for health.

It is important to note that the recommendations mentioned are not an exhaustive discussion. Various associations have issued recommendations focusing on different age groups such as children and older adults. Furthermore, associations such as the American Cancer Society, American Diabetes Association, and AHA have developed recommendations to prevent or rehabilitate from a specific chronic disease of interest.

In conclusion, the public health spectrum has focused on implementing physical activity recommendations for several decades in an effort to decrease the proportion of sedentary individuals and increase the proportion who achieves adequate levels of activity. The view has gradually shifted over time from a specific focus on improving cardiovascular fitness to improving overall health. In addition, the recommendations continue to shift toward catering to the large sedentary population by making the recommendations more generalized and flexible in frequency, intensity, duration, and mode, ensuring that the recommended volume of activity can be achieved by all individuals.

SUMMARY, CONCLUSIONS, AND WHERE DO WE GO FROM HERE?

We have provided an overview of physical activity and health from ancient times to the present. The review is not exhaustive, but does represent the transitions that have occurred and gives a summary of exercise physiology, physical activity epidemiology, and public health efforts. It now is abundantly clear that we have created a social and physical environment that makes regular physical activity unnecessary, and therefore have created a major public health problem. We must address this threat to overall health and function by giving serious attention and resources to combat the problem. We call for substantial shifts in the public health paradigm to a "Manhattan Project" approach (the undeterred efforts that resulted in the creation of the nuclear bomb from concept to actuality in only 4 years) or "Space flight" approach (the motivation to go from drawing board to a man on the moon in 9 years) to this critical public health issue. Small steps will not work.

STUDY QUESTIONS

1. Compare and contrast the contributions of Susruta, Hippocrates, and Galen to the development of exercise physiology and health.
2. Who deserved the honorary title "the father of Scandinavian exercise physiology," and why are these contributions important to the study of physical activity and health in the twenty-first century?

3. What methodological problems were seen by the early epidemiologists, for example, Morris, Paffenbarger, and Karvonen, in studying the relationship between occupational physical activity and coronary heart disease, and how did they try to overcome the problems?

4. Explain, using specific examples, how the beginnings of epidemiological research paved the way for future public health initiatives. What characteristics within these studies made them so significant?

5. Public health activities may include surveillance and monitoring, etiologic research, intervention research, and program implementation. Provide one or more examples for each category.

6. Identify an appropriate role for federal, state, and local governments regarding physical activity.

7. Explain the paradigm shift of physical activity recommendations. Why was this shift so important, in terms of a public health perspective?

REFERENCES

American College of Sports Medicine. 2006. *Guidelines for Graded Exercise Testing and Exercise Prescription*, 7th ed. Baltimore, MD: Lippincott Williams and Wilkins.

American College of Sports Medicine. 1978. Position statement on the recommended quantity and quality of exercise for developing and maintaining fitness in healthy adults. *Med. Sci. Sports Exerc.* 10: vii–vix.

American College of Sports Medicine Position Stand. 1990. The recommended quantity and quality of exercise for developing and maintaining cardiorespiratory and muscular fitness in healthy adults. *Med. Sci. Sports Exerc.* 22: 265–274.

Åstrand, P.-O. 1991. Influence of Scandinavian scientists in exercise physiology. *Scand. J. Med. Sci. Sports* 1: 3–9.

Blair, S. N. 2009. Physical inactivity: The biggest public health problem of the 21st century. *Br. J. Sports Med.* 43: 1–2.

Blair, S. N., H. W. Kohl, R. S. Paffenbarger et al. 1989. Physical fitness and all-cause mortality. A prospective study of healthy men and women. *JAMA* 262(17): 2395–401.

Bergström, J., L. Hermansen, E. Hultman et al. 1967. Diet, muscle glycogen and physical performance. *Acta Physiol. Scand.* 71: 140–50.

Berryman, J. W. 1992. Exercise and the medical tradition from Hippocrates through antebellum America: A review essay. In *Sport and Exercise Science: Essays in the History of Sports Medicine*, ed. J. W. Berryman and R. J. Park, 1–56. Urbana: Univ. of Illinois Press.

Berryman, J. W. 2003. Ancient and early influences. In *Exercise Physiology: People and Ideas*, ed. C. M. Tipton, 1–38. New York: Oxford University Press.

Berryman, J. W. 2010. Exercise is medicine: A historical perspective. *Curr. Sports Med. Rep.* 9: 195–201.

Farrell, S. W., G. M. Cortese, M. J. LaMonte et al. 2007. Cardiorespiratory fitness, difference measures of adiposity, and cancer mortality in men. *Obesity* 15: 3140–3149.

Fletcher, G. F., S. N. Blair, J. Blumenthal et al. 1992. Statement on exercise. Benefits and recommendations for physical activity programs for all Americans. A statement for health professionals by the Committee on Exercise and Cardiac Rehabilitation of the Council on Clinical Cardiology, American Heart Association. *Circulation* 86: 340–344.

Fox, S. M., and J. S. Skinner. 1964. Physical activity and cardiovascular health. *Am. J. Cardiol.* 14: 731–746.

Haskell, W. L., I. M. Lee, R. R. Pate et al. 2007. Physical activity and public health: Updated recommendation for adults from the American College of Sports Medicine and the American Heart Association. *Med. Sci. Sports Exerc.* 39: 1423–1434.

Heady, J. A., J. N. Morris, A. Kagan et al. 1961. Coronary heart disease in London busmen: A progress report with particular reference to physique. *Br. J. Prev. Med.* 15: 143.

Hill, A. V., and H. Lupton. 1923. Muscular exercise, lactic acid, and the supply and utilization of oxygen. *Q. J. Med.* 16: 135–171.

Institute of Medicine. 2002. *Dietary Reference Intakes For Energy, Carbohydrate, Fiber, Fat, Fatty Acids, Cholesterol, Protein and Amino Acids.* Washington, D.C.: National Academy Press.

Jakicic J. M., K. Clarke, and E. Coleman. 2001. Appropriate intervention strategies for weight loss and prevention of weight regain for adults. American College of Sports Medicine position stand. *Med. Sci. Sports Exerc.* 33: 214–256.

Karvonen, M. J. 1984. Physical activity and cardiovascular morbidity. *Scand. J. Work Environ. Health* 10: 389–395.

Karvonen, M. J. 1982. Physical activity in work and leisure time in relation to cardiovascular diseases. *Ann. Clin. Res.* 14: 118–123.

Karvonen, M. J. 1995. Prehistory of the North Karelia Project. In *The North Karelia Project 20 year results and experiences*, ed. P. Puska, J. Tuomilehto, A. Nissinen, and E. Vartiainen, 17–21. Helsinki: National Public Institute.

Karvonen, M. J., E. Kentala, and O. Mustala. 1957. The effects of training on heart rate; a longitudinal study. *Ann. Med. Exp. Biol. Fenn.* 35: 307–315.

Karvonen, M. J., P. M. Rautharju, E. Orma et al. 1961. Heart disease and employment: Cardiovascular studies on lumberjacks. *J. Occup. Med.* 3: 49–53.

Krogh, A. 1913. On the composition of the air in the tracheal system of some insects. *Scand. Arch. Physiol.* 29: 29–36.

Lalonde, M. 1974. A new perspective on the health of Canadians. A working document. Ottawa: Government of Canada.

Lee, C. D., S. N. Blair, and A. S. Jackson. 1999 Cardiorespiratory fitness, body composition, and all-cause and cardiovascular disease mortality in men. *Am. J. Clin. Nutr.* 69: 373–380.

Leon, A. S., and H. Blackburn. 1977. The relationship of physical activity to coronary heart disease and life expectancy. *Ann. N. Y. Acad. Sci.* 301: 561–578.

Liljestrand, G., and J. Lindhard. 1920. Uber das Minutvolumen des Herzens beim Schwimmen. Studien uber die Physiologie des Schwimmens. *Skand. Arch. Physiol.* 39: 64–77.

Morris, J. N., M. G. Everitt, R. Pollard R. et al. 1980. Vigorous exercise in leisure time: Protection against coronary heart disease. *Lancet* 2: 1207–1210.

Morris, J. N., J. A. Heady, P. A. B. Raffle et al. 1953. Coronary heart disease and physical activity of work (part 1 and part 2). *Lancet* 2: 1053–1057, 111–120.

National Center for Health Statistics. 2010. Selected Milestones in Physical Activity Research, Promotion and Surveillance. http://www.cdc.gov/nchs/nhis/physical_activity/pa_history .htm (accessed July 28, 2010).

National Physical Activity Plan. 2010. U.S. National Physical Activity Plan: 2010. http:// www.physicalactivityplan.org/theplan.htm (accessed August 28, 2010).

NIH Consensus Development Panel on Physical Activity and Cardiovascular Health. 1996. Physical activity and cardiovascular health. *JAMA* 276: 241–246.

Paffenbarger, R. S., M. E. Laughlin, A. S. Gima et al. 1970. Work activity of longshoremen as related to death from coronary heart disease and stroke. *N. Engl. J. Med.* 282: 1109–1114.

Paffenbarger, R. S., A. L. Wing, and R. T. Hyde. 1978. Physical activity as an index of heart attack risk in college alumni. *Am. J. Epidemiol.* 108: 161–175.

Pate, R. R., M. Pratt, S. N. Blair et al. 1995. Physical activity and public health: A recommendation from the Centers for Disease Control and Prevention and the American College of Sports Medicine. *JAMA* 273: 402–407.

Physical Activity Guidelines Advisory Committee. 2008. *Physical Activity Guidelines Advisory Committee Report, 2008*. Washington, DC: U.S. Department of Health and Human Services.

Pollock, M. L. 1973. The quantification of endurance training programs. *Exerc. Sport Sci. Rev.* 1: 155–188.

Powell, K. E., and R. S. Paffenbarger Jr. 1985. Workshop on epidemiologic and public health aspects of physical activity and exercise: A summary. *Public Health Rep.* 100: 118–126.

Powell, K. E., P. D. Thompson, C. J. Caspersen et al. 1987. Physical activity and the incidence of coronary heart disease. *Annu. Rev. Public Health* 8: 253–287.

Pratt, M., J. N. Epping, and W. H. Dietz. 2009. Putting physical activity into public health: A historical perspective from the CDC. *Prev. Med.* 49: 301–302.

Public Health Service. 1979. *Healthy people: The Surgeon General's Report on Health Promotion and Disease Prevention*. Department of Health, Education, and Welfare (PHS). Publication No. 79-55071.

Public Health Service. 1980. *Promoting Health Preventing Disease: Objectives for the Nation*. U.S. Department of Health and Human Services.

Rautaharju, P. M., M. J. Karvonen, and A. Keys. 1961. The frequency of arteriosclerotic and hypertensive heart disease among ostensibly healthy working populations in Finland. An electrocardiographic and clinical study. *J. Chronic Dis.* 13: 426–438.

Saris, W. H., S. N. Blair, M. A. van Baak et al. 2003. How much physical activity is enough to prevent unhealthy weight gain? Outcome of the IASO 1st Stock Conference and consensus statement. *Obes. Rev.* 4: 101–114.

Slattery, M. L., and D. R. Jacobs. 1988. Physical fitness and cardiovascular disease mortality: The US Railroad study. *Am. J. Epidemiol.* 127: 571–580.

Sui, X., S. P. Hooker, I. M. Lee et al. 2008. A prospective study of cardiorespiratory fitness and risk of type 2 diabetes in women. *Diabetes Care* 31: 550–555.

Taylor, H. L., E. Buskirk, and A. Henschel. 1955. Maximal oxygen intake as an objective measure of cardio-respiratory performance. *J. Appl. Physiol.* 8: 73–80.

Taylor, H. L., E. Klepetar, A. Keys et al. 1962. Death rates among physically active and sedentary employees of the railroad industry. *Am. J. Public Health Nation's Health* 52: 1697–1707.

Tipton, C. M. 2008a. Historical perspective: The antiquity of exercise, exercise physiology and the exercise prescription for health. *World Rev. Nutr. Diet* 98: 198–245.

Tipton, C. M. 2008b. Susruta of India, an unrecognized contributor to the history of exercise physiology. *J. Appl. Physiol.* 104: 1553–1556.

U.S. Department of Health and Human Services. 1996. *Physical Activity and Health: A report of the Surgeon General*. Atlanta, GA: U.S. Department of Health and Human Services. Centers for Disease Control and Prevention, National Center for Chronic Disease Prevention and Health Promotion.

U.S. Department of Health and Human Services. 2008. *Physical Activity Guidelines for Americans*. Available at: http://www.health.gov/paguidelines/ (accessed on July 10, 2010).

U.S. Department of Health and Human Services, U.S. Department of Agriculture. 2005. *Dietary Guidelines for Americans, 2005*. Washington, D.C.

World Health Organization (WHO). 1985. Primary prevention of coronary heart disease: Report on a WHO meeting. EURO Reports and Studies 98.

World Health Organization (WHO). 1995. Exercise for health. WHO/FIMS Committee on Physical Activity for Health. *Bull. World Health Organ.* 73: 135–136.

2 Physiological Adaptations to Moderate-Intensity Aerobic Exercise

Arthur S. Leon and Scott Brown

CONTENTS

INTRODUCTION

As evidenced by the writings of Hippocrates and Moses Maimonides, it has been recognized since antiquity that incorporation of regular physical activity (PA) into one's lifestyle, promotes health, well-being, and the quality—and perhaps the length—of one's life. These observations have been confirmed by scientific evidence accumulated primarily over the past three decades. The evidence is primarily from longitudinal observational studies supported by demonstration of multiple plausible biological mechanisms from animal studies and randomized clinical trials, particularly on the role of PA in the prevention of coronary heart disease (Shiroma and Lee 2010).

Table 2.1 lists many of the medical conditions reported to be benefited by regular, moderate-intensity PA, as supported by varying strengths of scientific support (Bouchard, Blair, and Haskell 2007; U.S. Department of Health and Human Services 1996, 2008). This topic is discussed in detail elsewhere in this text. Recently, evidence also has been accumulating of health hazards of prolonged sitting at work and during leisure time (e.g., the amount of time using a computer and/or watching television). This sedentary behavior is also a predictor of health problems, independent of one's PA status (Owen, Healy, and Matthews 2010; Shiroma and Lee 2010).

Both the acute physiologic responses and the long-term adaptations to chronic PA depend on the type, intensity, duration, and frequency or total volume of the activity. The major focus of this chapter is on the cardiovascular and musculoskeletal

TABLE 2.1

Medical Conditions Postulated to Be Reduced by Regular Moderate-Intensive Aerobic Physical Activity

Coronary heart disease

Strokes

Overweight, obesity, and the related metabolic syndrome

Type 2 diabetes mellitus

Essential hypertension

Osteoporosis and prevention of fall-related fractures

Mood and mental health disorders

Cognitive impairment and risk for senile dementia (Alzheimer's disease)

Risks of infection and immune dysfunctions

system's physiological responses to moderate-intensity, cardiorespiratory endurance or the so-called aerobic exercise. We will also briefly review some recent evidence of favorable brain adaptations to regular PA, which can improve mood and perhaps reduce risk of senile dementia (Alzheimer's disease). Examples of aerobic activities include jogging, running, brisk walking, calisthenics, cross-country skiing, cycling, and swimming. Moderate-intensity is defined as requiring 4 to 6 times one's resting energy expenditure (i.e., 4–6 METs [metabolic equivalent], where 1 MET is defined as the resting metabolic rate associated with an oxygen expenditure rate of about 3.5 mL/kg body weight per minute) (Bouchard, Blair, and Haskell 2007). This is generally equivalent to 60% to 80% of one's maximal heart rate (HR max), during all-out physical exertion. HR max can be determined directly by a maximal exercise test on a treadmill or cycle ergometer, or can be estimated using the formula: 220 bpm – age (years) ± 10 bpm.

The recommended frequency of exercise at this moderate-intensity is 3–5 days/ week for a minimum of 30 to 60 min/session or at least 150 min/week with a total energy expenditure of about 1000–2000 kcal/week (Shiroma and Lee 2010). The above exercise training prescription would be expected to provide the musculoskeletal, the cardiovascular, and the central nervous system's physiological adaptations discussed in this chapter, as well as other health benefits discussed elsewhere in this text. However, there is a great deal of variability between individuals in their responsiveness to training related to genetic factors (Bouchard et al. 1999). Although additional improvements in physical fitness and potential health benefits can be obtained by more strenuous and/or a larger volume (e.g., ≥4000 kcal/wk) of aerobic exercise training (Shiroma and Lee 2010), the potential risk of injury is also increased, as discussed later in this chapter.

ACUTE PHYSIOLOGIC RESPONSES

Initiation of aerobic activities requires immediate activation of the body's musculoskeletal, cardiovascular, and respiratory system (Rowell 1986). The primary function of the cardiovascular and respiratory systems is to provide the body, and particularly the skeletal muscles involved in the exercise, with an adequate supply of oxygen (O_2), and to eliminate from the body carbon dioxide and other metabolic waste products, including excess heat generated by muscle metabolism. The circulatory system also provides the muscles with nutrients (glucose and free fatty acids) as fuels for oxidative metabolism. Oxygen uptake increases with the intensity of exercise until a maximal volume uptake is achieved (VO_2 max). Hemodynamically, VO_2 max is the product of the maximal cardiac output and the difference between the O_2 content of arterial blood and mixed venous blood (arteriovenous O_2 difference), which reflects the extent of O_2 extraction, primarily by contracting muscles. The cardiac output is the total volume of blood pumped from the ventricles of the heart per minute during systole (the period of heart muscle/myocardial contraction) and is the product of HR times the stroke volume (SV), that is, the volume of blood ejected from the heart with each cardiac contraction during systole.

The pattern of arterial blood distribution to the different tissues of the body is also dramatically changed upon initiation of exercise (Rowell 1986). There is a major redistribution of the cardiac output to the muscles involved with the exercise associated with a reduction in blood flow to less metabolically active areas of the body, including inactive muscle, the gastrointestinal tract, and the kidneys. Changes in smooth muscle tone in arterioles (small arteries) are responsible for shunting blood flow to the active muscles from the less active organs, that is, a relaxation of smooth muscle in active skeletal muscles' arterioles results in vasodilatation and increased blood flow, whereas a constriction of smooth muscle in the less active tissues' arterioles reduces blood flow to these organs.

The excess heat generated by increased oxidative metabolism in active muscles also results in blood flow redistribution to the skin for its elimination during exercise, primarily by increased sweat evaporation from the skin surface. There also is a linear increase in systolic blood pressure (BP) with increasing intensity of physical exertion. This is related to the increase in cardiac output, which counteracts the BP-lowering effects of the reduced peripheral resistance to blood flow from the heart, caused by the associated dilatation of arterioles. The exercise-induced increase in both HR and systolic BP are major contributors to increased myocardial O_2 demands. Since even at rest, the heart muscles extract about 80% of the O_2 entering the myocardial capillaries (as compared to only 30–40% of O_2 uptake by skeletal muscle in the resting stage), an increase in myocardial O_2 demands during exercise can only be met by increasing coronary blood flow. Thus, a linear relationship exists between the product of HR times systolic BP and the metabolic O_2 demands of the myocardium, as well as with coronary blood flow requirements.

During the recovery period after each prolonged session of aerobic exercise, a number of important physiological adaptations occur. These include a reduction in BP for at least several hours during recovery, a phenomenon commonly referred to as "postexercise hypotension." In addition, there is an accelerated uptake for many hours of glucose from the blood by the exercised muscles, independent of insulin activity, which at rest is required for glucose uptake by muscles and other tissues. This appears to be due to both improved cell insulin receptor sensitivity and the effect of increased muscle contractions on levels at cell membranes of a glucose transporter protein (GLUT-4), required for muscle glucose uptake (Bouchard, Blair, and Haskell

2007). Another contributor to accelerated muscle glucose uptake during exercise recovery is an exercise-induced depletion of muscle glycogen stores, which results in an increase in activity of glycogen synthase, the enzyme required for glycogen resynthesis. Glycogen is a long-chained carbohydrate composed entirely of glucose, which is a necessary fuel for sustaining muscular contractions. The exercise-induced accelerated glucose uptake by skeletal muscle is especially important for individuals with an absolute or a relative deficiency of insulin due to insulin resistance (i.e., with prediabetes or type 1 or type 2 diabetes mellitus).

LONG-TERM CARDIOVASCULAR ADAPTATIONS

Aerobic exercise conditioning results in improved cardiorespiratory fitness, as evidenced by a usual 10% to 20% in VO_2 max. The extent of improvement is inversely related to the initial level of VO_2 max, and is directly related to the skeletal muscle mass used in the conditioning program, the intensity and volume of exercise, and the duration of the training program (Rowell 1986), as well as genetic determinants (Bouchard et al. 1999). Twenty weeks of moderate-intensity training generally appears optimal for improving VO_2 max. Both central (heart) and peripheral circulatory adjustments usually contribute to the exercise-induced increase in VO_2 max. These include an increase in maximal cardiac output and/or an increase in peripheral arterial oxygen extraction (arteriovenous O_2 difference) and in its metabolic utilization.

Since maximal HR is unaffected by exercise training, an increase in maximal cardiac output is entirely related to an increase in SV. This increase in SV, in turn, is generally due to enhanced myocardial contractility, which is usually associated with an increase in the return of venous blood to the heart during diastole (between heart beats), and the resulting increase in the end-diastolic blood volume in the ventricles of the heart (the so-called "preload volume"). In those regularly performing a very high volume of exercise (e.g., marathon running), these changes generally result in dilatation of the left ventricle, followed by the development of cardiac hypertrophy (increased ventricular muscle wall mass). Atrial dimensions also are increased by long-term intense exercise training (Hauser et al. 1985).

An increase in VO_2 max with exercise training is generally accompanied by a reduction in HR and BP, both at rest and during submaximal exercise. Thus, after aerobic exercise conditioning, an individual not only has greater cardiorespiratory exercise endurance, but also has a lower HR times systolic BP product at rest and during submaximal exercise, indicating a reduction in myocardial O_2 requirements, and therefore a reduction in coronary blood flow requirements. This reduction in myocardial O_2 demands is an important adaptation especially in the presence of reduced coronary blood flow reserve, resulting from atherosclerotic buildup of plaque in coronary artery linings. Thus, an exercise-trained individual with underlying coronary artery disease is less likely during physical exertion or emotional stress to experience myocardial ischemia (insufficient heart muscle O_2 supply), resulting in angina pectoris (chest pain) or a serious ventricular rhythm disturbance (ventricular tachycardia or ventricular fibrillation), a common cause of unexpected, out-of-hospital, sudden cardiac death (SCD). In addition to reducing coronary blood flow requirements, aerobic exercise training can also increase coronary blood flow capacity by multiple mechanisms. These include an increase in the luminal area and elasticity of major coronary arteries, an increase in myocardial capillary density (i.e., an increased number of coronary capillaries for each heart muscle fiber), and possibly an increase in collateral artery blood flow to ischemic areas of the heart (Leon and Bronas 2009). Furthermore, the associated increase in coronary flow during exercise stimulates endothelial cells (the single layer of cells lining the lumen of arteries) to increase their synthesis of nitric oxide, a potent vasodilator, as well as other vasodilators, further augmenting coronary flow capacity. Improved endothelial function in peripheral arteries, along with improved artery compliance (elasticity), also contributes to the exercise-induced BP reduction by decreasing peripheral resistance to blood flow. The above-mentioned cardiovascular adaptations support the growing body of evidence that a regular moderate volume and intensity of aerobic exercise, and the associated improvement in aerobic fitness, reduce the risk of fatal or nonfatal myocardial infarctions (heart attacks) (Shiroma and Lee 2010). There also is evidence that regular moderate-intensity exercise reduces the rate of development and progression of atherosclerosis by multiple mechanisms, including improved artery endothelial function, reduced inflammation, and by decreasing other cardiovascular disease risk factors (Leon and Bronas 2009). Risk factors, which can be favorably impacted by exercise training, include overweight/obesity, elevated BP, levels of blood glucose, and one's blood lipid profile. In addition, regular exercise reduces the risk of a thrombotic (blood clot) occlusion in a diseased coronary artery after disruption of a plaque (antithrombotic effect). Furthermore, there is limited evidence that exercise also can improve the electrical stability of the heart, reducing risk of fatal ventricular rhythm disturbances (antiarrhythmic effect).

Although a high volume of exercise (defined here as ≥ 2 hours per session) and vigorous exercise (greater than 6 METS energy expenditure or greater than 80% of HR max) result in a greater increase in VO_2 max and work capacity than a more moderate intensity and volume of exercise, they also are associated with a higher risk of injuries (Bouchard, Blair, and Haskell 2007). These include not only musculoskeletal injuries, but temporarily a much greater risk of a fatal ventricular rhythm disturbance then during rest or lower intensity exercise. Risk of SCD during vigorous exercise in young athletes is rare and generally related to underlying inherited cardiovascular anomalies (Maron 2003). In middle-aged and older individuals, SCD during exercise is usually associated with underlying, generally silent coronary artery disease. Habitually physically inactive (sedentary) individuals are at a considerable greater risk of sudden death when they perform strenuous physical exertion than are those who are habitually moderately active (and more physically fit). However, it should be noted that even habitually moderately active individuals are temporarily at increased risk of SCD during strenuous physical exertion if they have underlying coronary artery disease (Bouchard, Blair, and Haskell 2007). Prolonged physical exertion (>2 hours), such as training for and running a marathon, is also commonly followed by elevation in blood levels of protein biomarkers derived specifically from heart muscle (e.g., troponins; Shave, Baggish, and George 2010). Controversy exists as to whether these elevations in cardiac biomarkers are actually due to exercise-induced myocardial damage or result from an increase in heart muscle cell membrane permeability during prolonged exercise.

In contrast to the apparent antiatherosclerotic effects of a regular, moderate volume of aerobic exercise, a recent study reported at the 2010 annual meeting of the American College of Cardiology suggests that a regular high volume of exercise (such as repeated marathon running) may have a proatherogenic effect on coronary arteries (Schwartz et al., personal communication, 2010). This study compared the severity of atherosclerosis in the coronary arteries, identified by noninvasive computer tomography coronary angiography (coronary CT scans), of 25 middle-aged men (average age of 60 years), who had run at least one marathon a year for the past 25 years, with the coronaries of 23 matched sedentary men. Despite lower levels of body fat, resting HR and BP, and a more favorable blood lipid profile, the marathon runners as a group had significantly more severe atherosclerosis and a higher calcium score in their coronaries. It was hypothesized that the more favorable cardiovascular disease risk factor profile in the runners was counteracted by metabolic and mechanical damage to the endothelial linings of their coronary arteries, related to their high volume of regular long-distance running, which promoted the progression and severity of coronary atherosclerosis These disturbing findings require confirmation.

LONG-TERM MUSCULOSKELETAL ADAPTATIONS

As mentioned, exercise training increases O_2 uptake by active skeletal muscles. An increase in muscle capillary density (capillaries per muscle fiber) contributes to this increase in O_2 uptake (Rowell 1986). In addition, an exercise-induced increase in muscle myoglobin levels accelerates the transport of O_2 from capillaries to cell mitochondria (Bouchard, Blair, and Haskell 2007). Mitochondria are cellular structures containing the enzymes required for oxidative metabolism of fatty acids and glucose. In addition, there is a training-induced increase in the number of mitochondria per cell and in their enzymatic activity. Furthermore, exercise-conditioned skeletal muscle fiber also have a significant increase in their cross-sectional areas and in their stores of fuels used for oxidative metabolism, that is, glycogen and fat/triglycerides, a source of free fatty acids.

Exercise training also both improves cell sensitivity to insulin and increases muscle synthesis of GLUT-4, which, as mentioned earlier, is required for glucose transport across muscle cell membranes (Bouchard, Blair, and Haskell 2007). Thus, exercise training can markedly improve the metabolic capacity of skeletal muscle for glucose uptake and oxidative energy generation. These skeletal muscle adaptations (along with weight reduction) are postulated to contribute to reduced risk of type 2 diabetes in physically active, as compared to matched sedentary people, including in those with prediabetic conditions.

Although much research has been done on skeletal muscle responses to exercise, there is only limited information on its effects on tendons, which connect the muscles to bones. The available data indicate that exercise training increases tendon strength, especially at their insertion site to the bones, as well as the strength of other related connective tissue structures. However, overuse can cause painful injuries at tendon insertion sites in addition to skeletal muscle damage.

It is well established that daily weight-bearing activities are critical in order for adolescents to achieve their genetically determined, potential peak bone mass.

Furthermore, weight-bearing exercise helps reduce the rate of bone loss with aging, thus reducing the development of osteoporosis (weak porous bones prone to fragility fractures). Strength training and high impact physical activities (e.g., stair climbing, steps' aerobics, and jumping in place) have even a greater impact than walking or running for achieving peak bone mass during adolescence, and reducing the rate of bone loss and increased risk of osteoporosis with aging. In contrast, nonweight-bearing aerobic activities, such as high volume of daily swimming or cycling, have no impact or a negative impact on bone mass and strength (Kohrt et al. 2004).

BRAIN ADAPTATIONS

Ancient Greek philosophers, as early as the 4th century BC, recognized the importance of regular PA as a way of maintaining a clear mind, improve mental processing, and for attenuating the decline in mental powers associated with advanced age. Initial scientific studies confirming favorable effects of PA on mental processing can be traced back to more than a century ago; however, the vast majority of research and published studies on this topic occurred during the past four decades (Poon, Chodzko-Zajko, and Tomporowski 2006). This research has focused on the effects of aerobic exercise training on mood, tolerance to stress, anxiety, depression, and cognitive functions, as well as on biomarkers of brain functions. In addition, favorable mental changes with exercise have been linked to brain structural changes and increased capillarization in areas of the brain associated with memory and learning ability, for example, the hippocampus. These data have provided a compelling body of supportive evidence in humans on how regular aerobic activities reduce mental stress, anxiety, and depression (Bouchard, Blair, and Haskell 2007). Furthermore, a recent study suggests that even a single exercise session appears to help in anger management (Thom et al. 2010). An elevation in mood and a general feeling of well-being are particularly evident immediately after each aerobic exercise session.

It is also postulated that regular exercise can reduce the rate of decline in cognitive functions associated with aging, and thus reduce risk of developing senile dementia (Alzheimer's disease) (Komulainen et al. 2010; Zoeller 2010). Supporting evidence for this hypothesis comes from both animal research and human observational epidemiologic studies. In cross-sectional observational studies, healthy older adults with high cardiorespiratory fitness for their age almost universally performed better on cognitive function tests, then their contemporaries who were unfit. Physically fit subjects were also more likely on brain imaging to demonstrate an increased volume of both white and gray matter in several areas of the brain involved in cognitive functioning, as compared to unfit subjects (Poon, Chodzko-Zajko, and Tomporowski 2006). However, it cannot be ruled out that participants in these observational studies who had a high aerobic capacity may have been genetically predisposed for both higher cognitive function and a high aerobic capacity. Nevertheless, the consistency of these findings is robust. However, controlled exercise intervention studies in humans have generally had mixed results. Only a limited number of randomized, controlled trials in aging individuals have demonstrated a positive effect on cognitive functions or a delay in decline in these functions induced by regular moderate-intensity exercise (generally a walking program). At present, large-scale, better-designed, randomized trials are in progress to evaluate the effects of aerobic exercise on cognitive function changes with aging (e.g., Komulainen et al. 2010).

Neuroscientific studies have also demonstrated a number of plausible physiologic mechanisms by which exercise improves mood and reduces symptoms of anxiety and depression. An early postulated mechanism implicated the role of endogenous (brain and/or pituitary gland synthesized) opiates, such as endorphin, as being responsible for these mental health benefits of exercise. However, research has not supported this hypothesis. More plausible physiological pathways proposed to be responsible for the affective benefits of exercise are alternations in activity of brain monamine (amino acid-derived) neurotransmitters, for example, norepinephrine, dopamine, and serotonin activity (Bouchard, Blair, and Haskell 2007). Unfortunately, testing of this hypothesis is limited by difficulty in measuring brain levels of these neurohormones.

A plausible mechanism postulated to be related to improved cognitive functions attributed to exercise is increased cerebral blood flow, and thereby increasing the supply of O_2 and glucose to the brain. Glucose is a nutrient essential for brain oxidative metabolism to provide energy to sustain its functions. It should be noted that although the brain comprises only about 2% of the total body weight, it uses 20–25% of the total body O_2 uptake, and 25% of the total circulating blood glucose to meet its energy requirements. The previously noted cardiovascular adaptations and improved aerobic fitness with exercise training facilitate the circulatory delivery of O_2 and glucose to the brain. In a recent publication from the longitudinal Framingham Heart Study, positive associations were found between the cardiac index (cardiac output per body surface area) and brain volume, as assessed by brain magnetic resonance imaging (Jefferson et al. 2010). In addition, the study investigators demonstrated improved neuropsychological functions associated with the level of cardiac index. The previously mentioned antiatherosclerotic effects of moderate-intensity aerobic exercise also undoubtedly help the cerebral arteries maintain optimal circulation to the brain. Furthermore, exercise conditioning is postulated to reduce the risk of a thrombotic occlusion of a diseased cerebral artery. A cerebral thrombotic artery occlusion results in ischemic damage and necrosis to the area of the brain supplied by the artery (i.e., a stroke). Reduced cerebral blood flow due to diseased arteries also can cause the so-called "vascular dementia," accompanied by cognitive disturbances resembling those of Alzheimer's disease. Furthermore, as mentioned earlier, animal research shows that exercise training can enhance cerebral blood supply by increasing capillary density, at least in some areas of the brain.

Exercise training also increases the brain levels of neurotropic factors (Poon, Chodzko-Zajko, and Tomporowski 2006; Zoeller 2010). These factors are proteins synthesized by brain neurons (brain cells) that function to help maintain, protect, and promote the growth of neurons, and synapses responsible for communications between neurons (synapogenesis), the best studied of which is the so-called brain-derived neurotropic factor (BDNF). Several laboratories have reported that providing rats free access to running wheels daily for 1 week or longer increases the brain levels of the BDNF. In these studies, this increase was associated with increased neurogenesis (growth of new neurons) in the hippocampus, an area of the brain important for memory and other cognitive functions. Furthermore, a study in mice, selectively bred for deposition of beta amyloid protein in the brain, found that after exercise training the mice had a significantly reduced deposition of beta amyloid plaques. The relevance of the latter finding to the development of the so-called senile dementia in humans is that beta amyloid deposition in the brain is associated with the development of Alzheimer's disease. In addition, in humans, regular PA has been shown to increase blood levels of BDNF. In turn, a low blood level of BDNF in epidemiologic studies has been observed to be predictive of cognitive impairment and increased risk of future dementia. Another relevant finding of the relationship of BDNF to risk of cognitive impairment is that low blood levels of BDNF also are commonly associated with several risk factors for cardiovascular disease, including strokes.

CONCLUSIONS

Physiological adaptations in both heart and skeletal muscles contribute to the improvements in cardiorespiratory endurance with aerobic exercise training. These adaptations result in an increase in stroke volume of the heart, and in the arteriovenous O_2 difference related to the increased O_2 uptake by active skeletal muscle. In addition, exercise training is associated with an increase in blood supply to both myocardial and skeletal muscles. Furthermore, after exercise training the heart becomes more efficient as a pump because of a reduction in HR, BP, and thereby myocardial O_2 demands and coronary blood flow requirements during submaximal physical exertion. Thus, the risk of myocardial ischemia during physical exertion is reduced in someone with underlying advanced coronary artery disease. These anti-ischemic effects (i.e., increased coronary blood flow and reduced myocardial O_2 demands), associated with a moderate-intensity and volume of aerobic exercise training, may be accompanied by antiatherosclerotic, antithrombotic, and antiarrhythmic adaptations. These adaptations associated with regular exercise and improved fitness are postulated to be responsible for the reduced risk of a fatal or nonfatal heart attack due to coronary artery disease, as well as reduced risk of brain strokes due to cerebrovascular disease. However, a recently reported study in which middle-aged men who ran marathons regularly for 25 years of more, were demonstrated by noninvasive imaging of their coronary arteries to have greater severity of atherosclerosis than age-matched healthy sedentary men. This suggests that regular vigorous prolonged exercise training may have adverse effects on coronaries. Confirmation is required of these adverse coronary artery findings in marathon runners. However, in support of this hypothesis, marathon runners following a race have also been commonly found to have elevated blood biomarkers associated with myocardial injury (e.g., troponins). This is postulated to be due to ischemic damage resulting from reduced ability to meet the increased myocardial O_2 demands during prolonged exercise, perhaps because of subclinical coronary artery disease, in addition to an associated reduction in blood volume due to hypohydration. Strenuous physical exertion is also associated with a temporary increase in risk of ventricular rhythm disturbances, which can cause unexpected SCD in those with subclinical (silent) coronary artery disease; however, this risk during strenuous exercise is much greater in habitually sedentary, middle-aged, and older people than in those who are moderately active. The risk of musculoskeletal injury is also much higher with strenuous exercise, as compared to more moderate-intensity exercise.

Skeletal muscle adaptations to exercise training, in addition to the vascular changes previously elaborated, include an increase in muscle glucose uptake from the blood and its storage as glycogen. An accelerated blood glucose disposal by muscle, in addition to an exercise-induced reduction in body weight, are postulated to contribute significantly to the reported reduced risk of type 2 diabetes in regular exercisers.

Alterations of brain monoamine neurotransmitter activity are postulated to be responsible for the positive effects of even single sessions of aerobic exercise on mood, anxiety, depression, and perhaps also on suppression of anger. Furthermore, the antiatherosclerotic and antithrombotic effects of moderate exercise are postulated to reduce risk of cerebral artery disease-related vascular dementia, as well as of strokes causing ischemic brain damage. Both animal and human studies reveal that exercise training also increases brain neurotropic factors, including BDNF, that promote brain health. In addition, animal research suggests that regular exercise can also reduce brain deposition of beta amyloid plaque, which has been associated with development of senile dementia, that is, Alzheimer disease. Much additional research is needed to confirm these encouraging findings.

STUDY QUESTIONS

1. Outline an exercise prescription for a moderate-intensity walking program to include heart rate training zone, duration of sessions, and frequency per week for a healthy 50-year-old adult.
2. Identify two major hemodynamic contributors to an increase in VO_2 max with exercise training. What is the optimum amount of physical activity needed to make these hemodynamic adaptations?
3. Describe three physiological adaptations in skeletal muscle with regular aerobic exercise that contribute to improved functional capacity and reduced risk of type 2 diabetes. Create appropriate training programs that can create these physiological adaptations.
4. List five cardiovascular system adaptations to regular aerobic exercise that help reduce risk of nonfatal or fatal coronary heart disease. Compare differences in the adaptations with light-, moderate-, and vigorous-intensity physical activity.
5. Explain three of the postulated mechanisms for the apparent mental health and cognitive function-enhancing effects of an aerobic exercise program.

REFERENCES

Bouchard, C., P. An, T. Rice et al. 1999. Familial aggregation of VO_2 max response to exercise training results: From the HERITAGE Family Study. *J. Appl. Physiol.* 87: 103–108.
Bouchard, C., S. Blair, and W. Haskell. (eds.). 2007. *Physical Activity and Health.* Champaign, IL: Human Kinetics.
Hauser, A. M., R. H. Dressendorfer, M. Vos et al. 1985. Symmetric cardiac enlargement in highly trained endurance athletes: A two dimensional echocardiographic study. *Am. Heart J.* 109: 1038–1044.

Kohrt, W. M., S. A. Bloomfield, K. D. Little et al. 2004. American college of sports medicine position stand: Physical activity and bone health. *Med. Sci. Sports Exerc.* 36: 1985–1996.

Komulainen, P., M. Kivipelto, T. Lakka et al. 2010. Exercise fitness and cognition—a randomized controlled trial in older individuals. *Eur. Geriatr. Med.* 1: 257–272.

Jefferson, A., J. Himali, A. Beiser et al. 2010. Cardiac index is associated with brain aging. *Circulation* 122: 690–697.

Leon, A. S., and U. G. Bronas. 2009. Pathophysiology of coronary heart disease and biological mechanisms for the cardioprotective effects of regular aerobic exercise. *Am. J. Lifestyle Med.* 3: 379–385.

Maron, B. 2003. Sudden death in young athletes. *N. Engl. J. Med.* 346: 1064–1075.

Owen, N., G. Healy, C. Matthews et al. 2010. Too much sitting: The population health science of sedentary behavior. *Exerc. Sports Sci. Rev.* 38: 105–113.

Poon, L., W. Chodzko-Zajko, and P. Tomporowski. 2006. *Active Living, Cognitive Functioning and Aging.* Champaign, IL: Human Kinetics.

Rowell, L. 1986. *Human Circulation Regulation during Physical Stress.* New York: Oxford University Press.

Shave, R., A. Baggish, and K. George. 2010. Exercise-induced cardiac troponin elevation. *J. Am. Coll. Cardiol.* 56: 169–176.

Shiroma, E., and I.-M. Lee. 2010. Physical activity and cardiovascular health. *Circulation* 122: 743–752.

Thom, N., P. O'Conner, B. Clementz et al. 2010. The effects of an acute bout of moderate intensity exercise on anger and EEG responses during elicitation of angry emotions. *Med. Sci. Sports Exerc.* 42: S42.

U.S. Department of Health and Human Services. 2008. *Physical Activity Guidelines for Americans.* Atlanta, GA: Department of Health and Human Services, Centers for Disease Control and Prevention, National Center for Chronic Disease Prevention and Health Promotion.

U.S. Department of Health and Human Services. 1996. *Physical Activity and Health: A Report of the Surgeon General.* Atlanta, GA: U.S. Department of Health and Human Services, Centers for Disease Control and Prevention, National Center for Chronic Disease Prevention and Health Promotion.

Zoeller, R. Jr. 2010. Exercise in cognitive function: Can working out train the brain too? *Am. J. Lifestyle Med.* 4: 397–408.

3 The Unique Influence of Sedentary Behavior on Health

Genevieve N. Healy

CONTENTS

INTRODUCTION

This book is primarily about the several benefits of physical activity, and how to promote and support regular participation in physical activity. This chapter addresses something conceptually different: sedentary behavior. Sedentary behaviors can broadly be considered as those tasks that require very little energy expenditure and that involve sitting or reclining. Although often considered as simply reflecting the low end of the physical activity continuum, sedentary behaviors are considered to produce physiological responses distinct from those associated with physical activity (Hamilton, Hamilton, and Zderic 2007; Owen et al. 2010). Sedentary behaviors are very common and occur throughout the day and across every domain. Over the past few years, there has been a rapidly accumulating body of evidence regarding their prevalence and their influence on health outcomes. This chapter introduces the concept of sedentary behavior across five sections: (1) What is it? (2) How is it measured? (3) How common is it, and who is at risk? (4) How is it related to health? (5) How can we change it?

WHAT IS SEDENTARY BEHAVIOR?

DEFINITION

The word sedentary is derived from the word Latin word *sedere* meaning "to sit." Sedentary behaviors involve sitting or reclining resulting in little or no physical activity energy expenditure. If we think of activity as being a multiple of the resting metabolic rate (1 MET), then sedentary behaviors are those activities that expend between 1 and 1.5 METS, whereas an activity such as walking requires 3–4 METS. Behaviors classified as being sedentary include sitting for television viewing, computer use, driving, reading, socializing, work, public transport, and playing electronic games. As the term "sedentary" encompasses both sitting and reclining, the broader term sedentary is used in this chapter, except when sitting is specifically measured.

SEDENTARY BEHAVIOR AND PHYSICAL ACTIVITY

As you will read elsewhere in this book, Physical Activity Guidelines in the United States recommend that for health benefits, adults should accumulate at least 30 min of moderate-intensity physical activity on most, preferably all, days of the week. Importantly, this recommendation is in addition to routine activities of daily living that are of light-intensity, such as grocery shopping or taking out the trash (Haskell et al. 2007).

Traditionally, terms such as sedentary lifestyle, sedentariness, and inactive have been used to describe adults who do not meet these Physical Activity Guidelines. However, the term sedentary behavior refers to something different—those behaviors that involve prolonged sitting or reclining and minimal energy expenditure. An individual can be both physically active (i.e., meeting the physical activity guidelines) and highly sedentary (a phenomenon termed "the active couch potato"). Conversely, an individual may be inactive (i.e., not meeting the physical activity guidelines), but have low levels of sedentary time. For example, a parent of a young child may find very little time to do any exercise, but (s)he also may have very little time to be sedentary. In comparison, an office worker may do exercise outside of work hours, but may be sedentary for 9 h at work each day. As such, it is important to take a whole-of-day approach to physical activity promotion where both time spent in physical activity and time spent in sedentary behavior is considered. The following two case studies are used to further illustrate this point.

Case Study 1

On a typical day, Henry wakes up at 7 a.m., sits down to eat breakfast for 20 min, gets ready for work, drives to work (40 min), sits at his office-based work for most of the day (9 h), drives home, walks his dogs for 45 min, sits down to eat dinner (20 min), watches television for 3 h, then goes to bed.

Case Study 2

Lucy is the mother of 2-year-old Jake. On a typical day, Lucy is up at 6 a.m. feeding Jake and getting him dressed. The morning generally consists of household chores such as the dishes and vacuuming and a walk to the local park across the street. While Jake has his midday sleep, Lucy does the washing and prepares dinner. In the afternoon, Jake plays in the backyard while Lucy does some gardening. After dinner, Lucy puts Jake to bed, and then tidies up his toys before watching television for an hour before bed.

LEARNING QUESTIONS

1. Who would be considered to be meeting the physical activity guidelines?
2. Who do you think is more sedentary?

MEASUREMENT OF SEDENTARY BEHAVIOR

KEY POINTS

- Sedentary behaviors occur frequently through the day and across all domains.
- Most commonly measured by self-report questionnaire.
- Questionnaire measures have good reliability, but poor-to-modest validity.
- Objective measures such as accelerometer and inclinometers can reduce the error associated with self-report, but do not provide domain-specific information.
- A combination of self-report and objective measures provides the most useful information.

Sedentary behaviors occur throughout the day and across all domains (work, leisure time, domestic, and travel). Time spent in sedentary behavior is typically assessed during waking hours (i.e., sleep is not included in the calculation), and can be measured by both self-report and by more objectively derived measures. In addition to measuring the total time spent in sedentary behaviors, sedentary behaviors can be assessed individually and collectively in the context of the domains in which they occur. The measurement of time spent in sedentary behaviors is subject to the same considerations as other health behaviors: the applicability, acceptability, sensitivity, specificity, reliability, and validity of the measure.

Self-Report Measures

Time spent in sedentary behavior is most commonly measured by self-report questionnaires. Questionnaires can be implemented on a large scale, are relatively inexpensive to administer and analyze, and do not alter the behavior under investigation. Questionnaire measures are also able to measure both overall sitting time and individual sedentary behaviors (such as TV viewing). However, although they have generally shown good test–retest reliability (i.e., the measures are measuring a similar thing each time), their validity (how accurate the measure is) is generally poor to modest (Clark et al. 2009).

Learning Point

If you think across the whole day, or a whole week, it is probably very difficult to accurately remember all the times and locations that you were sedentary. This is the sitting question used in the International Physical Activity Questionnaire (IPAQ).

During the last 7 days, how much time did you usually spend sitting on a weekday?

_____ Hours per weekday
_____ Minutes per weekday

1. How well do you think you could answer this question?
2. Do you think this question would be more difficult for some people to answer than others?

Methods such as 24-h recalls (i.e., the participant remembers as much as possible about the previous days' activities) have now been adapted from the dietary literature to help to more accurately measure physical activity and sedentary behavior. This method can help to reduce reporting errors such as long-term averaging. Here, the participant uses a program to help record activities undertaken the previous day. The activities are generally recorded in short time intervals, such as 5 min. Even so, these time intervals may not be short enough to pick up short breaks in sedentary time. For example, person A may record that they watched television (TV) from 6:00 p.m. to 6:30 p.m. Person B may record the same thing, but unlike person A, they got up briefly during each of the commercial breaks. Twenty-four hours recalls can also have a substantially higher participant burden than brief questionnaires.

OBJECTIVE MEASURES

Objective measures of sedentary time eliminate errors associated with self-report and can provide information about not only total sedentary time and its dose–response relationship with health outcomes, but also the manner in which sedentary time is accumulated. Figure 3.1 illustrates the sedentary behavior patterns of two people: both with the same amount of total sedentary time, but very different in how they accrue their sedentary time (Healy 2007). Here, the "prolonger" is someone who is typically happy to remain seated for long periods, whereas the "breaker" is one of those people who finds it difficult to sit still—even if it is only to stand up and move about briefly for short periods. More interruptions or breaks in sedentary time have been beneficially linked to health outcomes (Healy et al. 2008a, 2011). However, these small "microbreaks" are very difficult to recall via self-report methods.

Accelerometers are the most commonly used instrument to objectively derive free-living sedentary time. These are small mechanical devices typically attached around the hip and worn for a number of consecutive days. Accelerometers measure the intensity, duration, and frequency of walking and running movements. The absence of these movements can be used to derive sedentary time. They have been used in large population based studies including the U.S. National Health and Nutrition Examination Survey (NHANES)—where more than 14,000 people had accelerometer readings taken in the years 2003–2006 (Matthews et al. 2008). Accelerometers have also been used as the criterion measure for the validation of physical activity and sedentary behavior questionnaires (Clark et al. 2009). However, their use as a criterion measure for sedentary time needs to be considered with caution as they are unable to distinguish between types of sedentary behavior (e.g., TV viewing vs. computer use), or different postures (e.g., sitting vs. standing still). Devices that tell what postural alignment (sitting/standing) the body is in (such as inclinometers) are now more readily available and could be considered a more appropriate criterion for the validation of self-report sedentary time measures.

A key limitation of these objective measures (accelerometers and inclinometers) is their cost: they are more expensive and resource-intensive than self-report

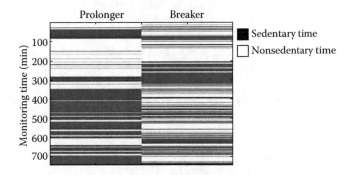

FIGURE 3.1 Accumulation pattern of sedentary (<100 cpm) and nonsedentary (≥100 cpm) time for two participants with identical total sedentary time for 1 day of accelerometer recording. (From Healy, G.N., *Physical Activity, Sedentary Time and Blood Glucose in Australian Adults*, University of Queensland, Brisbane, 2007. With permission.)

measures. They also have a greater participant burden, which may impact on studies that require repeated and/or long-term wear. Additionally, they do not provide information about the specific sedentary behavior or the domain in which it is occurring. This contextual information is useful for the development of intervention targets and public health messaging on how to reduce sedentary time. As such, a combination of both self-report and objective measures is likely to provide the most accurate and informative sedentary behavior data.

SUMMARY

Questionnaire measures are the most common method for measuring time spent in sedentary behaviors; however, they do have their limitations. Further research is required to determine the most reliable and valid questions to measure sedentary time, and also to see whether there are differences between population groups on these measures. The increasing affordability of objective measures, particularly those that measure postural alignment, offer exciting new possibilities for sedentary behavior measurement.

HOW COMMON IS IT, AND WHO IS AT RISK? SEDENTARY BEHAVIOR PREVALENCE, TRENDS, AND CORRELATES

KEY POINTS

- On average, more than 50% of the day is spent sedentary. Highest levels are observed in older adults.
- TV viewing is the most common leisure time sedentary behavior.
- For children and adolescents, less than 2 h/day of screen time is recommended. Most children and adolescents report watching more than this.
- High TV viewing time is correlated with not being in paid employment, having a lower income, lower education, and older age.

Unlike physical activity, there is less evidence in the literature on population levels of total sedentary time or time spent in specific sedentary behaviors, particularly in relation to trends across time. To some extent, surrogate measures such as car ownership, vehicle miles, and computer and television ownership can be used to highlight the rising potential for time spent sedentary. This section gives an overview of how much time is spent sedentary—both throughout the whole day and in specific sedentary behaviors. It also looks at the characteristics of those who have high levels of sedentary time.

HOW COMMON ARE SEDENTARY BEHAVIORS?

The largest population-based study using accelerometer measures of sedentary time is NHANES. Data from this study reported that, on average, U.S. children and adults spend more than half (55% or 460 min/day) of their waking hours sedentary (Matthews et al. 2008). Similarly high levels of accelerometer-derived sedentary time have been reported in Australian adults (57% or 504 min/day; Healy et al. 2007, 2008c), Swedish adults (459 min/day; Hagstromer, Oja, and Sjostrom 2007), and Chinese adults (509 min/day; Peters et al. 2010). The remainder of waking hours is mostly spent in light-intensity, incidental activity, with only a small proportion of time spent in moderate-vigorous intensity activity (Healy et al. 2008c; Hagstromer, Oja, and Sjostrom 2007).

Estimates of self-reported sitting time are slightly lower than those derived from accelerometers. Using the same sitting question from the IPAQ (as per the "Learning Point" in "Measurement of Sedentary Behavior" section), daily time spent sitting was compared for 49,493 adults aged 18–65 years across 20 countries (Bauman et al. 2011). Average sitting time was 346 min/day, with the highest rates observed in Taiwan, Norway, Hong Kong, Saudi Arabia, and Japan (440 min/day). Interestingly, self-reported rates from the United States were 330 min/day—far lower than the objectively derived estimates. This suggests that sitting rates across countries may be even higher than what is currently reported.

When specific sedentary behaviors are examined, TV viewing time is both the most commonly measured (Clark et al. 2009) and the most prevalent leisure-time sedentary behavior (Biddle et al. 2009). For example, TV viewing time occupied one-third to one-half of all sedentary behavior time for Scottish adolescents, with similar findings observed in Hungarian (Hamar et al. 2010) and British (Gorely et al. 2009) youths.

Given its high prevalence, TV viewing time has been targeted in public health guidelines. Specifically, the American Academy of Pediatrics (2001) recommends that children and youths spend no more than 2 h/day in front of screens. However, a survey of 41 countries across Europe and North America (the Health Behavior in School Age Children Survey), asking 11-, 13-, and 15-year-olds to report their television viewing time (including DVDs and videos), found that the proportion who exceeded this level was 61%, 70%, and 68%, respectively (Currie et al. 2008). The highest levels were reported in Bulgaria (11- and 13-year-olds) and Slovakia (15-year-olds), with proportions in these countries exceeding 80%, whereas the lowest levels were reported in Switzerland for all three age groups (Currie et al. 2008).

For adults, data from the United States reports a dramatic rise in TV ownership from 1950 to 2000 that was matched by an approximate doubling of average viewing hours per day from an estimated 4.5 to nearly 8 h/day (Brownson et al. 2005). Although TV viewing time declined in Canada over the periods of 1986 to 2005, this was matched by a rapid increase in home computer use and Internet availability such that actual screen time is on the rise (Shields and Tremblay 2008).

Compared to these leisure-time sedentary behaviors, relatively less is known about the prevalence of sedentary time in the work and travel domains. The last decade has seen rapid declines in work-related activity in both men and women (Brownson et al. 2005), and for many adults, the workplace is a common setting for prolonged sedentary time. Findings from Australia and the Netherlands have shown that working adults report between 2 and 4 h of sitting at work per day, and workdays are associated with less standing and more sitting than leisure days (Brown, Miller, and Miller 2003; Jans, Proper, and Hildebrandt 2007; McCrady and Levine 2009).

Why might this be so? Well, one reason is that the number of work tasks focused around sitting at a computer has increased markedly over the past few decades. For example, in Australia, the proportion of businesses with internet access rose from 29% in 1994 to 90% in 2008/2009 (Australian Bureau of Statistics 2010). The increased time spent in front of the computer and the availability of e-mail has meant that many of those previous office-based tasks that involved intermittent standing and some physical activity, such as filing or walking over to see a colleague, are no longer required.

The last decade has also seen marked increases in vehicle miles per person and rapid declines in household-related activity in women (Brownson et al. 2005). Some may argue that despite these changes, we are still spending nearly half of our day not sedentary. Unfortunately, we may not have bottomed out yet, and we have the potential to get far more sedentary—particularly given the pace of technological innovation (Hamilton, Hamilton, and Zderic 2007). As such, it becomes even more important to have reliable and valid measures of population levels of sedentary behaviors so that trends across time and the impact of any health promotion campaigns can be monitored.

CHARACTERISTICS OF THOSE WITH HIGH SEDENTARY TIME

It is important to understand not only how sedentary the population is on average, but also whether there are specific groups that have higher rates of sedentary time than others. Using objective (accelerometer) measures of sedentary time, the most sedentary groups in the United States were older adolescents and older adults (≥60 years). Gender and race/ethnicity differences were observed with women being more sedentary than men before the age of 30 years, with this pattern reversed after 60 years, whereas Mexican–American adults were significantly less sedentary than U.S. adults of other race/ethnicities (Matthews et al. 2008).

When specific sedentary behaviors are examined, time use surveys from both the United States and Australia show that TV viewing time is higher within older age groups and that on average men watch more TV than women (Australian Bureau of Statistics 1997; Bureau of Labor Statistics 2008). Among adolescents, exceeding the 2 h/day screen time recommendation is more common among those in less affluent households and those living in Eastern Europe (Currie et al. 2008). Similarly, in a longitudinal study in British adolescents ($N = 5863$; 11–12 years at baseline), sedentary behavior levels (including watching TV and playing video games) were higher among those with low socio-economic status (Brodersen et al. 2007). Race/ethnicity differences in TV viewing time are also reported, with high levels of TV viewing time observed among Blacks compared to Whites or Hispanics (Sidney et al. 1996).

The characteristics of those who watch high levels of TV are consistent across U.S. (Bowman 2006), Canadian (Shields and Tremblay 2008), and Australian adults (Clark et al. 2010): low educational attainment, not employed, and low income (Shields and Tremblay 2008; Bowman 2006; Clark et al. 2010). High body mass index (BMI) (Bowman 2006) is also a common characteristic of those with high TV viewing time; however, as discussed later, the causal direction of this relationship has not been elucidated. The sociodemographic characteristics of those with high levels of other sedentary behaviors have been less well studied. In Canadian adults, the characteristics of frequent computer users included high educational attainment and young age, as well as not being employed (Shields and Tremblay 2008). Environments can also play a role, with the walkability of a neighborhood (street connectivity, residential density, access to destinations) associated with TV viewing time (Owen et al. 2010).

Summary

Sedentary behaviors occur across the day and across every domain. In 2003–2004, the U.S. population aged 6 years and older spent over half of their waking hours sedentary. With the rapid proliferation of computer-based activities at the home, school, and work settings, as well as environmental factors such as urban sprawl and traffic congestion, it can be expected that this rate may now be even higher, particularly among those sociodemographic groups at high risk.

SEDENTARY BEHAVIOR AND HEALTH OUTCOMES

Key Points

- The physiological response to sedentary behavior may be different to the response to a lack of exercise.
- Sedentary behaviors are linked with several health outcomes including early death, obesity, cardiovascular disease, and cancer.
- Detrimental associations with health are observed even in those who are physically active.

This section gives a general overview of the physiology underpinning sedentary behavior and the relationship of sedentary behavior with major health outcomes including premature mortality, obesity, cardiovascular disease, and cancer. Although the majority of epidemiological studies have used self-report measures of sedentary behavior, there is an emerging evidence linking objectively measured (via accelerometers and by heart rate) sedentary time with these health outcomes and other factors such as bone health and depression. Importantly, for the majority of studies, the presented findings are independent of several other risk factors, including moderate-vigorous intensity physical activity levels. To date, most research has come from cross-sectional studies.

Physiology

In terms of energy expenditure, there is a relatively small differential between sitting and static standing. However, although energy expenditure is important for preventing weight gain, being sedentary may impart other deleterious health-related consequences. During standing, postural muscles (predominately those of the lower limbs) are continually contracting in order to keep the body upright and prevent loss of balance. Frequent contractions in these large muscle groups are largely absent while sedentary. Animal studies have shown that this leads to changes in two key physiological responses that can promote poor metabolic health. First, skeletal muscle lipoprotein lipase (LPL) production is suppressed. The LPL enzyme is necessary for breaking down blood fats (i.e., triglycerides) in the body. Suppression of LPL induced through being sedentary can lead to elevated triglyceride levels. Second, the breaking down and use of glucose (blood sugar) is reduced, thereby contributing to elevations within the blood. The decline in LPL activity observed with being sedentary does not appear to exist when incidental, light-intensity activity (including standing) is introduced (Hamilton, Hamilton, and Zderic 2007). Importantly, the LPL response is different for sedentary behavior and physical activity. For sedentary behavior, the reduction in LPL response is largely restricted to the oxidative (red) muscle fibers, whereas increases in LPL due to physical activity are mostly observed in the glycolytic (white) muscle fibers (Hamilton, Hamilton, and Zderic 2007). Furthermore, the decreases in LPL activity observed with sedentary behavior are more than four times greater than the increases in LPL activity observed after vigorous exercise (Hamilton, Hamilton, and Zderic 2007). To date, this "inactivity physiology" research has only been carried out in animal models. It is important to replicate these studies with human participants to further understand and distinguish the unique physiological effects of prolonged sedentary time.

SEDENTARY BEHAVIOR AND EARLY DEATH

Sedentary time, assessed as either daily sitting time (Katzmarzyk et al. 2009), leisure time sitting (Patel et al. 2010), time spent sitting in cars (Warren et al. 2010), or television viewing time (Dunstan et al. 2010; Wijndaele et al. 2011), is associated with higher mortality risk—particularly from cardiovascular disease. Figure 3.2 shows the hazard ratios (or relative risks) and 95% confidence intervals for cardiovascular disease mortality of these various sedentary measures from four different studies. Values greater than 1 show an increased risk for cardiovascular disease mortality. As can be seen, the risks for early death are remarkably similar across the different studies and sedentary behavior measures, particularly for total sitting, sitting in cars, and television viewing time. All of these studies showed a dose–response relationship—that is, the longer the time spent in the behavior, the higher the risk for early death. These relationships were observed even after taking into account other factors that may have contributed to early death, such as medical history, age, and other health behaviors including physical activity levels.

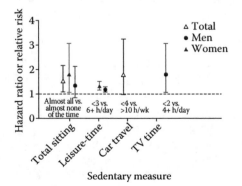

FIGURE 3.2 Cardiovascular disease mortality risk for four different sedentary behavior measures for men, women, and overall.

SEDENTARY BEHAVIOR AND OBESITY

There is substantial evidence linking sedentary behavior with obesity, both in children and in adults, although most of this is cross-sectional. The majority of research has looked at the specific sedentary behavior of TV viewing time. For children, a review concluded that there was sufficient evidence to recommend setting a limit to the time spent watching TV—especially for younger children (Rey-Lopez et al. 2008). Detrimental links between TV viewing time and obesity have also been observed in adults. For example, in a group of 50,277 U.S. women (not obese at baseline) who were followed up over 6 years, each 2 h/day increase in TV viewing time was associated with a 23% increase in obesity (Hu et al. 2003).

When total sedentary time across the day is examined, a similar relationship is observed. For example, in 5424 children aged 12 years, the odds of being obese were 32% higher for every hour per day spent sedentary (Mitchell et al. 2009). Importantly, this study used high-quality measures of both obesity (dual-energy X-ray emission absorptiometry) and sedentary time (accelerometers), and took into account several other risk factors.

However, the link between sedentary time and obesity appears to differ across countries. Figure 3.3 shows the relationship between self-reported sitting time (as measured by the IPAQ question reported in the subsection "Learning Point";

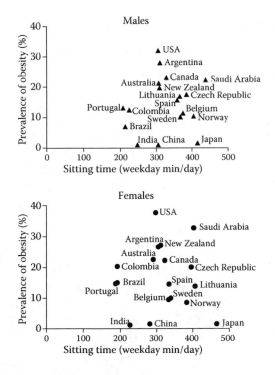

FIGURE 3.3 Prevalence of obesity (BMI ≥ 30 kg m^{-2}: (https://apps.who.int/infobase/Comparisons.aspx) by mean sitting time estimates (weekday min/day) for 20 countries for the year 2002.

Bauman et al. 2011), and the prevalence of obesity (BMI ≥30 kg m^{-2}) for the year 2002 (as reported by the World Health Organization, https://apps.who.int/infobase/Comparisons.aspx). It is important to note that this is an ecological study—that is, the unit of analysis is the population, not the individual. For some countries, such as Saudi Arabia and Portugal, the relationship is as expected: high sitting time, high prevalence of obesity and vice versa. However, for other countries such as Japan, the prevalence rates of obesity are very low despite the high self-reported sitting time. There are several risk factors for obesity, and it likely that the link between sedentary behavior and obesity is bidirectional (Ekelund et al. 2008)—that is, sedentary behavior can lead to obesity and obesity can lead to sedentary behavior. Continued monitoring of population levels of sedentary behavior and obesity rates will help to further clarify their relationship.

SEDENTARY BEHAVIOR AND CARDIOVASCULAR AND METABOLIC HEALTH

In addition to obesity, sedentary behaviors have been detrimentally linked to other cardiovascular disease risk factors including elevated triglycerides, blood glucose, insulin, and systolic blood pressure, and low levels of "good" cholesterol (high-density lipoprotein cholesterol) (Owen et al. 2010; Healy et al. 2011). Interestingly, the pattern of sedentary time (or how a person accumulates their sedentary time) also appears to be important for cardiovascular and metabolic health. More frequent breaks or interruptions to sedentary time, even as short as 1 min and as light in intensity as standing up, were associated with lower waist circumference, BMI, triglycerides, and 2-h plasma glucose (Healy et al. 2008a, 2011).

Again, the majority of the evidence available is in relation to TV viewing time. This behavior has been linked to an increased risk of type 2 diabetes (Hu et al. 2003) and acute coronary syndrome in adults (Burazeri, Goda, and Kark 2008), as well as the metabolic syndrome in both adolescents (Mark and Janssen 2008) and adults (Dunstan et al. 2005). For example, in the Nurses' Health Study, each 2 h/day increase in TV viewing time was associated with a 14% increase in type 2 diabetes, whereas each 2 h/day increase in sitting at work was associated with a 7% increase (Hu et al. 2003). These relationships were observed regardless of exercise levels.

SEDENTARY BEHAVIOR AND CANCER

The relationship of sedentary behavior with obesity and poor metabolic health is thought to play a role in the link between sedentary behavior and cancer. Time spent in sedentary behavior is associated with an increased risk of colorectal, endometrial, ovarian, and prostate cancer, as well as cancer mortality in women and weight gain in colorectal cancer survivors (Lynch 2010). Again, these relationships were independent of moderate-vigorous physical activity levels, although they were more pronounced in those who were inactive. For example, the risk for endometrial cancer in those who were inactive (did vigorous physical activity fewer than three times per week) and who sat for 9 h or more per day was more than double that of those who were active and sat less than 3 h/day (Moore et al. 2010).

HEALTH RISKS FOR THE "ACTIVE COUCH POTATO"

The majority of the studies examining the health risks of sedentary behavior have looked at the relationships independent of time spent in moderate-vigorous intensity activity. However, to further understand the independence of these two behaviors, some studies have also looked at the relationship in those that would typically be considered active (at least 150 min/week of moderate intensity activity and/or 20 min of vigorous-intensity activity three times a week) and at low risk for the consequences of physical inactivity. Even among these active adults, detrimental dose–response associations of time spent sedentary (either measured through TV viewing time or time spent sitting) were observed with several cardiovascular disease risk factors, such as waist circumference, systolic blood pressure, blood glucose, and triglycerides (Healy et al. 2008b), as well as the metabolic syndrome (Dunstan et al. 2005), and endometrial cancer (Moore et al. 2010). This "active couch potato" phenomenon further reinforces sedentary behavior as a unique health risk, and emphasizes the importance of measuring both this, and physical activity level in lifestyle assessments.

SUMMARY

There is a rapidly growing body of evidence linking sedentary behavior with several health outcomes, including premature mortality, cardiovascular disease, and cancer. Most of the research to date is cross-sectional—that is, measured at one point in time. However, more and more prospective research, where people are followed up over time, is emerging and showing similar findings. Importantly, most of the detrimental associations observed are independent of how much moderate-vigorous intensity activity people do, but those who are inactive and who have high levels of sedentary time are at the highest risk of poor health.

INTERVENING ON SEDENTARY BEHAVIOR

KEY POINTS

- Intervention studies provide important information regarding cause and effect.
- Approaches to reduce time spent in sedentary behavior are likely to differ from those aimed at increasing exercise time.
- To date, most of the intervention work has been conducted with children and adolescents.
- It is important to think about what targets to set, what behaviors to address, and how to overcome any barriers.

If we think of evidence in terms of a pyramid, most of the building blocks we have for sedentary behavior are based on cross-sectional studies. This evidence is fairly consistent across several population groups and health outcomes. Importantly, there are also some long-term data showing links with premature mortality, type

2 diabetes, and cardiovascular disease. Taken together, this evidence is strongly suggestive that sedentary time is an important health risk behavior. However, to be able to say that sedentary time causes these health outcomes, intervention evidence is required. Compared to the number of physical activity interventions, there have been very few sedentary behavior interventions and these have primarily been conducted with children and adolescents. It is important that more interventions are conducted—but several key questions need to be considered. These include targets to set, behaviors to address, and barriers to overcome.

WHAT TARGETS SHOULD WE SET?

In the United States, the recommended level of screen time for children and adolescents is no more than 2 h/day (American Academy of Pediatrics 2001). However, what type of targets should be set for other behaviors? Is one single bout of sitting for 4 h better or worse than 6 h of sitting broken up across the day? Should the recommendation be general, or be different for different population groups? Some sedentary time each day is needed for the body to rest, so the intervention cannot be simply to "stop sitting." Instead, a dual message targeting both time spent sedentary in a single bout (e.g., try to get up and move at least every 30 min) and limiting sedentary time overall (e.g., try to not to be sedentary for more than 6 h/day) may be required. As more intervention studies are conducted, the feasibility, acceptability, and effectiveness of these messages will become more evident. It is also important to measure any health, social, or economic changes arising from the sedentary behavior intervention.

WHAT BEHAVIORS SHOULD WE ADDRESS?

If the evidence on sedentary time and health is considered across the work, leisure, domestic, and travel domains, or just as overall sedentary time, the majority of evidence is in relation to leisure time and specifically, on TV viewing time. So, should TV viewing be our primary target for intervention? Interventions to reduce TV viewing time have been successful in both children and adults (DeMattia, Lemont, and Meurer 2007; Kamath et al. 2008; Otten et al. 2009). However, for most people, TV viewing makes up only a small proportion of their day. Additionally, the problem may not be the TV viewing, but more the sitting/lying down while watching TV and/or the unhealthy eating while watching TV. If a participant does not want to miss their favorite TV show, it may be more successful to recommend that they get up during advertisement breaks or use the TV to change the channel (instead of the remote) rather than recommending to turn the TV off. It is also important to monitor changes in other sedentary behaviors: if TV viewing time is reduced, but time spent on the computer is increased—are there any benefits?

A settings-based approach may be useful for both intervening on sedentary behavior, and also for increasing the knowledge about the health effects of prolonged sedentary time. For example, the school setting has been successfully used to deliver interventions that not only targeted reducing sedentary behavior while at school, but also in the home environment through tasks such as active homework.

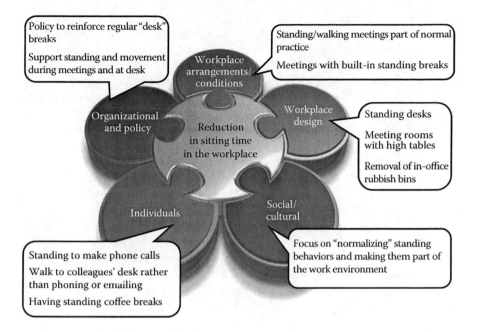

FIGURE 3.4 Practical examples that can be used to address various elements that impact on reducing workplace sitting time.

For working adults, the majority of waking hours are spent at the workplace, and thus the workplace may provide a useful setting in which to implement change, particularly since workdays are associated with less standing and more sitting than leisure days (McCrady and Levine 2009). In terms of health, occupational sedentary time has been linked to an increased risk of type 2 diabetes and mortality (van Uffelen et al. 2010). However, despite these links, there is currently a dearth of evidence on the effectiveness of workplace interventions for reducing sedentary time (Chau et al. 2010). Successful workplace interventions are likely to incorporate both behavioral (such as standing meetings) and environmental (such as open-access stairwells) aspects, and be implemented not only the individual level, but also at the organizational level (e.g., having policies and management buy-in to support regular breaks from sitting). Figure 3.4 gives an example of how these different elements may fit together to reduce sitting time in an office-based workplace.

WHAT ARE SOME OF THE BARRIERS?

For those who have not, or cannot embrace, an organized or structured program of physical activity, reducing sedentary behavior may be a more feasible and achievable approach for increasing movement and energy expenditure. For example, an older adult with chronic disease who has never done any formal exercise may find it very difficult to start a physical activity program such as regular walking. As an initial first goal, it may be easier for them to get up more regularly from the couch, do more of their domestic chores standing, and use behavioral cues such as standing while on the telephone. Although these are relatively small changes, if carried out throughout the day they have the potential to substantially increase energy expenditure, enhance mobility, and also give confidence to the participant that they can be more active. Importantly, for those with limited financial resources or available time, a reduction in sedentary behavior can be achieved with minimal financial or additional time requirements (e.g., registration fees, transportation, equipment, prolonged interruptions of work or domestic tasks).

However, there are some barriers to reducing sedentary time. Although many daily tasks can be carried out in a standing, rather than a seated position, there are situations where this is not practical. For example, driving a car or truck requires sitting. Here, the solution may be to have regular breaks while driving (this also assists with driver fatigue), and for the breaks to be active, not seated. Another example may be for a taxi driver to hop out of the taxi to let passengers in and out.

A key barrier to reducing sedentary time is social norms. Our environment is designed to encourage sedentary behavior and standing up at events or in the office may feel strange. An important aspect of this is education. Knowing the benefits of standing may encourage others to join you such that regular changes in posture between sitting and standing become the "norm." This concept is supported by occupational health and safety guidelines, which recommend regular changes in postures and work variety.

SUMMARY

Achieving reductions in time spent in sedentary behavior are likely to require different approaches than those used to increase time spent in exercise. As sedentary behavior occurs across every domain, there are opportunities to intervene throughout the day. Furthermore, reductions can be achieved with minimal financial or time requirements. However, as the environment is strongly conducive to sedentary behaviors, it may be difficult to implement even these small changes. A mixture of a broad message (e.g., limit sitting time), as well as specific intervention targets (e.g., get up every 30 min; no more than 2 h of screen time per day), may be helpful. Furthermore, although interventions may be conducted within a specific setting, or target a particular behavior, it is important to recommend changes across the whole day. Solutions should be discussed regarding common barriers to reducing sedentary time.

CONCLUSION

Over the past few decades, humans have engineered our environment so that we can be more sedentary. However, until recently, the extent and the impact of sedentary behavior has largely been unrecognized, with public health campaigns primarily promoting the several benefits of moderate-vigorous intensity physical activity. Regular participation in exercise is crucial for several health outcomes. However, for most people, it makes up a very small proportion of the day.

This chapter provided a brief overview of sedentary behavior: what it is, how it is measured, its prevalence and risk factors, its relationship to health, and how to intervene on it. Of key importance is that being sedentary, or doing too much sitting or reclining with minimal energy expenditure, should be considered separately from being inactive—that is, not meeting the physical activity guidelines. This distinct relationship was observed in the inactivity physiology studies and epidemiological findings. It also impacts on how interventions may be designed to reduce time spent in sedentary behavior.

The field of sedentary behavior research is in its relative infancy. What we know is that on average, people spend more than half of their day sedentary, and that prolonged time spent in sedentary behaviors is linked to several health outcomes, including early death, cardiovascular disease, diabetes, and cancer. We know that groups vulnerable to high sedentary time include older adults, those who are unemployed, and those with low education, and that interventions have successfully reduced time spent in sedentary behavior in children and adolescents.

However, there remain several research questions to address (Owen et al. 2010). These include: (1) determining the most valid and reliable self-report and objective measures of sedentary time for epidemiological, behavioral, and population-health studies; (2) understanding the environmental determinants of prolonged sedentary time; (3) understanding the physiological mechanisms underpinning the associations observed; and (4) examining the feasibility and effectiveness of interventions to reduce sedentary time across different groups (older, younger) and across different settings (workplace, domestic, transit, leisure time). To address these questions, it is important that sedentary behavior is acknowledged as a unique health risk behavior on the physical activity public health agenda.

STUDY QUESTIONS

1. Discriminate the difference between in behaviors in being sedentary and being physically inactive.
2. Identify limitations for using accelerometers to derive sedentary time and construct alternate ways to measure sedentary time to overcome these limitations.
3. Identify the population groups most at risk of high sedentary time, and suggest ways in which they can reduce time spent in sedentary behaviors.
4. Briefly describe the physiological benefits of standing, rather than sitting.
5. In 2002, which three countries had the highest levels of sitting time? Which three had the lowest? Contrast the differences between the countries that could explain the differences in sitting time.
6. Briefly outline how you would design an intervention aimed at reducing workplace sitting time in office workers. Intervention aspects to take into account include study design, intervention content and targets, and type and length of the intervention.

REFERENCES

American Academy of Pediatrics. 2001. Children, adolescents, and television. *Pediatrics* 107(2): 423–426.
Australian Bureau of Statistics. 2010. Summary of IT Use and Innovation in Australian Business, 2008–09. Report No. 8166.0.

Australian Bureau of Statistics. 1997. *How Australians Use Their Time*. In: Government C, editor. Commonwealth Government, Canberra, Australia.

Bauman, A., B. E. Ainsworth, J. F. Sallis et al. 2011. The descriptive epidemiology of sitting a 20-country comparison using the International Physical Activity Questionnaire (IPAQ). *Am. J. Prev. Med.* 41(2): 228–235.

Biddle, S. J., T. Gorely, S. J. Marshall et al. 2009. The prevalence of sedentary behavior and physical activity in leisure time: A study of Scottish adolescents using ecological momentary assessment. *Prev. Med.* 48: 151–155.

Bowman, S. A. 2006. Television-viewing characteristics of adults: Correlations to eating practices and overweight and health status. *Prev. Chronic Dis.* 3: A38.

Brodersen, N. H., A. Steptoe, D. R. Boniface et al. 2007. Trends in physical activity and sedentary behaviour in adolescence: Ethnic and socioeconomic differences. *Br. J. Sports Med.* 41: 140–144.

Brown, W. J., Y. D. Miller, and R. Miller. 2003. Sitting time and work patterns as indicators of overweight and obesity in Australian adults. *Int. J. Obes. Relat. Metab. Disord.* 27: 1340–1346.

Brownson, R. C., T. K. Boehmer, and D. A. Luke. 2005. Declining rates of physical activity in the United States: What are the contributors? *Annu. Rev. Public Health* 26: 421–443.

Burazeri, G., A. Goda, and J. D. Kark. 2008. Television viewing, leisure-time exercise and acute coronary syndrome in transitional Albania. *Prev. Med.* 47(1): 112–115.

Bureau of Labor Statistics. 2008. American Time Use Survey. http://www.bls.gov/news .release/atus.nr0.htm (accessed July 16, 2011).

Chau, J. Y., H. P. van der Ploeg, J. G. van Uffelen et al. 2010. Are workplace interventions to reduce sitting effective? A systematic review. *Prev. Med.* 51: 352–356.

Clark, B. K., T. Sugiyama, G. N. Healy et al. 2009. Validity and reliability of measures of television viewing time and other non-occupational sedentary behaviour of adults: A review. *Obes. Rev.* 10(1): 7–16.

Clark, B. K., T. Sugiyama, G. N. Healy et al. 2010. Socio-demographic correlates of prolonged television viewing time in Australian men and women: The AusDiab study. *J. Phys. Activity Health* 7: 595–601.

Currie, C., S. N. Gabhainn, E. Godeau et al. 2008. Inequalities in young people's health. Health behaviour in school-aged children: International report from the 2005/2006 survey. World Health Organisation.

DeMattia, L., L. Lemont, and L. Meurer. 2007. Do interventions to limit sedentary behaviours change behaviour and reduce childhood obesity? A critical review of the literature. *Obes. Rev.* 8(1): 69–81.

Dunstan, D. W., E. L. M. Barr, G. N. Healy et al. 2010. Television viewing time and mortality: The AusDiab study. *Circulation* 121(3): 384–391.

Dunstan, D. W., J. Salmon, N. Owen et al. 2005. Associations of TV viewing and physical activity with the metabolic syndrome in Australian adults. *Diabetologia* 48(11): 2254–2261.

Ekelund, U., S. Brage, H. Besson, et al. 2008. Time spent being sedentary and weight gain in healthy adults: Reverse or bidirectional causality? *Am. J. Clin. Nutr.* 88(3): 612–617.

Gorely, T., S. J. Biddle, S. J. Marshall et al. 2009. The prevalence of leisure time sedentary behaviour and physical activity in adolescent boys: An ecological momentary assessment approach. *Int. J. Pediatr. Obes.* 4: 289–298.

Hagstromer, M., P. Oja, and M. Sjostrom. 2007. Physical activity and inactivity in an adult population assessed by accelerometry. *Med. Sci. Sports Exerc.* 39: 1502–1508.

Hamar, P., S. Biddle, I. Soos et al. 2010. The prevalence of sedentary behaviours and physical activity in Hungarian youth. *Eur. J. Public Health* 20: 85–90.

Hamilton, M. T., D. G. Hamilton, and T. W. Zderic. 2007. The role of low energy expenditure and sitting on obesity, metabolic syndrome, type 2 diabetes, and cardiovascular disease. *Diabetes* 56: 2655–2667.

Haskell, W. L., I. M. Lee, R. R. Pate et al. 2007. Physical activity and public health: Updated recommendation for adults from the American College of Sports Medicine and the American Heart Association. *Circulation* 116: 1081–1093.

Healy, G. N. 2007. *Physical Activity, Sedentary Time and Blood Glucose in Australian Adults*. Brisbane: University of Queensland.

Healy, G. N., D. W. Dunstan, J. Salmon et al. 2007. Objectively measured light-intensity physical activity is independently associated with 2-h plasma glucose. *Diabetes Care* 30: 1384–1389.

Healy, G. N., D. W. Dunstan, J. Salmon et al. 2008a. Breaks in sedentary time: Beneficial associations with metabolic risk. *Diabetes Care* 31: 661–666.

Healy, G. N., D. W. Dunstan, J. Salmon et al. 2008b. Television time and continuous metabolic risk in physically active adults. *Med. Sci. Sports Exerc.* 40: 639–645.

Healy, G. N., K. Wijndaele, D. W. Dunstan et al. 2008c. Objectively measured sedentary time, physical activity, and metabolic risk: The Australian Diabetes, Obesity and Lifestyle Study (AusDiab). *Diabetes Care* 31: 369–371.

Healy, G. N., C. E. Matthews, D. W. Dunstan et al. 2011. Sedentary time and cardio-metabolic biomarkers in US adults: NHANES 2003–06. *Eur Heart J*, 32(5): 590–597. doi:10.1093/eurheartj/ehq451.

Hu, F. B., T. Y. Li, G. A. Colditz et al. 2003. Television watching and other sedentary behaviors in relation to risk of obesity and type 2 diabetes mellitus in women. *JAMA* 289: 1785–1791.

Jans, M. P., K. I. Proper, and V. H. Hildebrandt. 2007. Sedentary behavior in Dutch workers: Differences between occupations and business sectors. *Am. J. Prev. Med.* 33: 450–454.

Kamath, C. C., K. S. Vickers, A. Ehrlich et al. 2008. Clinical review: Behavioral interventions to prevent childhood obesity: A systematic review and metaanalyses of randomized trials. *J. Clin. Endocrinol. Metab.* 93: 4606–4615.

Katzmarzyk, P. T., T. S. Church, C. L. Craig et al. 2009. Sitting time and mortality from all causes, cardiovascular disease, and cancer. *Med. Sci. Sports Exerc.* 41: 998–1005.

Lynch, B. M. 2010. Sedentary behavior and cancer: A systematic review of the literature and proposed biologic mechanisms. *Cancer Epidemiol. Biomarkers Prev.* 19: 2691–2709.

Mark, A. E., and I. Janssen. 2008. Relationship between screen time and metabolic syndrome in adolescents. *J. Public Health* 30: 153–160.

Matthews, C. E., K. Y. Chen, P. S. Freedson et al. 2008. Amount of time spent in sedentary behaviors in the United States, 2003–2004. *Am. J. Epidemiol.* 167: 875–881.

McCrady, S. K., and J. A. Levine. 2009. Sedentariness at work: How much do we really sit? *Obesity* 17: 2103–2105.

Mitchell, J. A., C. Mattocks, A. R. Ness et al. 2009. Sedentary behavior and obesity in a large cohort of children. *Obesity* (Silver Spring) 17: 1596–1602.

Moore, S. C., G. L. Gierach, A. Schatzkin et al. 2010. Physical activity, sedentary behaviours, and the prevention of endometrial cancer. *Br. J. Cancer* 103: 933–938.

Otten, J. J., K. E. Jones, B. Littenberg et al. 2009. Effects of television viewing reduction on energy intake and expenditure in overweight and obese adults: A randomized controlled trial. *Arch. Intern. Med.* 169: 2109–2115.

Owen, N., G. N. Healy, C. E. Matthews et al. 2010. Too much sitting: The population health science of sedentary behavior. *Exerc. Sport Sci. Rev.* 38: 105–113.

Patel, A. V., L. Bernstein, A. Deka et al. 2010. Leisure time spent sitting in relation to total mortality in a prospective cohort of US adults. *Am. J. Epidemiol.* 172: 419–429.

Peters, T. M., S. C. Moore, Y. B. Xiang et al. 2010. Accelerometer-measured physical activity in Chinese adults. *Am. J. Prev. Med.* 38: 583–591.

Rey-Lopez, J. P., G. Vicente-Rodriguez, M. Biosca et al. 2008. Sedentary behaviour and obesity development in children and adolescents. *Nutr. Metab. Cardiovasc. Dis.* 18: 242–251.

Shields, M., and M. S. Tremblay. 2008. Screen time among Canadian adults: A profile. *Health Rep.* 19: 31–43.

Sidney, S., B. Sternfeld, W. L. Haskell et al. 1996. Television viewing and cardiovascular risk factors in young adults: The CARDIA study. *Ann. Epidemiol.* 6: 154–159.

van Uffelen, J. G. Z., J. Wong, J. Y. Chau et al. 2010. Associations between occupational sitting and health risks: A systematic review. *Am. J. Prev. Med.* 39: 379–388.

Warren, T. Y., V. Barry, S. P. Hooker et al. 2010. Sedentary behaviors increase risk of cardiovascular disease mortality in men. *Med. Sci. Sports Exerc.* 42: 879–885.

Wijndaele, K., S. Brage, H. Besson et al. 2011. Television viewing time independently predicts all-cause and cardiovascular mortality: The EPIC Norfolk Study. *Int. J. Epidemiol.* 40: 150–159.

4 Physical Activity in Chronic Disease Prevention

Jared P. Reis and Bethany Barone Gibbs

CONTENTS

INTRODUCTION

In this chapter, we explore the role of physical activity and fitness in preventing major chronic diseases, including cardiovascular disease, cancer, pulmonary, and musculoskeletal conditions. Obesity and diabetes, two additional major chronic conditions, will not be discussed in this chapter, since they will be reviewed in detail in other areas. The research presented in this chapter is primarily acquired from the epidemiological literature; however, when appropriate, a brief discussion of biologic mechanisms will make use of research emanating from clinical trials and laboratory investigations.

To avoid confusion, it is important to differentiate between many of the terms commonly used throughout the scientific literature. Physical activity is a behavior that includes skeletal movement resulting in energy expenditure, whereas physical fitness is the outcome of that behavior. Physical fitness is a broad term that encompasses many physiological attributes, including aerobic power or cardiorespiratory fitness, muscular fitness (strength and endurance), body composition, flexibility, speed, and balance. Exercise is defined as planned, structured, and repetitive bodily movement performed to improve or maintain one or more components of physical fitness. Physical activity can be measured using subjective questionnaires, logs, recalls, and several objective electronic devices, whereas cardiorespiratory fitness, for example, can be measured with a graded treadmill exercise test. For the most part, this chapter presents data on physical activity rather than information on physical fitness. The primary reason for this is the small number of studies that have measured fitness. When discussing physical fitness, this chapter focuses on cardiorespiratory fitness and muscular fitness.

PHYSICAL ACTIVITY, FITNESS, AND CARDIOVASCULAR DISEASE

Cardiovascular disease is the leading cause of death among men and women in the United States and many developed countries throughout the world (Figure 4.1). Cardiovascular disease is a global term that refers generally to a class of diseases including the heart and/or blood vessels. Individual forms of cardiovascular disease include heart disease, stroke, hypertension, rheumatic fever, congenital heart defects, heart failure, and peripheral vascular disease. In this chapter, we focus on some of the more common forms of cardiovascular disease that are important in the context of physical activity and fitness, and where most of the scientific evidence has accumulated.

PHYSICAL ACTIVITY, FITNESS, AND RISK OF CORONARY HEART DISEASE

There is now compelling and consistent evidence from a number of populations that leisure-time physical activity plays a causal role in the development of coronary heart disease (Wannamethee and Shaper 2001). There appears to be a linear dose–response relationship between total physical activity and coronary heart disease, at least up to a certain level. In other words, as the overall dose (frequency, intensity, and duration) of physical activity increases, the risk of developing heart disease

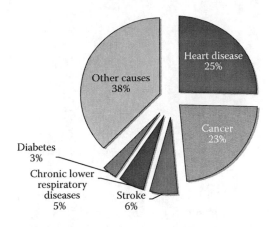

FIGURE 4.1 Distribution of leading causes of death in the United States, 2007.

subsequently decreases. Most of the epidemiologic studies investigating the relationship between physical activity and heart disease have been conducted in men; however, there is now evidence from a number of studies within large samples of women showing that physical activity is inversely associated with risk for coronary heart disease. Furthermore, although there was a long-standing belief that vigorous intensity activity was required to reduce one's risk for developing heart disease, it is now widely accepted that moderate intensity activities, such as gardening and brisk walking, are sufficient.

In a relevant study that determined the association of walking with the development of severe coronary heart disease among a large sample of female health professionals, walking was inversely associated with the risk of heart disease (Manson et al. 1999). Women who reported the most walking (≥3 h/week brisk walking) reduced their risk of heart disease by 35% compared to women who reported walking infrequently, and the magnitude of the reduction in heart disease was similar to that of vigorous physical activity. In the same study, walking pace was similarly associated with decreased risk of coronary events. As shown in Figure 4.2, even women who walked at an average pace (2–2.9 mph) had a significant reduction in their risk for coronary heart disease.

PHYSICAL ACTIVITY, FITNESS, AND RISK OF STROKE

Although the body of literature examining whether physical activity or fitness plays a role in preventing stroke is less extensive than that of heart disease, there is now evidence from a number of studies suggesting a causal link. This area of study has been the subject of numerous in-depth reviews and meta-analyses of the published scientific evidence. In one of these carefully conducted meta-analyses, moderate-intensity physical activity compared with inactivity during leisure time and work lowered the risk of stroke by 36% and 15%, respectively (Wendel-Vos et al. 2004). The protective influence of physical activity was apparent for stroke subtypes, including ischemic strokes (when a blood vessel supplying blood to the brain becomes blocked) and

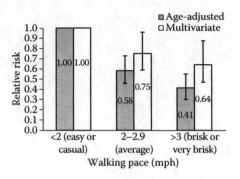

FIGURE 4.2   Age-adjusted and multivariate relative risks of coronary events (nonfatal myo-cardial infarction or death from coronary causes) according to walking pace among women in the Nurses' Health Study. Compared to women who walked at a casual pace, women who walked at an average or brisk pace had significant reductions in their risk for coronary heart disease.

hemorrhagic strokes (when a blood vessel to the brain becomes weakened and bursts open). In one of the few published studies on cardiorespiratory fitness, high fit men had 68% and moderate fit men had 63% lower risk for stroke mortality than low fit men (Lee and Blair 2002). This association could not be accounted for by a number of factors, such as smoking, alcohol use, body composition, hypertension, diabetes, and a family history of heart disease. Thus, similar to coronary heart disease, physical activity and fitness both appear to be important modifiable factors in the prevention of stroke.

PHYSICAL ACTIVITY, FITNESS, AND RISK OF HYPERTENSION

Hypertension is clinically defined as a systolic blood pressure ≥140 mm Hg and/or a diastolic blood pressure ≥90 mm Hg when properly measured on each of at least two or more occasions. Although not recognized as a major risk factor for cardiovascular disease until the latter portion of the last century, hypertension is now considered a well-established, major cardiovascular disease risk factor. It has been estimated that as many as 1 billion people worldwide have hypertension, with 7.1 million deaths per year attributed to this condition (World Health Report 2002). The risk of developing hypertension increases with age. Approximately 9 out of 10 people who do not develop hypertension by the age of 55 years will eventually develop the condition before they die (Vasan et al. 2002).

It is important to note that an abnormally elevated blood pressure is responsive to lifestyle interventions, including physical activity; weight, stress, alcohol, and sodium reduction; and potassium supplementation. Furthermore, even small reductions in an abnormally elevated blood pressure result in a decrease in the risk of death from heart disease and stroke. For example, diastolic blood pressure reductions of 7.5 and 10 mm Hg are, respectively, associated with a 46% and 56% lower risk of stroke and a 29% and 37% decrease in risk for coronary heart disease (MacMahon et al. 1990).

Epidemiologic studies have shown that physical activity and fitness are inversely associated with blood pressure. Low fit and physically inactive persons are more likely to develop hypertension. In a long-term study of men who completed a preventive medical examination, those who had higher levels of cardiorespiratory fitness had a significantly lower risk of developing hypertension during the next 18 years than less fit men (Chase et al. 2009). Furthermore, this inverse association between fitness and the incidence of hypertension was evident among men regardless of their baseline level of physical activity.

Intervention studies have confirmed these epidemiologic findings. In a recent meta-analysis of 54 randomized controlled trials, aerobic exercise significantly reduced systolic blood pressure by 3 to 6 mm Hg and diastolic blood pressure by 2 to 4 mm Hg (Whelton et al. 2002). Furthermore, the blood pressure–lowering effects of aerobic exercise were apparent among hypertensive participants and those with normal blood pressure and in overweight and normal weight participants, suggesting that the effects of exercise on blood pressure are independent of one's initial level of blood pressure and body weight. It is interesting to note that the exercise-related reduction in blood pressure was greater than the reported effects of other common strategies to lower blood pressure discussed earlier, including sodium and alcohol reduction, as well as potassium supplementation, highlighting the important role of physical activity in the primary prevention of hypertension.

PHYSICAL ACTIVITY AND SUBCLINICAL CARDIOVASCULAR DISEASE

An important public health priority involves identifying novel methods for detecting cardiovascular disease before the development of clinical signs and symptoms. The objective of this research into subclinical cardiovascular disease is to identify individuals at an increased risk of developing clinical disease so that appropriate interventions can be instituted. To this end, a number of sophisticated technologies have been developed, including techniques to measure the ankle brachial pressure index to identify the presence of peripheral vascular disease, computed tomography to detect coronary artery calcified plaque, ultrasonography to measure the thickness of the carotid arteries, echocardiography and magnetic resonance imaging to detect abnormal heart structure and function, and methods to measure arterial stiffness. In the following sections, we highlight research that has investigated the role of physical activity in the development of subclinical cardiovascular disease, and where most of the recent scientific evidence has accumulated.

Peripheral Vascular Disease

Lower-extremity peripheral vascular disease is a manifestation of atherosclerosis resulting in the obstruction of blood flow to the lower extremities, significant morbidity, and elevated risks of all-cause and cardiovascular disease mortality. In one of the few studies that have examined the association between physical activity and peripheral vascular disease risk, increased moderate and vigorous activity and intentional exercise were positively associated with ankle brachial index among women (Bertoni et al. 2009). A higher ankle brachial index reflects less obstruction to blood flow in the lower extremities and therefore less atherosclerosis in the arteries supplying blood to the legs. In a similar study of older adults without clinical cardiovascular disease, greater intensity and duration of physical activity over the prior 2 weeks was also positively associated with ankle brachial index (Siscovick et al. 1997). Thus, accumulating evidence suggests that higher levels of physical activity may positively influence the risk for developing peripheral vascular disease.

Coronary Artery Calcified Plaque/Carotid Intima-Media Thickness

Coronary artery calcified plaque identified via computed tomography and increased carotid intima-media thickness are strong, independent risk factors for cardiovascular disease. In a recent systematic review of more than 20 published studies, investigators determined that the majority of cross-sectional observational studies suggest higher levels of physical activity are inversely associated with carotid intima-media thickness; however, structured lifestyle interventions that have included physical activity have not consistently shown less progression over time (Kadoglou, Iliadis, and Liapis 2008). Thus, physical activity seems to be inversely related to carotid intima-media thickness, but does not appear to play an important role in *reducing* the thickness or limiting the thickening of the carotid arteries.

Similar inconsistent results have also been observed in studies of physical activity and coronary artery calcified plaque. In a sample of asymptomatic adults with at least two risk factors for metabolic syndrome (a clustering of risk factors for cardiovascular disease, including hypertension, obesity, high cholesterol, and elevated glucose concentrations), those who regularly engaged in long-duration physical activity (>30 min for ≥3 times/week) had a lower prevalence of coronary artery calcified plaque compared to those who were sedentary or participated in moderate-duration physical activity (<30 min for 1–2 times/week) (Desai et al. 2004). In another study, higher levels of cardiorespiratory fitness among adults aged 18–30 years at baseline were significantly associated with a lower prevalence of coronary artery calcified plaque observed 15 years later (see Figure 4.3) (Lee et al. 2009). However, a number of studies have reported no association between physical activity and coronary artery calcified plaque (Folsom et al. 2004; Taylor et al. 2002). Therefore, additional studies are necessary to determine whether physical activity influences markers of subclinical cardiovascular disease such as coronary artery calcified plaque and carotid intima-media thickness.

Physical Activity versus Cardiorespiratory Fitness

Cardiorespiratory fitness is frequently found to be more strongly associated with cardiovascular disease and other health-related outcomes than is physical activity. For example, Figure 4.4 shows a stronger inverse dose–response association with risk for myocardial infarction across increasing categories of cardiorespiratory fitness measured with a maximal bicycle ergometer test than across similar categories of leisure-time physical activity measured via questionnaires among middle-aged men in the Kuopio Ischemic Heart Disease Risk Factor Study (Lakka et al. 1994). The fact that fitness is more strongly associated with cardiovascular disease may lead one to conclude that fitness is the more important exposure than is physical activity. However, in some ways, this is an invalid conclusion since physical activity

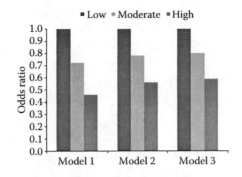

FIGURE 4.3 Odds ratio for the presence of 15 year coronary artery calcified plaque by low, moderate, and high baseline cardiorespiratory fitness among white and black adults. Model 1 adjusts for age, sex, race, clinical center, and education. Model 2 additionally adjusts for smoking, waist girth, alcohol intake, and physical activity. Model 3 adjusts for variables in Model 2 in addition to systolic blood pressure, antihypertensive medication use, diabetes, and fasting insulin. Compared to low fit adults, those who were moderately or highly fit had lower odds of developing coronary artery calcified plaque.

performed over the past several weeks or months is a major determinant of cardio-respiratory fitness, and therefore physical activity is the fundamental exposure of interest. One reason fitness may be a stronger predictor of health-related outcomes is that fitness is assessed using more precise and objective measures, such as a maximal exercise test, than physical activity. Thus, fitness can be measured with less random error and is not susceptible to problems related to memory and recall. Physical activity, on the other hand, is generally measured with greater error using subjective measures, such as self-report questionnaires or recalls. These more imprecise measures have the potential to lead to higher rates of misclassification of physical activity levels than the more precise fitness measures. This type of misclassification tends to bias the results toward finding no association or weaker associations

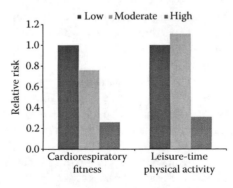

FIGURE 4.4 Relative risk for myocardial infarction among men according to levels of cardiorespiratory fitness and leisure-time physical activity. Figure shows a stronger inverse dose–response association with risk for myocardial infarction across increasing categories of cardiorespiratory fitness measured when a maximal bicycle ergometer test was observed than across similar categories of leisure-time physical activity measured via questionnaire.

between physical activity behaviors and cardiovascular disease. Another possibility is that other genetic and environmental factors might be associated with both fitness and health, making fitness levels appear to be more important than it is, or fitness levels may be an indirect marker for physical activity and health.

RESISTANCE-BASED PHYSICAL ACTIVITY

Although the majority of the available epidemiologic studies have investigated the role of aerobic physical activity or cardiorespiratory fitness in the prevention of chronic conditions, there are a number of recent studies reporting the beneficial influence of resistance-based physical activity or muscular strength in the prevention of cardiovascular disease. These studies have been complicated, however, by the difficulty in determining the separate influence of aerobic- and resistance-based activity because of their high degree of correlation. Those more likely to engage in aerobic activities are also more likely to participate in resistance-based physical activities. In a 19-year study of men aged 20–80 years at baseline who were initially free of metabolic syndrome, muscular strength measured by one-repetition maximum testing for the leg press and bench press was inversely associated with the development of metabolic syndrome (Jurca et al. 2005). Compared to men in the lowest 25% of muscular strength, men in the highest 25% had a 34% lower risk of metabolic syndrome. When the researchers additionally accounted for the cardiorespiratory fitness of these men, the association between muscular strength and metabolic syndrome was substantially reduced, but remained modestly statistically significant. Although this is a promising new area of research, additional studies are necessary to examine the independent role of resistance-based physical activity or muscular strength in the primary prevention of cardiovascular disease and to understand the biologic mechanisms underpinning these associations.

SEDENTARY BEHAVIOR

Accumulating research is beginning to show that sedentary behaviors, which involve sitting and are in the energy expenditure range of 1.0–1.5 METs (metabolic equivalent) (typically television viewing, computer and game console use, workplace sitting, and sitting while commuting), may have independent adverse health consequences beyond that of simply being physically inactive. This research area asserts that too much sitting is distinct from too little exercise. Higher amounts of television viewing have been positively associated with metabolic risk factors for cardiovascular disease independently of time spent in moderate and vigorous physical activity as well as adiposity. In a recent study of Australian adults, high levels of television viewing time were significantly associated with increased all-cause and cardiovascular disease mortality independent of other risk factors such as smoking, blood pressure, cholesterol, waist circumference, diet, and leisure-time physical activity (Dunstan et al. 2010). Each 1-h increase in television time was associated with an 11% and an 18% increase in the risk of all-cause and cardiovascular disease mortality, respectively. These findings have generally been confirmed in studies that have used objective electronic motion sensors that provide a continuous depiction of time spent in sedentary and active pursuits. These motion sensors are not susceptible to some of the measurement error inherent in self-report questionnaires or problems related to measuring only a single sedentary activity such as television viewing. Although this is another exciting and promising area of research, additional epidemiologic studies, laboratory-based investigations to understand biologic mechanisms, and intervention trials are needed to understand the independent role of sedentary behavior in the etiology of cardiovascular disease.

PHYSICAL ACTIVITY AND CANCER

Cancer is second only to heart disease as a leading cause of death among men and women in the United States and is among the top causes of mortality in developed countries. Cancer is a class of diseases defined by abnormal and uncontrolled cell growth, and more than 100 types of cancer have been identified. The most common sites of incident (newly diagnosed) cancer as well as causes of cancer mortality in the United States are lung, prostate, and colorectal cancers among men, and lung, breast, and colorectal cancers among women (American Cancer Society 2010). The following section will review current evidence, which indicates that regular physical activity may be associated with decreased risk for some types of cancer.

COLON AND RECTAL CANCER

Colon and rectal cancer together make up the third most common newly diagnosed cancer and the third leading cause of cancer death among all U.S. adults (American Cancer Society 2010). Both the colon and the rectum are parts of the large intestine, and cancers of these sites are often grouped together (as colorectal cancer). However, the associations of physical activity with colon and rectal cancer appear to differ between sites and are therefore discussed separately below.

Numerous research studies have demonstrated that more physical activity is associated with a decrease in colon cancer risk across various study designs and populations, and it is now commonly accepted that regular exercise can reduce the risk of developing colon cancer. When combining results from 52 studies comparing most versus least active individuals, colon cancer risk was reduced by 24%, and this finding was consistent for men and women (Wolin et al. 2009). Another meta-analysis found evidence of a dose–response relationship between physical activity and colon cancer, where risk decreased progressively from the 20th to the 95th percentile of physical activity among both men and women (Harriss et al. 2007). For example, in the NIH–AARP (National Institutes of Health–American Association of Retired Persons) Diet and Health Study of 488,720 men and women between the ages of 50 and 71 years over an average follow-up period of 7 years, increased frequency of physical activity was associated with a decreased risk of colon cancer in men with a suggestive trend toward reduced risk among women (see Figure 4.5) (Howard et al. 2008). This association was observed after adjusting for many other demographic factors including age, education, race, and family history, along with lifestyle factors such as smoking, alcohol use, and diet. Interestingly, this large cohort study also showed that participation in moderate/low intensity physical activity as well as

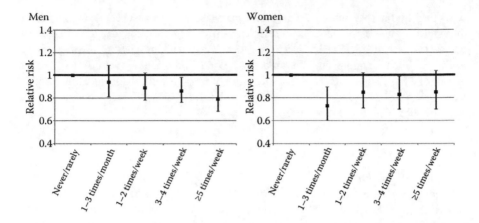

FIGURE 4.5 Adjusted relative risk and 95% confidence intervals of colon cancer with increasing frequency of physical activity in men (*p* for trend = 0.001) and women (*p* for trend = 0.38) in NIH–AARP Diet and Health Study. Data were adjusted for age, smoking, alcohol consumption, education, race, family history of colon cancer, total energy and energy-adjusted intake of red meat, calcium, whole grains, fruit, and vegetables. Figure shows an increased frequency of physical activity lowered the risk of developing colon cancer among men with a suggestive trend among women.

vigorous physical activity were each associated with a 19% and 18% reduction in the development of colon cancer in men, respectively, with similar, although nonsignificant, patterns among women.

Although the pathways through which physical activity reduces colon cancer risk are unknown, one possible mechanism is reduced transit time of fecal matter through the large bowel minimizing contact of cancer causing materials with intestinal tissues. Other potential pathways include decreased inflammation of colonic tissues that could decrease cell damage and subsequent development of cancerous cells, improved insulin sensitivity with decreased insulin and insulin-like growth factors (IGF) that could accelerate abnormal cell growth, and better immune function (Harriss et al. 2007).

Alternatively, physical activity is not consistently associated with decreased rectal cancer risk. A meta-analysis combining results from eight studies found that being physically active was not associated with any decrease in risk of rectal cancer in men or women (Harriss et al. 2009). The reasons for the different associations between physical activity and colon or rectal cancer are not clear, but may result because the colon is more affected by the aforementioned biological mechanisms as compared to the rectum and that cancer promoting agents may have less contact with tissue in the rectum.

Breast Cancer

Among women, breast cancer is the most common newly diagnosed cancer and the second leading cause of cancer death in the United States (American Cancer Society

2010). Consistent evidence supports an inverse dose–response association between physical activity and breast cancer risk by menopausal status, across types, doses, and timing of physical activity, and independently of weight (Pan and DesMeules 2009). A recent systematic review that combined results from 62 studies found that the most physically active women had a 25–30% reduced risk of breast cancer (Friedenreich and Cust 2008). These authors additionally identified greater decreases in risk among women engaging in vigorous, recreational, and lifelong or recent physical activity (Friedenreich and Cust 2008). Furthermore, greater risk reduction was seen among groups of women with normal body mass index (BMI), women that were postmenopausal, had no family history of breast cancer, that had children, nonwhite racial groups, and in women with hormone receptor negative tumors. Most studies also reported a dose–response association, where more physical activity resulted in greater risk reduction for breast cancer.

For example, the French E3N cohort study evaluated more than 90,000 women enrolled in a specific national health insurance plan (Tehard et al. 2006). Women were divided into five levels of vigorous recreational physical activity based on self-report: inactive, <1 h/week, 1–2 h/week, 3–4 h/week, and ≥5 h/week. Compared to inactive women, the risk was decreased by 10% with <1 h/week, by 12% with 1–2 h/week, by 18% with 3–4 h/week, and by 38% with ≥5 h/week (p for trend <0.0001). This trend was observed after taking into account BMI, menopausal status, use of hormone replacement therapy or oral contraceptives, first-degree family history of breast cancer, and other important confounders that could alter the relationship studies. The pattern of decreasing breast cancer risk with increasing levels of leisure-time physical activity was strongest for vigorous physical activity, but was also observed for moderate and total (walking + moderate + vigorous) leisure-time physical activity (Figure 4.6).

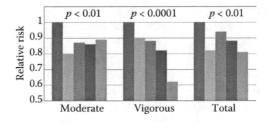

FIGURE 4.6 Relative risk of breast cancer (p for trend) associated with increasing levels of moderate recreational physical activity (inactive, 0, 1–4, 5–13, ≥14 h/week), vigorous recreational physical activity (inactive, 0, 1–2, 3–4, ≥5 h/week), and total recreational physical activity (inactive, <16.0, 16.0–22.3, 22.3–33.8, ≥33.8 MET h/week) in the E3N Cohort, France, 1990–2002. Relative risks adjusted for BMI, menopausal status, HRT use, age at menarche, age at first full-term pregnancy, parity, marital status, use of oral contraceptives, first-degree family history of breast cancer, personal history of benign breast disease, and work status. Figure shows a pattern of decreasing breast cancer risk with increasing levels of leisure-time physical activity that was strongest for vigorous physical activity, but was also observed for moderate and total (walking + moderate + vigorous) leisure-time physical activity.

Breast cancer risk is thought to be improved through physical activity by several pathways. These include reduced sex steroid hormone levels such as estrogen and progesterone, favorable changes in insulin and IGF, decreased levels of inflammation, increased immune system function, and through improved body composition and maintenance of a healthier weight (Friedenreich and Cust 2008; Lee 2007).

Prostate Cancer

Prostate cancer is the most common type of cancer in men and the second leading cause of cancer-related death among men in the United States (American Cancer Society 2010). Associations between physical activity and risk of prostate cancer are less consistent than those for colon or breast cancer. This phenomenon may result from different etiologies of organ-confined or nonadvanced prostate cancer compared to advanced or fatal prostate cancer as well as differing effects by age and exercise intensity.

Examination of the relationship between physical activity and prostate cancer in large, observational studies reveals, on average, no significant association (Lee 2007). However, subgroup analyses find that vigorous physical activity may have a beneficial influence on risk of advanced prostate cancer, particularly among older men (Pan and DesMeules 2009). For example, in an analysis of 47,620 men from the Health Professionals Follow-Up Study, no association was observed between total or vigorous physical activity and total prostate cancer risk. However, older men (≥65 years) engaging in approximately 3 h of vigorous physical activity per week, compared to no vigorous physical activity, had a modest increase in the risk of nonadvanced prostate cancer by 25%, but a decreased risk of advanced prostate cancer by 67%. No associations were observed in younger men (<65 years) (Giovannucci et al. 2005). High vigorous physical activity was also associated with decreased risk of fatal prostate cancer in the older group. Although the reasons for these associations are poorly understood, discussion of potential biological pathways of risk reduction highlights important points that may influence the relationship of physical activity and prostate cancer risk.

First, the lack of association in young men may result from a stronger genetic influence in earlier-onset prostate cancers. On the other hand, later prostate cancer in older men may be less strongly influenced by genetic factors and more susceptible to risk reduction through environmental factors such as physical activity (Giovannucci et al. 2005). Second, the greater risk of nonadvanced disease may result from an increased tendency for men who engage in vigorous physical activity to get screened for prostate cancer (Lee 2007). Nonadvanced or organ-confined prostate cancer is often subclinical (with no symptoms), but has been detected at greater rates in the past few decades with the introduction of screening for prostate cancer by a blood test measuring prostate-specific antigen (PSA). Health-conscious men could be more likely to engage in physical activity *and* undergo PSA screening, which could potentially increase detection of nonadvanced cancer in these men. Last, the significant, inverse associations in older men for advanced disease were only observed with high levels of physical activity. Vigorous exercise in particular may decrease androgen levels through increased binding of circulating testosterone, and lower levels of testosterone have been associated with decreased prostate cancer cell growth. Furthermore, vigorous exercise may reduce other factors known to promote prostate cancer carcinogenesis (e.g., IGF and leptin) by improving insulin sensitivity and decreasing inflammation, which could also inhibit cancerous cell growth. It is possible that lower levels of these factors could reduce risk of advanced cancer in older men (Newton and Galvao 2008).

LUNG CANCER

Although lung cancer is the second most common newly diagnosed type of cancer among men and women in the United States, it is the leading cause of cancer deaths for all adults accounting for 29% and 26% of cancer deaths for men and women, respectively (American Cancer Society 2010). Studies of physical activity and lung cancer must be interpreted with caution because cigarette smoking is a strong risk factor for lung cancer and is inversely related to physical activity (Lee 2007). However, current evidence suggests that physical activity may have a role in lung cancer prevention.

A meta-analysis combining results from nine studies found that, compared to low leisure-time physical activity, moderate leisure-time physical activity was associated with a 13% lower risk of lung cancer and high leisure-time physical activity with 30% lower risk (Tardon et al. 2005). Because of the tendency for physically active and nonsmoking behaviors to cluster, results from studies that restrict analyses within smoking groups (e.g., nonsmokers, former smokers, light smokers, or heavy smokers) may be the best evidence of the influence of physical activity on lung cancer risk. An inverse association is often observed within these smoking groups, although less often among nonsmokers, potentially because of the very low absolute risk of lung cancer in this group (Lee 2007; Pan and DesMeules 2009).

For example, a recent report also from the NIH–AARP Diet and Health Study in more than 500,000 men and women investigated associations between physical activity and the development of lung cancer (Leitzmann et al. 2009). In this study, individuals were classified as current smokers who smoked >20 cigarettes/day, current smokers who smoked ≤20 cigarettes/day, former smokers who quit 1–9 years ago, former smokers who quit ≥10 years ago, or lifetime nonsmokers. In fully adjusted models, the risk of lung cancer was reduced by 22% comparing most to least active adults when pooling all smoking categories. Similar reductions in risk were observed in separate analyses of current and former smokers. However, no significant decline was observed among the never smokers, who had a very low rate of lung cancer compared to other categories.

Proposed biologic pathways through which physical activity may reduce the risk of lung cancer include improved pulmonary function, effects on IGF and insulin levels, and increased immune function (Tardon et al. 2005). Nevertheless, the combination of protection among current and former smokers with negative findings among never smokers from the NIH–AARP Diet and Health Study highlights the possibility that the observed inverse association between physical activity and lung cancer may result from an imperfect measurement of smoking and the strong coincidence of smoking and inactive lifestyle behaviors (Leitzmann et al. 2009).

ENDOMETRIAL CANCER

Endometrial cancer is the fourth most common newly diagnosed cancer in women in the United States, but ranks eighth in cancer mortality (American Cancer Society 2010). Most studies find that physical activity is associated with decreased endometrial cancer risk, with two recent systematic reviews of the literature estimating risk reduction between 20% and 30% (Cust et al. 2007; Voskuil et al. 2007). Many studies have also observed a dose–response association, where risk decreases with increasing amounts of physical activity. Furthermore, growing evidence suggests that physical activity may be associated with greater risk reduction in overweight and obese women compared to normal weight women, although these findings are still preliminary (Gierach et al. 2009; Patel et al. 2008). For example, in 42,672 postmenopausal women from the American Cancer Society Cancer Prevention Study II Nutrition Cohort (Patel et al. 2008), risk of endometrial cancer was similar when comparing the most and least active women with a BMI of <25.0 kg/m². However, risk of endometrial cancer was reduced by 41% when comparing the most to least active women who were overweight or obese (BMI ≥25.0 kg/m²). Optimal timing, dose, and type of physical activity for the greatest reduction in endometrial cancer risk remains unclear and more studies are needed to better characterize the association between physical activity and endometrial cancer risk.

Physical activity is known to have a beneficial effect on serum sex steroid levels (estrogen, testosterone, progesterone) as well as three established risk factors for endometrial cancer: obesity, insulin resistance, and hyperinsulinemia. Although not fully understood or directly tested, exercise may decrease risk of endometrial cancer through these biological pathways (Voskuil et al. 2007).

OTHER CANCERS

The associations between physical activity and risk of ovarian, kidney, and pancreatic cancer have been investigated in a number of observational studies, but results for these sites are inconsistent. In general, studies in cohorts do not show a reduced risk of these cancers with more physical activity, and therefore do not support a relationship between physical activity and decreased risk at this time (Pan and DesMeules 2009).

CARDIORESPIRATORY FITNESS AND CANCER

Limited studies have assessed the relationship of cardiorespiratory fitness with risk of cancer, but existing studies show promising results and encourage further research to confirm associations. For example, testing in the highest tertile of cardiorespiratory fitness reduced the risk of developing any type of cancer by 27% in a population-based cohort of 2268 men in Finland (Laukkanen et al. 2010). Figure 4.7 depicts the adjusted rate of all new cancers in this cohort by tertiles of cardiorespiratory fitness. The figure shows low fit men were at the highest risk, whereas high fit men were at the lowest. Similarly, in a study of 12,975 men in the Aerobic Center Longitudinal Study (ACLS), men in the highest versus lowest quartile of fitness had

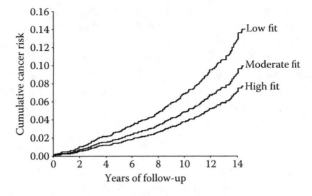

FIGURE 4.7   Multivariable-adjusted cumulative overall cancer incidence during an average follow-up of 12 years in men according to tertiles of cardiorespiratory fitness (low fit group <26.9 mL kg^{-1} min^{-1}, moderate fit group 26.9–33.2 mL kg^{-1} min^{-1}, and high fit group >33.2 mL kg^{-1} min^{-1}). Figure shows that low fit men had the highest risk of developing any new cancer during follow-up, whereas high fit men had the lowest risk.

a 74% decrease in the risk of prostate cancer after accounting for factors related to prostate cancer, including age, BMI, and smoking (Oliveria et al. 1996). In more than 38,000 men and women also from the ACLS, lung cancer risk was more than 50% lower for those with high and moderate levels of fitness compared to those with low fitness, and this finding was present among both current and former smokers (Sui et al. 2010).

Increased cardiorespiratory fitness is speculated to decrease cancer risk through biological mechanisms similar to those for physical activity, including decreased oxidative stress, improved immune function, and improved insulin metabolism (Laukkanen et al. 2010). The findings from the above-mentioned studies complement associations between physical activity and overall, prostate, and lung cancer, and additional studies are needed to better characterize the association between cardiorespiratory fitness and cancer risk.

PHYSICAL ACTIVITY AND PULMONARY CONDITIONS

In this section, we will review the role that physical activity and cardiorespiratory fitness may play in the primary prevention of pulmonary conditions, including asthma and chronic obstructive pulmonary disease. Asthma is a chronic inflammatory disease of the airways characterized by variable and recurring symptoms, airway obstruction, and bronchospasm. Although asthma is a chronic obstructive condition, it is not considered a part of chronic obstructive pulmonary disease since airway obstruction in asthma is generally reversible. However, if left untreated, asthma can result in chronic inflammation and irreversible obstruction. Symptoms of asthma include wheezing, coughing, chest tightness, and shortness of breath.

Very few studies have examined whether physical activity or increased fitness may prevent the development of asthma. In one study of 757 initially asymptomatic children who were followed for more than 10 years, baseline cardiorespiratory fitness measured via a maximal bicycle ergometer test was inversely associated with the development of asthma (Rasmussen et al. 2000). Children who developed asthma had a modestly lower mean fitness level at baseline compared to children who did not develop asthma. However, determining whether low physical activity actually preceded the development of asthma as opposed to the symptoms of asthma resulting in reduced physical activity and low fitness at baseline is complicated by the difficulty in identifying childhood asthma.

Chronic obstructive pulmonary disease refers to chronic bronchitis and emphysema, two often cooccurring conditions resulting in airway restriction and shortness of breath. In contrast to asthma, airflow restriction is rarely reversible and frequently becomes worse over time. Although physical activity may play an important role in improving function in patients with chronic obstructive pulmonary disease, there is limited evidence suggesting physical activity offers any protective influence. In a 22-year follow-up study of San Francisco longshoremen, cigarette smoking was associated with increased risk of death from myocardial infarction (heart attack), cancer, and chronic obstructive pulmonary disease, whereas low physical activity was associated with increased fatal myocardial infarction and stroke, but not mortality due to chronic obstructive pulmonary disease (Paffenbarger et al. 1978).

Thus, it is currently unknown whether physical activity and fitness play an important role in the prevention of asthma and chronic obstructive pulmonary disease. Additional research is needed in order to clarify these associations.

PHYSICAL ACTIVITY AND MUSCULOSKELETAL CONDITIONS

In this section, we will describe the influence that physical activity or fitness may have on the development of two major chronic musculoskeletal conditions: arthritis and osteoporosis. Although these conditions may not by themselves result in death and may not be mentioned in discussions regarding the leading causes of death in the United States, arthritis and osteoporosis are serious chronic health conditions that diminish quality of life and functional independence.

PHYSICAL ACTIVITY AND ARTHRITIS

Osteoarthritis is the most common form of arthritis affecting more than 21 million people in the United States, and in 2009, resulted in more than $40.1 billion in healthcare-related expenditures. Osteoarthritis, or degenerative joint disease, frequently affects the large weight-bearing joints, such as the knees, hips, and spine. Osteoarthritis is more common among women, older persons, Caucasians, overweight or obese persons, and those with a history of significant joint injuries. It is a disease of the articular cartilage (smooth white tissue that covers the ends of bones where they come together at joints) and the subchondral bone (located immediately below the articular cartilage). Clinical diagnosis is frequently made by observing specific radiographic features, including joint space narrowing, sclerosis (or thickening) of subchondral bone, and osteophyte (or excess bone) formation. Signs and symptoms of osteoarthritis include pain, swelling, crepitus (or a crackling sensation felt below the skin during joint movement and palpation), and restricted range of motion.

Select types of activities may contribute to the development of osteoarthritis. Activities with high-load joint stresses, especially those involving twisting and torsional types of stress have been associated with degenerative joint conditions. Examples of these activities include soccer, football, tennis, and certain track-and-field events. These forces over time may result in excessive wear to the hyaline cartilage of the joint, which can lead to osteoarthritis. In addition, activities with chronic and repetitive joint forces, including running, jumping, and throwing, may eventually lead to articular surface damage, initiating the development of osteoarthritis. However, some level of activity may also be necessary to promote optimal joint health. Loss of joint motion, either through injury or spinal cord transection, is known to be associated with muscle atrophy, loss of bone density, connective tissue stiffness, and other adverse effects on the musculoskeletal system.

Since the incubation period (the time it takes for the disease to develop) for the development of osteoarthritis can be upward of 30 years, there are very few studies that have systematically evaluated the influence of participation in various activities throughout a lifetime with the long-term development of osteoarthritis. The few available studies have produced mixed results. In one small study of young and middle-aged runners and nonrunners, no increase was observed in knee osteoarthritis by serial radiographs after nearly 10 years of follow-up (Lane et al. 1998). Similarly, in the Framingham Offspring Study, a community-based cohort of sons and daughters from the original Framingham Heart Study population, no association was observed in this middle-aged and elderly cohort between recreational walking, jogging, or high activity levels at baseline and incident radiograph-confirmed osteoarthritis diagnosed approximately 9 years later (Felson et al. 2007). However, other studies have shown higher levels of self-reported physical activity earlier in life to be associated with an increased risk of osteoarthritis later in life, although these findings may be influenced by the subjective recall of physical activity many years, sometimes decades, before the occurrence of osteoarthritis.

Although there are no experimental studies examining the dose–response association between physical activity and osteoarthritis, the collective studies seem to suggest that this relation is very likely to be nonlinear and is probably J-shaped. That is, the risk of osteoarthritis may be increased slightly with no or very limited activity and may be even greater at extreme levels of activity, whereas the optimal activity zone associated with the lowest risk may be somewhere in between. Additional long-term observational and experimental studies are needed to clarify the dose–response association.

Physical Activity and Osteoporosis

Osteoporosis is a disease in which bones become fragile due to a loss of bone mineral density over time. This loss of bone results in diminished mechanical strength, fragility, and an increased likelihood of fracture in response to severe stresses. Osteoporosis is a major public health problem, particularly among the older adult population. It is estimated that 55% or about 44 million adults aged 50 years and older in the United States have osteoporosis, and about 80% of those affected are women (National Osteoporosis Foundation 2002). Osteoporosis is responsible for millions of fractures every year, mostly of the lumbar spine, hip, and wrist, and in 2005, resulted in an estimated $19 billion in health care expenditures (National Osteoporosis Foundation 2002). Osteoporosis itself has no specific symptoms, and may not come to light until the occurrence of a fracture.

Numerous studies as well as systemic reviews of the literature are available describing the role that physical activity plays in the prevention and amelioration of osteoporosis. Physical activity has the potential to decrease the likelihood of developing osteoporosis during three critical periods over the life course. The first is during the period of attainment of peak bone mass, which generally occurs by late adolescence. Weight-bearing activities that involve running, jumping, and twisting during childhood and adolescence, particularly around puberty, help to develop peak bone mass. Numerous studies have shown that young adults who were more active earlier in life have greater peak bone mass than their more inactive peers.

During the second critical period, the second to the fifth decades of life, physical activity may help to maintain peak bone mass. Observational studies have shown greater bone mineral densities among active adults during this time (Brewer et al. 1983); however, intervention studies frequently show only a modest impact of exercise training on the addition of new bone or on changes in bone mineral density (Borer 2005). These findings highlight the importance of physical activity early in life.

In the third critical period, later adult life (after the fifth decade), physical activity is mostly important in the maintenance of bone mineral density and in slowing the rate of bone loss. The available studies suggest that increases in bone mineral density with exercise training during this period are usually very modest, but are often greater for those with the lowest bone values. Furthermore, some studies show greater-than-expected increases, suggesting that an appropriately designed exercise program can be an effective strategy for increasing bone mineral density in older adulthood.

There are several principles on the adaptation to bone in response to mechanical loading that are important to consider when using physical activity or exercise to prevent or ameliorate osteoporosis. Adaptive bone response requires dynamic rather than static mechanical stimulation. Bone-loading activities should consist of forceful and fast mechanical loads generated from muscular contraction or weight-bearing forces that load the bone at various angles. The load should be above a threshold intensity, and specific bones must be targeted for the best localized effect. The bone response is improved with brief but intermittent exercise, and because bone accommodates to customary loads over time, the magnitude of loads should be increased periodically to continually stimulate new bone formation. In addition, an adaptive bone response to exercise requires abundant availability of nutrient energy as well as calcium and vitamin D.

SUMMARY

Current evidence suggests that physical activity is causally associated with incident cardiovascular disease, including heart disease, stroke, and hypertension. Research is beginning to accrue on the role that physical activity may play in the development of subclinical cardiovascular disease as well as the influence of resistance training and sedentary behaviors in the etiology of cardiovascular disease. Strong scientific evidence suggests that physical activity has a protective, dose–response relationship with the risk of colon and breast cancers. Accumulating studies support a role for physical activity in the prevention of prostate, lung, and endometrial cancers, although these associations are in need of further study. It is very likely that physical activity plays only a minimal role in the development of pulmonary conditions, such as asthma and chronic obstructive pulmonary disease. Physical activity is important in improving quality of life and maintaining functional independence in osteoarthritis and osteoporosis, and very likely plays a beneficial role during all critical time points in the development of these conditions over the life course. Physical activity has a great potential to decrease the burden of cardiovascular disease, cancer, and major musculoskeletal conditions in the United States and other countries throughout the world, adding to the public health importance of increasing physical activity levels in the general population.

STUDY QUESTIONS

1. Define physical activity, physical fitness, and exercise, and compare how they may differ in reducing chronic disease risk factors.
2. Describe the leading causes of death in the United States, and explain how regular physical activity can reduce the risk for developing these conditions.
3. Which is typically more strongly associated with cardiovascular disease, cancer, and other health-related outcomes, physical activity or cardiorespiratory fitness? What are the possible reasons for this difference?
4. Compare the strength of evidence showing the benefits of physical activity on breast, prostate, colon, rectal, lung, and endometrial cancers. What are some possible reasons for these associations?
5. What are the most common fatal cancers among women in the United States? Among them, what is the most common newly diagnosed cancer among women?
6. What is likely to be the dose–response association between physical activity and osteoarthritis? How would you design a study to best describe and examine this association?

REFERENCES

American Cancer Society. 2010. *Cancer Facts and Figures 2010*. Atlanta, GA: American Cancer Society.

Bertoni, A. G., M. C. Whitt-Glover, H. Chung et al. 2009. The association between physical activity and subclinical atherosclerosis: The Multi-Ethnic Study of Atherosclerosis. *Am. J. Epidemiol.* 169: 444–454.

Borer, K. T. 2005. Physical activity in the prevention and amelioration of osteoporosis in women: Interaction of mechanical, hormonal and dietary factors. *Sports Med.* 35: 779–830.

Brewer, V., B. M. Meyer, M. S. Keele et al. 1983. Role of exercise in prevention of involutional bone loss. *Med. Sci. Sports Exerc.* 15: 445–449.

Chase, N. L., X. Sui, D. C. Lee et al. 2009. The association of cardiorespiratory fitness and physical activity with incidence of hypertension in men. *Am. J. Hypertens.* 22: 417–424.

Cust, A. E., B. K. Armstrong, C. M. Friedenreich et al. 2007. Physical activity and endometrial cancer risk: A review of the current evidence, biologic mechanisms and the quality of physical activity assessment methods. *Cancer Causes Control* 18: 243–258.

Desai, M. Y., K. Nasir, J. A. Rumberger et al. 2004. Relation of degree of physical activity to coronary artery calcium score in asymptomatic individuals with multiple metabolic risk factors. *Am. J. Cardiol.* 94: 729–732.

Dunstan, D. W., E. L. Barr, G. N. Healy et al. 2010. Television viewing time and mortality: The Australian Diabetes, Obesity and Lifestyle Study (AusDiab). *Circulation* 121: 384–391.

Felson, D. T., J. Niu, M. Clancy et al. 2007. Effect of recreational physical activities on the development of knee osteoarthritis in older adults of different weights: The Framingham Study. *Arthritis Rheum.* 57: 6–12.

Folsom, A. R., G. W. Evans, J. J. Carr et al. 2004. Association of traditional and nontraditional cardiovascular risk factors with coronary artery calcification. *Angiology* 55: 613–623.

Friedenreich, C. M., and A. E. Cust. 2008. Physical activity and breast cancer risk: Impact of timing, type and dose of activity and population subgroup effects. *Br. J. Sports Med.* 42: 636–647.

Gierach, G. L., S. C. Chang, L. A. Brinton et al. 2009. Physical activity, sedentary behavior, and endometrial cancer risk in the NIH–AARP Diet and Health Study. *Int. J. Cancer* 124: 2139–2147.

Giovannucci, E. L., Y. Liu, M. F. Leitzmann et al. 2005. A prospective study of physical activity and incident and fatal prostate cancer. *Arch. Intern. Med.* 165: 1005–1010.

Harriss, D. J., G. Atkinson, K. George et al. 2009. Lifestyle factors and colorectal cancer risk (1): Systematic review and meta-analysis of associations with body mass index. *Colorectal Dis.* 11: 547–563.

Harriss, D. J., N. T. Cable, K. George et al. 2007. Physical activity before and after diagnosis of colorectal cancer: Disease risk, clinical outcomes, response pathways and biomarkers. *Sports Med.* 37: 947–960.

Howard, R. A., D. M. Freedman, Y. Park et al. 2008. Physical activity, sedentary behavior, and the risk of colon and rectal cancer in the NIH–AARP Diet and Health Study. *Cancer Causes Control* 19: 939–953.

Jurca, R., M. J. Lamonte, C. E. Barlow et al. 2005. Association of muscular strength with incidence of metabolic syndrome in men. *Med. Sci. Sports Exerc.* 37(11): 1849–1855.

Kadoglou, N. P., F. Iliadis, and C. D. Liapis. 2008. Exercise and carotid atherosclerosis. *Eur. J. Vasc. Endovasc. Surg.* 35: 264–272.

Lakka, T. A., J. M. Venalainen, R. Rauramaa et al. 1994. Relation of leisure-time physical activity and cardiorespiratory fitness to the risk of acute myocardial infarction. *N. Engl. J. Med.* 330: 1549–1554.

Lane, N. E., J. W. Oehlert, D. A. Bloch et al. 1998. The relationship of running to osteoarthritis of the knee and hip and bone mineral density of the lumbar spine: A 9 year longitudinal study. *J. Rheumatol.* 25: 334–341.

Laukkanen, J. A., E. Pukkala, R. Rauramaa et al. 2010. Cardiorespiratory fitness, lifestyle factors and cancer risk and mortality in Finnish men. *Eur. J. Cancer* 46: 355–363.

Lee, C. D., and S. N. Blair. 2002. Cardiorespiratory fitness and stroke mortality in men. *Med. Sci. Sports Exerc.* 34: 592–595.

Lee, C. D., D. R. Jacobs Jr., A. Hankinson et al. 2009. Cardiorespiratory fitness and coronary artery calcification in young adults: The CARDIA Study. *Atherosclerosis* 203: 263–268.

Lee, I. M. 2007. Physical activity, fitness, and cancer. In *Physical Activity and Health*, ed. C. Bouchard, S. N. Blair, and W. L. Haskell. Champaign, IL: Human Kinetics.

Leitzmann, M. F., C. Koebnick, C. C. Abnet et al. 2009. Prospective study of physical activity and lung cancer by histologic type in current, former, and never smokers. *Am. J. Epidemiol.* 169: 542–553.

MacMahon, S., R. Peto, J. Cutler et al. 1990. Blood pressure, stroke, and coronary heart disease: Part 1. Prolonged differences in blood pressure: Prospective observational studies corrected for the regression dilution bias. *Lancet* 335: 765–774.

Manson, J. E., F. B. Hu, J. W. Rich-Edwards et al. 1999. A prospective study of walking as compared with vigorous exercise in the prevention of coronary heart disease in women. *N. Engl. J. Med.* 341: 650–658.

National Osteoporosis Foundation. 2002. *America's Bone Health: The State of Osteoporosis and Low Bone Mass in Our Nation.* Washington, DC: National Osteoporosis Foundation.

Newton, R. U., and D. A. Galvao. 2008. Exercise in prevention and management of cancer. *Curr. Treat. Options Oncol.* 9: 135–146.

Oliveria, S. A., H. W. Kohl 3rd, D. Trichopoulos et al. 1996. The association between cardiorespiratory fitness and prostate cancer. *Med. Sci. Sports Exerc.* 28: 97–104.

Paffenbarger Jr., R. S., R. J. Brand, R. I. Sholtz et al. 1978. Energy expenditure, cigarette smoking, and blood pressure level as related to death from specific diseases. *Am. J. Epidemiol.* 108: 12–18.

Pan, S. Y., and M. DesMeules. 2009. Energy intake, physical activity, energy balance, and cancer: Epidemiologic evidence. *Methods Mol. Biol.* 472: 191–215.

Patel, A. V., H. S. Feigelson, J. T. Talbot et al. 2008. The role of body weight in the relationship between physical activity and endometrial cancer: Results from a large cohort of US women. *Int. J. Cancer* 123: 1877–1882.

Rasmussen, F., J. Lambrechtsen, H. C. Siersted et al. 2000. Low physical fitness in childhood is associated with the development of asthma in young adulthood: The Odense schoolchild study. *Eur. Respir. J.* 16: 866–870.

Siscovick, D. S., L. Fried, M. Mittelmark et al. 1997. Exercise intensity and subclinical cardiovascular disease in the elderly. The Cardiovascular Health Study. *Am. J. Epidemiol.* 145: 977–986.

Sui, X., D. C. Lee, C. E. Matthews et al. 2010. Influence of cardiorespiratory fitness on lung cancer mortality. *Med. Sci. Sports Exerc.* 42: 872–878.

Tardon, A., W. J. Lee, M. Delgado-Rodriguez et al. 2005. Leisure-time physical activity and lung cancer: A meta-analysis. *Cancer Causes Control* 16: 389–397.

Taylor, A. J., T. Watkins, D. Bell et al. 2002. Physical activity and the presence and extent of calcified coronary atherosclerosis. *Med. Sci. Sports Exerc.* 34: 228–233.

Tehard, B., C. M. Friedenreich, J. M. Oppert et al. 2006. Effect of physical activity on women at increased risk of breast cancer: Results from the E3N cohort study. *Cancer Epidemiol. Biomarkers Prev.* 15: 57–64.

Vasan, R. S., A. Beiser, S. Seshadri et al. 2002. Residual lifetime risk for developing hypertension in middle-aged women and men: The Framingham Heart Study. *JAMA* 287: 1003–1010.

Voskuil, D. W., E. M. Monninkhof, S. G. Elias et al. 2007. Physical activity and endometrial cancer risk, a systematic review of current evidence. *Cancer Epidemiol. Biomarkers Prev.* 16: 639–648.

Wannamethee, S. G., and A. G. Shaper. 2001. Physical activity in the prevention of cardiovascular disease: An epidemiological perspective. *Sports Med.* 31: 101–114.

Wendel-Vos, G. C., A. J. Schuit, E. J. Feskens et al. 2004. Physical activity and stroke. A meta-analysis of observational data. *Int. J. Epidemiol.* 33: 787–798.

Whelton, S. P., A. Chin, X. Xin et al. 2002. Effect of aerobic exercise on blood pressure: A meta-analysis of randomized, controlled trials. *Ann. Intern. Med.* 136: 493–503.

Wolin, K. Y., Y. Yan, G. A. Colditz et al. 2009. Physical activity and colon cancer prevention: A meta-analysis. *Br. J. Cancer* 100: 611–616.

World Health Report. 2002. Reducing risks, promoting healthy life.

5 Physical Activity and Injury Prevention

Kenneth E. Powell

CONTENTS

INTRODUCTION

Injuries are the unhealthy side effects of physical activity (PA). The most important thing to know about them is that they do not outweigh the health benefits of regular PA from a population (i.e., public health) perspective. Epidemiologic studies of outcomes that encompass both positive and negative (i.e., injuries) events such as all-cause mortality, quality of life, and medical costs consistently show that it is healthier to be physically active than inactive.

Still, injuries lower the net benefit of PA for people who are physically active. In addition, they cause some people to stop being active and deter others from beginning (Finch, Owen, and Price 2001; Hootman et al. 2002; Koplan et al. 1982; Koplan, Rothenberg, and Jones 1995). Therefore, preventing injuries, even minor ones, is an important pathway for maximizing the benefits of regular PA.

The purpose of this chapter is to provide a framework for thinking about injuries caused by PA. We view PA broadly, encompassing transportational, occupational, and domestic PA as well as sports and recreation. The goal is to develop principles for preventing PA-related injuries in general rather than methods for preventing specific injuries. Musculoskeletal injuries are the most common and have been the topic of the most research, but the general principles derived apply to most—if not all—types of injuries.

SCOPE OF INJURIES AND PERSPECTIVE FOR PREVENTION

The scope of PA-related injuries is so broad and so varied that no truly useful and complete classification system exists. Injuries may be mild (e.g., blister from new walking shoe) or severe (e.g., fractured skull from bicycle collision). They may be acute (e.g., torn anterior cruciate ligament) or chronic (e.g., iliotibial band syndrome). Injuries include such diverse maladies as fractures, blisters, cardiac arrhythmias, heat injuries, and infectious diseases. They encompass events arising directly from the activity such as a collision between two football players, and events caused by external sources such as being hit by a car while walking or cycling.

As noted, our purpose is to develop general principles for the prevention of PA-related injuries. Current research on the prevention of PA-related injuries provides much valuable information but is commonly limited to

- Injuries associated with sports and recreation, omitting injuries associated with physically active transportation, occupation, and household activities.
- A specific sport such as soccer, skiing, or running.
- A specific injury such as stress fracture or medial meniscus tear.
- A specific level of injury severity, such as all injuries causing death or causing hospitalization.
- Competitive athletes. The frequency, duration, and intensity of the exposure and, sometimes, even the rules of the game differ markedly between competitive athletes and the general population. Extrapolation from the injury experiences of competitive athletes to the general population is potentially misleading.

Our perspective being a description of the factors that contribute to the risk of all types of PA-related injuries in the general population, we have sought research that

TABLE 5.1

Factors Possibly Associated with Physical Activity-Associated Injuries[a]

1. Aspects of physical activity itself
   a. Type of activity[b] (e.g., walking, soccer, gardening)
   b. Dose of activity[b] (e.g., volume, intensity, rate of change of dose)
   c. Auxiliary behaviors (e.g., stretching, warming up, and cooling down)
   d. Protective gear and equipment[b] (e.g., shoes, clothing, bicycle helmets, mouth guards, break away bases, reduced impact baseballs and softballs, wrist guards, ski binding adjustments)
2. Personal characteristics
   a. Demographic (e.g., age, sex, race/ethnicity, anatomical characteristics)
   b. Health status (e.g., prior musculoskeletal injury,[b] overweight and obesity, chronic diseases)
   c. Health behaviors (e.g., tobacco use)
3. Environmental conditions (e.g., safety from traffic[b] and crime, air pollution, very hot[b] or cold[b] temperatures)

[a] For a more thorough discussion of these and other factors, please see Physical Activity Guidelines Advisory Committee (2008b).
[b] A causal relationship between this item and PA-related injuries is firmly established.

takes a more general approach and have searched for general principles across the reports with limited scope. We begin with a table of potential risk factors (Table 5.1).

TYPE OF ACTIVITY

Probably the most important determinant of injury risk is the type of PA performed. For any given activity (e.g., football, cycling), the risk of injury can be modulated by other factors, such as protective equipment, environmental conditions, or personal characteristics. The activity itself, however, sets the stage. For musculoskeletal injuries, the risk is determined to a large extent by the frequency and force of collisions or contact with other people, the ground, or other objects. A categorization scheme for games and sports has been developed (Committee on Sports Medicine and Fitness 2001) that works reasonably well even though style and rules of play vary by age, location, and other factors:

- Collision sports (e.g., football, ice hockey, wrestling). Participants purposefully hit or collide with each other or inanimate objects.
- Contact sports (e.g., basketball, soccer). Participants make contact with each other but usually with less force.
- Limited-contact sports (e.g., baseball, ultimate Frisbee). Contact with other players or objects is infrequent or unintentional.
- Noncontact sports (e.g., running, swimming, tennis). Contact between participants is uncommon.

In general, the risk of injury is higher for collision or contact sports than for limited- or noncontact activities. Reported injury rates for college, secondary school,

and youth sports support the general validity of the categories (Physical Activity
Guidelines Advisory Committee 2008b). Most transportation, occupational, and
domestic activities are noncontact and can be assigned an appropriate category without much difficulty.

Information about PA-related injury rates for the general population, especially
studies based on the amount of exposure (e.g., time spent doing the activity), are

TABLE 5.2
Injuries per 1000 h of Participation by Activity, Finland

Activity	Injuries per 1000 h of Participation
Commuting activities	
– Walking	0.2
– Cycling	0.5
Lifestyle activities	
– Hunting, fishing, berry picking	0.3
– Home repair	0.5
– Gardening	1.0
Sports, noncontact	
– Golf	0.3
– Dancing	0.7
– Swimming	1.0
– Walking	1.2
– Rowing	1.5
– Pole walking	1.7
– Cross-country skiing	1.7
– Running	3.6
– Track and field sports	3.8
– Tennis	4.7
Sports, limited contact	
– Cycling	2.0
– Aerobics, gymnastics	3.1
– Horse riding	3.7
– Downhill skiing	4.1
– In-line skating	5.0
– Volleyball	7.0
– Squash	18.3
Sports, collision and contact	
– Karate	6.7
– Ice hockey	7.5
– Soccer	7.8
– Basketball	9.1
– Wrestling	9.1
– Judo	16.3

Source: Parkkari, J. et al., *Int. J. Sports Med.*, 25, 209–216, 2004. With permission.

sparse. The best so far is a survey of PA-related injury risk in the general population in Finland (Table 5.2) (Parkkari et al. 2004). The findings are based on a yearlong population-based random survey of Finns 15–74 years of age, 92% of whom agreed to record all PA sessions of 15 min or more and register all acute and overuse injuries that "caused a significant complaint to the subject" and that were related to the activities. Participation and related injuries were collected by telephone once every 4 months.

Reported PA-related injuries per 1000 h of participation ranged from 0.2 for walking as a commuting activity to 18.3 for squash. Injury rates were lower for commuting activities, lifestyle activities, and noncontact sports than for limited contact, contact, and collision sports. It is interesting to note that injury rates for walking and cycling during commuting activities (0.2 and 0.5, respectively) were less than the rates for walking and cycling performed as sports or recreation (1.2 and 2.0, respectively), indicating that the same activity done for different purposes may have different injury rates. Four other surveys of the general population also report appreciably lower injury rates among participants of noncontact activities such as walking, bicycling, gardening, golf, or swimming (Finch and Cassell 2006; Mummery et al. 1998; Mummery, Schofield, and Spence 2002; Powell et al. 1998).

Walking is the most commonly reported PA. Therefore, even though injury rates are low, the number of people injured while walking is probably large. Unfortunately, we have little information about the causes of walking-related injuries (Physical Activity Guidelines Advisory Committee 2008b).

CONCLUSIONS

Activities with fewer and less forceful contact with other people or objects have appreciably lower injury rates than collision or contact sports. Walking, gardening or yard work, bicycling or exercise cycling, dancing, swimming, and golf have the lowest injury rates.

DOSE OF ACTIVITY

The risk of injury may be related to dose in a variety of ways: total dose, frequency, duration, absolute intensity, relative intensity, change in total dose, relative size of change in total dose, and others. The dose, or volume, of activity is determined by the frequency, duration, and intensity of activity or activities performed during a specified period of time. For example, the dose of PA for a person who rides a bicycle to and from work for a weekly total of 50 miles at an average speed of 10 mph, and who does general gardening at home for 3 h every weekend, is about 2520 MET min/week. This assumes a MET (metabolic equivalent) value of 6 for bicycling at 10 mph and a MET value of 4 for general gardening. Dose is sometimes described simply by the number of minutes per week an activity is performed (e.g., 150 min/week of moderate intensity PA), or, for activities such as running or walking, by the number of miles per week.

Absolute intensity is the amount of energy or force required to perform an activity. The intensity of aerobic activities can be quantified in METs, kilocalories, and other scales. If one adjusts for differences in body weight (e.g., measure energy expenditure in METs instead of kilocalories), the rate of energy expenditure is similar for all persons. For example, running at 6 mph similarly requires about 6 METs for all persons.

Relative intensity is the proportion of one's capacity used to perform an activity. Not all persons have the same capacity or level of physical fitness. Capacity differs for many reasons, such as age, sex, genetics, and routine activity levels. Therefore, all people running at 6 mph have a similar rate of absolute energy expenditure but their relative energy expenditure varies. When doing any specific activity (e.g., running at 10 mph), individuals with high levels of fitness (i.e., capacity) use a smaller percentage of their capacity than persons with lower fitness. Relative intensity can be described as percent of aerobic capacity (VO_{2max}), percent of maximal heart rate, or other similar measures. It can also be described by how hard an individual perceives an activity to be: very light, light, moderate, hard, very hard, or maximal.

The relative size of increase in PA is calculated by dividing the amount of increase by the usual amount. For example, a person who adds 10 min/week of walking to a usual weekly total of 30 min has increased the amount of PA by 33% ($10 \div 30 = 0.33$), whereas a person who adds 10 min/week to a usual total of 150 min has the amount by only 7% ($10 \div 150 = 0.07$).

A direct relation between injury risk and the following three is reasonably well established:

- Total dose of PA
- Relative size of increase in total dose, if total dose is increasing
- Relative intensity of effort

TOTAL DOSE

Evidence of the direct relationship between dose of activity and risk of injury is demonstrated by the results from seven high quality studies of running injuries (Physical Activity Guidelines Advisory Committee 2008b). All reported increases in the risk of injury as the number of miles per week increased regardless of definition of injury. Injuries in all studies were self-reported but definitions varied, including seeking medical care, stopping running for ≥7 days, modifying usual running program, and simply considered an injury by the runner. Individuals who were running 40 miles/week or more (speed of running assumed to be 10 min/mile at an intensity of 10 METs = 4000 or more MET min/week) were 2 to 3 times more likely than individuals who ran 5 to 10 miles/week (500–1000 MET min/week) to have had a running injury in the past 12 months (Blair, Kohl, and Goodyear 1987; Colbert, Hootman, and Macera 2000; Hootman et al. 2001; Koplan et al. 1982; Macera et al. 1989; Marti et al. 1988; Walter et al. 1989) (Figure 5.1). The trends were similar for males and females and for runners of different ages. Frequency, duration, and absolute intensity (in this case, speed) were infrequently and inconsistently associated with risk of injury, suggesting that risk of injury is more closely related to total dose than any single component. Similar findings have been reported for triathletes (Shaw et al. 2004; Vleck and Gorbutt 1998).

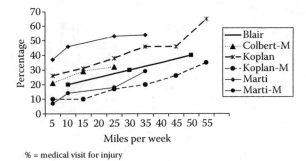

FIGURE 5.1   Percentage of recreational runners injured by average number of miles run per week. (Adapted from U.S. Department of Health and Human Services, DDPHP Publication No. 40036, 2008.)

RELATIVE SIZE OF INCREASE

Studies of military recruits and experimental subjects provide evidence that the risk of injury is related to the relative size of increase in PA.

Military recruits are young healthy adults who undergo 2 to 3 months of rigorous, often vigorous, aerobic and muscular training. Typically, recruits expend about 3000 MET min/week, or approximately 3–6 times the currently recommended amount for the general population (Jones et al. 1993; Physical Activity Guidelines Advisory Committee 2008b). Recruits experience high levels of overuse musculoskeletal injuries during this period (11–37% for men, 22–67% for women) (Gilchrist, Jones, and Sleet 2000). Low levels of prior PA and physical fitness are two of the most consistently observed risk factors for injuries during basic training. This means that recruits who have the largest gap between their PA levels before and during basic training are most likely to be injured (Institute of Medicine 2007; Physical Activity Guidelines Advisory Committee 2008b; see below for discussion of female sex as a risk factor for PA-related injuries). Students in physical education (PE) classes (de Loës, Jacobsson, and Goldie 1990) and participants in aerobic dance classes (Garrick, Gillien, and Whiteside 1986) also have been shown to be more likely to be injured if they are less physically active outside of class.

EXPERIMENTAL STUDIES

Some older and a few recent experimental trials provide information about dose and risk of injury. In most early experimental studies, subjects were relatively inactive males 25 to 60 years of age and they were exposed to vigorous PA. The subjects experienced high injury rates, nearly 50% (Mann et al. 1968; Kilbom et al. 1969; Saltin et al. 1969). A small but nicely designed trial tested the effects of different doses of running on the incidence of injuries (Pollock et al. 1977) (Figure 5.2). Six groups of 23–26 middle-aged men were assigned different doses of running: three groups ran for 30 min on 1, 3, or 5 days/week, and three other groups ran for 15, 30, or 45 min on 3 days/week. The incidence of injuries was highest among those men

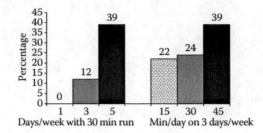

FIGURE 5.2 Percentage of subjects with injury by dose of running. (Adapted from Pollock, M.L. et al., *Med. Sci. Sports*, 9, 31–36, 1977.)

running 30 min 5 days/week and 45 min 3 days/week. This implicates frequency, duration, and total dose in the genesis of PA-related injuries but most strongly implicates relative size of increase.

In both early and recent publications, researchers have noted a higher frequency of injuries during the first weeks of an intervention (Mann et al. 1968; Ready et al. 1999). Because the gap between usual and current dose is likely to be largest at the onset of an activity program, these observations are consistent with the risk of injuries being directly related to the relative size of the increase.

The finding that the relative size of increase is directly related to the risk of injury is consistent with the overload and adaptation principle of exercise science (American College of Sports Medicine 2000). The overload and adaptation principle states that function is improved when tissues (e.g., muscles) and organs (e.g., heart) are exposed to an overload (i.e., a stimulus greater than usual) and provided time to recover and adapt. Repeated exposures to a tolerable overload are followed by adaptation of the tissues and organs to the new load and improvements in performance and function. Too large an overload or insufficient time for adaptation, however, leads to injury and malfunction.

RELATIVE INTENSITY OF EFFORT

The intensity of any specific PA can be described in absolute or relative terms. Absolute intensity is the amount of energy or force required to perform an activity; relative intensity is the proportion of one's capacity required to perform the activity. High relative intensities occur among people who are already regularly physically active, who are performing at or near capacity, and who make an extra effort (e.g., competitive athletes). Even though the size of the increase in activity may be small, individuals who strain to perform at top capacity increase their risk of injury. Studies of youth, high school, and collegiate athletes demonstrate that injury rates during games are about 2–4 times higher than during practices (Physical Activity Guidelines Advisory Committee 2008b). This is true for non- and limited-contact sports as well as contact and collision sports. Among recreational runners, speed of running was unrelated to injury when other factors (e.g., total weekly distance) were taken into account but injuries were more common among runners who described themselves as competitive runners than those who described themselves as recreational or noncompetitive

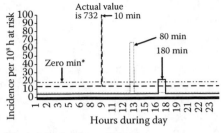

*Usual min/week of vigorous PA is zero

FIGURE 5.3 Risk of sudden cardiac arrest by usual min/week of vigorous PA. (Adapted from U.S. Department of Health and Human Services, DDPHP Publication No. 40036, 2008.)

(Marti et al. 1988; Walter et al. 1989). Similar findings have been reported for gymnasts (Leaf, Keating, and Kolt 2003) and triathletes (Vleck and Gorbutt 1998).

High relative intensities also occur among inactive and unfit people who perform an activity at an absolute intensity that is unusual for them (e.g., shoveling snow, running after a bus). Studies of the risk of PA-related sudden adverse cardiac events (e.g., heart attacks, arrhythmias) demonstrate the added risk of a high relative intensity. Although the risk of PA-related sudden adverse cardiac events is very small, estimated to be about 10^{-6} to 10^{-8} per hour of vigorous activity, the outcome is severe, the publicity of such events is often high, and they tend to make people fear the risk of activity rather than appreciate its benefits. An adverse event that does happen is noticed more easily than one that does not.

All individuals have a higher rate of sudden adverse cardiac events during vigorous physical activities than at other times. The magnitude of that risk, however, is inversely related to routine volume of vigorous activity (Siscovick et al. 1984) (Figure 5.3). In Figure 5.3, the horizontal lines represent the average risk for each group during most of the day. The vertical bars indicate the risk during vigorous activity. The highest horizontal line is the average risk for people who reported no routine vigorous activity and for whom a relative risk during vigorous activity cannot be calculated. Similar findings have been reported in several articles (Lee and Sattelmair 2009; Physical Activity Guidelines Advisory Committee 2008b).

Because cardiovascular fitness is directly related to one's regular PA habits, people who routinely participate in more vigorous PA usually have a higher VO_{2max} than individuals who are vigorously active less often. As a result, the relative intensity during vigorous PA is higher for those who routinely do less vigorous PA than for those who do more.

CONCLUSIONS

The risk of PA-related injury is related to the total dose of activity, rapid increases in total dose, and a high relative intensity of activity. Most of the evidence to support these conclusions comes from PA exposures well above the currently recommended volume for substantial health benefits. The routine PA of military recruits, recreational runners and triathletes, and competitive athletes far exceeds the recommended dose of 500–1000 MET min/week (U.S. Department of Health and Human Services 2008). Risks of injury at or around that recommended level are lower but have been poorly documented and quantified in recent clinical trials (Physical Activity Guidelines Advisory Committee 2008b). As a result, guidelines for inactive people who want to increase their routine PA lack firm empirical support. The principle of overload and adaptation indicates that inactive people should add small amounts, allow time for adaptation, and limit themselves to light to moderate relative intensity. Expert opinion suggests that adding an activity of relatively light or moderate intensity (e.g., walking) for 5–15 min on 2–3 days/week should be safe (Physical Activity Guidelines Advisory Committee 2008b; U.S. Department of Health and Human Services 2008). The speed of adaptation slows with age, so older adults should add increments no more often than every 2–4 weeks. It is better to progress slowly and establish PA as a regular behavior than to suffer injury and drop out because the goal was approached too rapidly. Every increase, no matter how small, is helpful (U.S. Department of Health and Human Services 2008). There are risks to PA, but the risks of sedentarism are greater.

OTHER RISK FACTORS FOR PA-RELATED INJURIES

In addition to risks associated with type and dose of PA, there are other risk factors, some with injury prevention potential (Table 5.1). A few of the more interesting ones are mentioned below; more information is available elsewhere (Physical Activity Guidelines Advisory Committee 2008b). Personal characteristics (e.g., demographic) influence the type and dose of PA and, thereby, influence the risk of injury. This section is not concerned with whether these characteristics influence the choice of activity but whether the potential risk factor directly influences the risk of injury: Do people with different characteristics (e.g., old or young) but doing the same amount and type of activity have the same risk of activity-related injury?

ACTIVITY-RELATED BEHAVIORS

Common elements of activity programs such as stretching, warming up, and cooling down are commonly assumed to help prevent injuries. They do when all are included in an activity program, but supportive scientific evidence for each behavior alone is scant (Physical Activity Guidelines Advisory Committee 2008b; Thacker et al. 2004).

PROTECTIVE GEAR

Proper protective equipment has been shown to reduce the rate of injuries in a variety of activities. Comfortable shoes, bicycle helmets, football helmets, mouth guards, full face shields in hockey, wrist guards for in-line skating, binding adjustments in skiing, and other protective gear have been shown to reduce injuries (Gilchrist, Saluja, and Marshall 2007).

AGE

Slower reflexes, decline in balance, less elasticity of connective tissue, and other physiological changes of aging would appear to place older people at greater risk of PA-related injuries. Studies of military recruits confirm higher injury rates among older recruits even though the oldest recruits are in their mid to upper 20s (Heir and Eide 1997; Jones et al. 1993). Surveys of active adults of all ages, however, report lower injury rates among older than younger persons (Carlson et al. 2006; Finch and Cassell 2006; Parkkari et al. 2004; Powell et al. 1998; Uintenbroek 1996). This surprising finding presumably arises from a confounding of age with exposure—the fact that older individuals cannot and do not attempt to perform at levels comparable to younger persons.

SEX

Aside from a few specific types of injuries (e.g., stress fractures and tears of the anterior cruciate ligament appear to be more common among females) females and males appear to have equivalent risk of PA-related injury (Physical Activity Guidelines Advisory Committee 2008b). Sport-specific injury rates for college athletes are equivalent for males and females, and male and female military recruits have similar injury rates if the rates are adjusted for physical fitness.

RACE/ETHNICITY

The influence of race and ethnicity on PA-related injuries has been uncommonly reported (Physical Activity Guidelines Advisory Committee 2008b). When it has been reported there are usually no differences among race and ethnic groups. However, certain health conditions that are more common in one race or ethnic group may predispose that group to higher risk of specific problems. For example, sickle cell trait is more common among African Americans; individuals with the trait are more likely than those without to suffer rhabdomyolysis and sudden death.

PRIOR MUSCULOSKELETAL INJURIES

Prior injury is one of the most consistently reported and strongest risk factors for future injury, with the risk generally reported to be about 2-fold (Physical Activity Guidelines Advisory Committee 2008b). Reinjury may occur because the original injury has not healed or the wound and surrounding structures have been inadequately rehabilitated (Hootman and Powell 2009), or because the primary risk factor has not been modified (e.g., structural or training defect).

OVERWEIGHT/OBESITY

The mechanical and metabolic consequences of obesity suggest that overweight/obese persons may be at greater risk than normal weight persons for PA-related injuries. However, because overweight/obese persons are also more likely inactive, it has been impossible to tell if the risk is due to overweight/obesity or inactivity (Powell 2010).

CHRONIC DISEASES

For many chronic diseases such as atherosclerotic heart disease, diabetes, arthritis, or chronic lung disease, participation in an appropriately designed PA program is therapeutically beneficial. However, many people with chronic diseases are inactive and, therefore, unfit. Most people with a chronic disease can safely add several minutes of walking or other light to moderate intensity activity to their everyday activities (Physical Activity Guidelines Advisory Committee 2008b). Just like people without chronic disease, they are susceptible to injury if they increase the total dose of activity too quickly or if they perform activity at a high level of relative intensity.

SAFETY FROM TRAFFIC

Injury rates of pedestrians and cyclists in the United States are 2- to 4-fold higher than those in Germany and the Netherlands (Pucher and Dijkstra 2003). Two important features of safe walking and biking are lower traffic speed and separation from traffic. Neighborhoods can be modified to reduce traffic speed and to assure separation between pedestrians, cyclists, and motor vehicles. Mechanisms to slow traffic, sometimes referred to as traffic calming, include (1) vertical deflections (e.g., speed bumps), (2) horizontal deflections (e.g., bends), (3) road narrowing, and (4) medians, four-way stops, and small roundabouts (Loukaitou-Sideris 2005; Retting, Ferguson, and McCartt 2003; Tester et al. 2004). Mechanisms to separate pedestrians and cyclists from traffic include installation and maintenance of (1) sidewalks and bicycle lanes, (2) pedestrian over- and underpasses, and (3) fences or parkways between sidewalks and streets (Lott and Lott 1976; Retting, Ferguson, and McCartt 2003). Methods of reducing the risk at crossings—areas shared by pedestrians, bicyclists, and motor vehicles—include the installation of traffic signals, pedestrian prompting devices (e.g., signs), in-pavement flashing lights to warn drivers when pedestrians are present, traffic signals with exclusive walk signal phasing, refuge islands, raised medians, and improved nighttime lighting (Retting, Ferguson, and McCartt 2003; Zegeer et al. 2000, 2001).

AIR POLLUTION

The adverse health effects of both air pollution and inactivity are well established. The balance between the risks and benefits of being physically active in air polluted at levels commonly experienced in the United States is not established (Physical Activity Guidelines Advisory Committee 2008b). People are commonly urged to avoid "prolonged or heavy exertion" near heavy traffic, industrial sites, and on days when air pollution is judged to be severe. Such recommendations may be reasonable for individuals who can easily modify the location or time for exercise. However, they may be a barrier to regular PA for people with less flexible daily demands. In addition, they take into account only short-term adverse effects of PA in polluted air.

The long-term benefits of regular PA in polluted air may outweigh the short-term risks. Lower mortality rates among more active than less active individuals in a polluted industrial community have been reported (Wong et al. 2007). Regular PA in a polluted environment may ameliorate the adverse effects of pollution just as it reduces the adverse health effects of obesity and diabetes.

OTHER ASPECTS OF INJURY PREVENTION

So far, in this chapter, we have considered risk factors for PA-related injuries in general, such as type of activity, dose and changes in dose, and personal and environmental factors. This section considers two interesting aspects of PA-related injuries less tightly connected to specific risk factors: medical clearance and risk of injuries unrelated to PA.

MEDICAL CLEARANCE

Given that PA-related injuries do occur and that some of these injuries can be severe or even life threatening (e.g., sudden cardiac arrest), recommendations for PA have often included the restriction that certain people—usually people with known medical conditions and people above a certain age—should not perform vigorous activities without permission from a medical care provider (National Institutes of Health 1996; Pate et al. 1995). Current Guidelines for Americans (U.S. Department of Health and Human Services 2008) have dropped the age restriction but do suggest that people with "chronic conditions or symptoms" should develop an activity plan with their healthcare provider. That seems reasonable enough. It is worth noting, however, that there is no evidence that persons who consult a healthcare provider receive more benefits or suffer fewer adverse effects than persons who do not. It is also possible that official recommendations to seek medical advice before increasing one's regular PA practices may reduce participation in regular moderate PA, because it implies that being active is less safe and provides fewer benefits than being inactive (Buchner 2003).

RISK OF INJURY NOT ASSOCIATED WITH PA

Physically active people have more PA-related injuries than sedentary people because they spend more time being physically active. For other types of injury, however, PA may be protective. For example, regularly active older adults are less likely than inactive older adults to suffer fall-related injuries (Physical Activity Guidelines Advisory Committee 2008a). This raises the question whether physically active persons may have fewer overall injuries than inactive persons in spite of the fact that they have more PA-related injuries. Only two population-based studies have examined this issue. One reported that people who ran or participated in sports activities were about 50% more likely to report an injury (activity-related or not) than people who reported walking for exercise or were sedentary (Hootman et al. 2001). The other reported no significant differences in overall injury rates (activity-related or not) between inactive people, irregularly active people, and people who met current recommendations for PA (Carlson et al. 2006). More studies of this type are needed, but it is possible that regular PA may cause some injuries and prevent others, and that physically active people may have no more injuries than sedentary individuals.

CONCLUSION

Injuries detract from the health benefits of regular PA because they are negative health events and because they prevent and discourage people from becoming more active. There is a wide range of types and severities of PA-related injuries. Injuries are related to the type and dose of activity. The incidence of injury is higher during collision and contact sports than during limited and noncontact activities. The incidence of injuries is directly related to the total dose of activity, the relative size of increase in the routine dose, and to the relative intensity of effort.

The risk of injury at recommended doses of PA (i.e., 150–300 min/week at moderate intensity) has been poorly quantified but appears to be low. People increasing their routine PA to achieve personal health goals or other reasons can minimize their risk of injury by adding small increments and allowing sufficient time for adaptation. The addition every 2–4 weeks of 5–15 min of relatively light or moderate intensity PA on 2–3 days/week is considered a safe rate of increase. The less active one has been, the smaller the increment and pace of increase should be. Prior injury and failure to use appropriate protective gear are other well-established causes of injury. The positive or negative value of preparticipation medical screening has not been determined. It is possible that physically active people may have overall injury rates no higher than those of inactive people.

STUDY QUESTIONS

1. The author asserts that preventing even minor injuries is important. Why does he say that? Do you agree? How would you measure the public health impact of PA-related injuries? Would you include the burden of diseases people develop because an injury caused them to be less active?
2. Propose a taxonomy (method of classifying) for activity-related injuries.
3. Make a list of at least 10 transportation, occupational, or household physical activities and place them into the appropriate collision/contact/limited contact/noncontact categories.
4. Recreational runners and military recruits have a much higher total dose of physical activity than recommended for the general public for health benefits. Do you think that the risk factors for injury for runners and military recruits are likely to apply to the general public?
5. The author of this chapter comments, "An adverse event that does happen is noticed more easily than one that does not." Do you agree? If the statement is correct, what are the implications for public health activities, most of which are designed to prevent bad things from happening.
6. The author asserts that type and dose of PA are influenced by demographic factors such as age and sex. Do you agree? If so, how do the choices influence the types and rates of injuries?

7. In general, females are smaller and have a smaller muscle mass than males. As a result, their maximal physical capacity is less than males. If injury rates for females and males are equivalent only after adjusting for physical fitness, do you think that females and males should be considered to have equal risk of PA-related injury?

8. Do you think that telling people ≥60 years of age to consult their medical care provider before increasing their PA levels would have a net health benefit or a net health loss? Why?

9. How might regular PA prevent non-PA–related injuries (e.g., motor vehicle collision or occupational injuries)?

REFERENCES

American College of Sports Medicine (ACSM). 2000. *ACSM's Guidelines for Exercise Testing and Prescription*, 6th edition, ed. B. A. Franklin, 138–139. Baltimore: Lippincott, Williams and Wilkins.

Blair, S. N., H. W. Kohl, and N. N. Goodyear. 1987. Rates and risks for running and exercise injuries: Studies in three populations. *Res. Q. Exerc. Sport* 58: 221–228.

Buchner, D. M. 2003. Physical activity to prevent or reverse disability in sedentary older adults. *Am. J. Prev. Med.* 25(Sii): 214–215.

Carlson, S. A., J. M. Hootman, K. E. Powell et al. 2006. Self-reported injury and physical activity levels: United States 2000 to 2002. *Ann. Epidemiol.* 16: 712–719.

Colbert, L. H., J. M. Hootman, and C. A. Macera. 2000. Physical activity-related injuries in walkers and runners in the Aerobics Center Longitudinal Study. *Clin. J. Sport Med.* 10: 259–263.

Committee on Sports Medicine and Fitness. 2001. Medical conditions affecting sports participation. *Pediatrics* 107: 1205–1209.

de Loës, M., B. Jacobsson, and I. Goldie. 1990. Risk exposure and incidence of injuries in school physical education at different activity levels. *Can. J. Sport Sci.* 15: 131–136.

Finch, C., and E. Cassell. 2006. The public health impact of injury during sport and active recreation. *J. Sci. Med. Sport* 9: 490–497.

Finch, C., N. Owen, and R. Price. 2001. Current injury or disability as a barrier to being more physically active. *Med. Sci. Sports Exerc.* 33: 778–782.

Garrick, J. G., D. M. Gillien, and P. Whiteside. 1986. The epidemiology of aerobic dance injuries. *Am. J. Sports Med.* 14: 67–72.

Gilchrist, J., B. H. Jones, and D. A. Sleet. 2000. Exercise-related injuries among women: Strategies for prevention from civilian and military studies. *MMWR Recommend. Rep.* 49(RR02): 13–33.

Gilchrist, J., G. Saluja, and S. W. Marshall. 2007. Interventions to prevent sports and recreation-related injuries. In *Handbook of Injury and Violence Prevention*, ed. L. S. Doll, S. E. Bonzo, D. A. Sleet, J. A. Mercy, and E. N. Haas, 117–136. New York: Springer.

Heir, T., and G. Eide. 1997. Injury proneness in infantry conscripts undergoing a physical training programme: Smokeless tobacco use, higher age, and low levels of physical fitness are risk factors. *Scand. J. Med. Sci. Sports* 7: 304–311.

Hootman, J. M., C. A. Macera, B. E. Ainsworth et al. 2001. Association among physical activity level, cardiorespiratory fitness, and risk of musculoskeletal injury. *Am. J. Epidemiol.* 154: 251–258.

Hootman, J. M., C. A. Macera, B. E. Ainsworth et al. 2002. Epidemiology of musculoskeletal injuries among sedentary and physically active adults. *Med. Sci. Sports Exerc.* 34: 838–844.

Hootman, J. M., and K. E. Powell. 2009. Physical activity, fitness, and musculoskeletal injury. In *Physical Activity Epidemiology*, ed. I. M. Lee, 263–280. New York: Oxford University Press.

Institute of Medicine (IOM). 2007. *Adequacy of Evidence for Physical Activity Guidelines Development: Workshop Summary.* Washington, DC: National Academies Press.

Jones, B. H., D. N. Cowan, J. P. Tomlinson et al. 1993. Epidemiology of injuries associated with physical training among young men in the army. *Med. Sci. Sports Exerc.* 25: 197–203.

Kilbom, A., L. H. Hartley, B. Saltin et al. 1969. Physical training in sedentary middle-aged and older men: I. Medical evaluation. *Scand. J. Clin. Lab. Invest.* 24: 315–322.

Koplan, J. P., K. E. Powell, R. K. Sikes et al. 1982. An epidemiologic study of the benefits and risks of running. *JAMA* 248: 3118–3121.

Koplan, J. P., R. B. Rothenberg, and E. L. Jones. 1995. The natural history of exercise: A 10-yr follow-up of a cohort of runners. *Med. Sci. Sports Exerc.* 27: 1180–1184.

Leaf, J. R., J. L. Keating, and G. S. Kolt. 2003. Injury in the Australian sport of calisthenics: A prospective study. *Aust. J. Physiother.* 49: 123–130.

Lee, I.-M., and J. Sattelmair. 2009. Risk of acute cardiac events with physical activity. In *Epidemiologic Methods in Physical Activity Studies*, ed. I.-M. Lee, 246–262. New York: Oxford University Press.

Lott, D. F., and D. Y. Lott. 1976. Effect of bike lanes on ten classes of bicycle–automobile accidents in Davis, California. *J. Safety Res.* 8: 171–179.

Loukaitou-Sideris, A. 2005. Transportation, land use, and physical activity: Safety and security issues. Background paper for TRB Special Report 282. Does the Built Environment Influence Physical Activity? Examining the Evidence. http://trb.org/downloads/sr282papers/sr282Sideris.pdf (accessed August 29, 2010).

Macera, C. A., R. R. Pate, K. E. Powell et al. 1989. Predicting lower-extremity injuries among habitual runners. *Arch. Int. Med.* 149: 2565–2568.

Mann, G. V., J. L. Garrett, A. Farhi et al. 1968. Exercise to prevent coronary heart disease. *Am. J. Med.* 46: 12–27.

Marti, B., J. P. Vader, C. E. Minder et al. 1988. On the epidemiology of running injuries: The 1984 Bern Grand-Prix study. *Am. J. Sports Med.* 16: 285–294.

Mummery, W. K., G. Schofield, and J. C. Spence. 2002. The epidemiology of medically attended sport and recreational injuries in Queensland. *J. Sci. Med. Sport* 5: 307–320.

Mummery, W. K., J. C. Spence, J. A. Vincenten et al. 1998. A descriptive epidemiology of sport and recreation injuries in a population-based sample: Results from the Alberta Sport and Recreation Injury Survey (ASRIS). *Can. J. Public Health* 89: 53–56.

National Institutes of Health (NIH). 1996. NIH consensus development on physical activity and cardiovascular health. Physical activity and cardiovascular health. *JAMA* 276: 241–246.

Parkkari, J., P. Kannus, A. Natri et al. 2004. Active living and injury risk. *Int. J. Sports Med.* 25: 209–216.

Pate, R. R., M. Pratt, S. N. Blair et al. 1995. Physical activity and public health: A recommendation from the Centers for Disease Control and Prevention and the American College of Sports Medicine. *JAMA* 273: 402–407.

Physical Activity Guidelines Advisory Committee. 2008a. Physical Activity Guidelines Advisory Committee Report: 2008, Part G Section 6: Functional Health. Washington, DC: U.S. Department of Health and Human Services. http://www.health.gov/paguidelines/Report/pdf/CommitteeReport.pdf (accessed August 29, 2010).

Physical Activity Guidelines Advisory Committee. 2008b. Physical Activity Guidelines Advisory Committee Report: 2008, Part G Section 10: Adverse events. Washington, DC: U.S. Department of Health and Human Services. http://www.health.gov/paguidelines/Report/pdf/CommitteeReport.pdf (accessed August 29, 2010).

Pollock, M. L., L. R. Gettman, C. A. Milesis et al. 1977. Effects of frequency and duration of training on attrition and incidence of injury. *Med. Sci. Sports* 9: 31–36.

Powell, K. E. 2010. Adverse events from physical activity in obese persons. In *Physical Activity and Obesity*, ed. C. Bouchard and P. T. Katzmarzyk, 323–326. Champaign, IL: Human Kinetics.

Powell, K. E., G. W. Heath, M.-J. Kresnow et al. 1998. Injury rates from walking, gardening, weightlifting, outdoor bicycling, and aerobics. *Med. Sci. Sports Exerc.* 30: 1246–1249.

Pucher, J., and L. Dijkstra. 2003. Promoting safe walking and cycling to improve public health: Lessons from The Netherlands and Germany. *Am. J. Public Health* 93: 1509–1516.

Ready, A. E., G. Gergeron, S. L. Boreskie et al. 1999. Incidence and determinants of injuries sustained by older women during a walking program. *J. Aging Phys. Activity* 7: 91–104.

Retting, R. A., S. A. Ferguson, and A. T. McCartt. 2003. A review of evidence-based traffic engineering measures designed to reduce pedestrian–motor vehicle crashes. *Am. J. Public Health* 93: 1456–1463.

Saltin, B., L. H. Hartley, A. Kilbom et al. 1969. Physical training in sedentary middle-aged and older men: II. Oxygen uptake, heart rate, and blood lactate concentration at submaximal and maximal exercise. *Scand. J. Clin. Lab. Invest.* 24: 323–334.

Shaw, T., P. Howat, M. Trainor et al. 2004. Training patterns and sports injuries in triathletes. *J. Sci. Med. Sport* 7: 446–450.

Siscovick, D. S., N. S. Weiss, R. H. Fletcher et al. 1984. The incidence of primary cardiac arrest during vigorous exercise. *N. Engl. J. Med.* 311: 874–877.

Tester, J. M., G. W. Rutherford, Z. Wald et al. 2004. A matched case-control study evaluating the effectiveness of speed humps in reducing child pedestrian injuries. *Am. J. Public Health* 94: 646–650.

Thacker, S. B., J. Gilchrist, D. F. Stroup et al. 2004. The impact of stretching on sports injury risk: A systematic review of the literature. *Med. Sci. Sports Exerc.* 36: 371–378.

Uintenbroek, D. G. 1996. Sports, exercise, and other causes of injuries: Results of a population survey. *Res. Q. Exerc. Sport* 67: 380–385.

U.S. Department of Health and Human Services (USDHHS). 2008. *Physical Activity Guidelines for Americans*. U.S. Department of Health and Human Services, 2008. ODPHP Publication No. U0036. Also available at: http://www.health.gov/paguidelines/pdf/paguide.pdf.

Vleck, V. E., and G. Gorbutt. 1998. Injury and training characteristics of male elite, development squad, and club triathletes. *Int. J. Sports Med.* 19: 38–42.

Walter, S. D., L. E. Hart, J. M. McIntosh et al. 1989. The Ontario cohort study of running-related injuries. *Arch. Int. Med.* 149: 2561–2564.

Wong, C.-M., C.-Q. Ou, T.-Q. Thach et al. 2007. Does regular exercise protect against air pollution-associated mortality? *Prev. Med.* 44: 386–392.

Zegeer, C. V., C. Seiderman, P. Lagerway et al. 2000. *Pedestrian Facilities Users' Guide—Providing Safety and Mobility*. Washington, D.C., Federal Highway Administration.

Zegeer, C. V., J. R. Stewart, H. H. Huang et al. 2001. Safety effects of marked versus unmarked crosswalks at uncontrolled locations. *Transport. Res. Rec.* 1723: 56–68.

6 Physical Activity in Treatment of Chronic Conditions

J. Larry Durstine, Keith Burns, and Ryan Cheek

CONTENTS

INTRODUCTION

Current aging trends indicate that Americans are living longer (Arias 2010). In the past 100 years, life expectancy in the United States has increased from less than 50 years to more than 76 years (Arias 2010). Unfortunately, the prevalence of chronic diseases and disabilities is also rising and now represents the major cause of death and disability not only in the United States but worldwide (Centers for Disease Control and Prevention 2004). These chronic conditions include cardiovascular diseases (CVD), cancer, type 2 diabetes, obesity, and respiratory diseases and accounts for 59% of the 57 million annual deaths due to chronic diseases and conditions. Globally, this figure accounts for 46% of the world disease burden (World Health Organization 2003). The good news is that by incorporating daily physical activity and exercise as part of one's lifestyle, both primary and secondary prevention disease rates are likely reduced. Primary prevention is the process of preventing diseases and conditions in an attempt to prevent them from occurring. Secondary prevention is the process of administering treatment to persons with diagnosed diseases and conditions in an attempt to reverse the effects of the disease. These lifestyle changes have now become an important part of the medical disease management plan (Moore et al. 2009).

Epidemiologists during the twentieth century established numerous factors associated with risk for many different chronic diseases and conditions. For example,

CVD is one of the earliest conditions where risk factors were identified, and has primary determinants that include high cholesterol, high blood pressure, obesity, cigarette smoking, and lack of regular exercise. In addition, strong scientific evidence supports the incorporation of healthy lifestyles such as good dietary habits and daily physical activity and exercise as having positive influences on many risk factors regardless of the disease. When considering secondary prevention, chronic disease management plans should include behavioral change programs to reduce risk factors as part of the medical management protocol (Artinian et al. 2010). Behavioral change programs usually reduce the severity or prevalence of risk factors within several weeks but up to several months. By consuming a healthy diet or with daily physical activity and exercise, primary disease prevention programs can achieve reductions in heart disease by 80%, in cancer by 33%, and in type 2 diabetes by 90% (World Health Organization 2003). Daily physical activity and exercise are known to positively impact many chronic health conditions such as high cholesterol and hypertension. In addition, daily physical activity and exercise have been shown to relieve symptoms of depression and anxiety and improve mood (Dudgeon et al. 2004). Thus, present scientific information support the importance of daily physical activity and exercise in both the primary and secondary prevention of most chronic conditions (Durstine, Peel, and LaMonte 2009).

Formulating a physical activity and exercise program for healthy persons to meet primary prevention goals is based on well-established scientific principles leading to the development of the American College of Sports Medicine (ACSM) physical activity guidelines and the 2008 U.S. activity guidelines (American College of Sports Medicine 2010; U.S. Department of Health and Human Services 2008). In this regard, the essence of a physical activity or exercise program is developed by knowing the individual's interests, health needs, and clinical status. In the medical management plan for persons with a chronic condition, the same exercise principles are used. When designing physical activity and exercise regimens to meet a patient's specific needs, special consideration is given to the patient's present health status and the need for exercise monitoring (Moore, Marsh, and Durstine 2009). In secondary disease prevention, supervised exercise becomes an important part of the medical management plan and the completion of the rehabilitation process (Thompson et al. 2003).

In the past 25 years, much new scientific information concerning daily physical activity and exercise programming for the secondary prevention of many chronic diseases and disabilities has been developed and is now reported in the literature. Chronic diseases such as diabetes, dyslipidemia, and chronic obstructive pulmonary disease (COPD) have been extensively studied, and methods for an exercise prescription have been developed. At the same time, there is still much to learn about exercise programming for individuals with many other chronic conditions and diseases such as Crohn's disease and various forms of cancer. Although exercise prescription principles are best scientifically defined for patients with coronary heart disease (CHD), the exercise professional uses these scientifically defined activity guidelines with their clinical exercise management experiences to best develop safe physical activity and exercise programming for patients with other less-defined chronic conditions.

EXERCISE IS MEDICINE™—EVIDENCE-BASED GUIDELINES

Exercise Is Medicine™ is an initiative promoting daily physical activity and exercise as part of every person's lifestyle because of the many associated health benefits. Thus, daily physical activity and exercise should be viewed as a medication. The notion Exercise Is Medicine™ is easily demonstrated by simple comparisons between exercise adaptations, medications, and their intended actions. For example, when comparing exercise training adaptations and beta blockers (a common drug used to treat numerous health conditions, such as hypertension), both elicit a comparable reduction in resting heart rate. However, exercise does not have the side effects often seen with beta blocker use. Another example is found when examining blood levels of C-reactive protein (CRP), which many scientists believe is a general marker of inflammation. Chronic low levels of blood CRP are associated with increased CHD risk (Libby and Ridker 2006). Regular exercise will lower blood CRP. Also keep in mind that statins, a class of medications widely used to lower blood cholesterol, also reduce blood CRP (Libby and Ridker 2006). In 2004, Milani, Lavie, and Mehra compared cardiac patients undergoing 3 months of cardiac rehabilitation with exercise training and cardiac patients not involved in cardiac rehabilitation. Patients completing cardiac rehabilitation had significantly lower blood CRP levels than patients not undergoing rehabilitation. Most importantly, some cardiac rehabilitation patients were taking a statin to reduce cholesterol, whereas other rehabilitation patients were not. Regardless of whether patients were taking a statin, all rehabilitation patients underwent exercise training as part of their medical management and rehabilitation plan. After rehabilitation, all patients had reduced blood CRP levels. The magnitude in CRP change after rehabilitation was similar whether taking a statin or not taking a statin (Milani, Lavie, and Mehra 2004). Thus, exercise training is as effective in reducing blood CRP and reducing inflammation as the stain medication statin, and both likely provide additional secondary disease prevention health benefits.

Daily physical activity and exercise are useful in the medical management of various health conditions including dyslipidemia, high blood pressure, and type 2 diabetes. For example, high blood pressure remains a primary global health concern and is associated with an increased incidence of all cause cardiovascular mortality, stroke, CHD, heart failure, peripheral arterial disease, and renal insufficiency (Pescatello et al. 2004). Generally, higher levels of physical activity and physically fitness are associated with a reduced incidence of high blood pressure in white men. These effects are likely similar for both men and women although few studies exist for women, and few studies exist examining whether differences exist between ethnicities (Pescatello et al. 2004).

The medications of choice in the treatment of chronic conditions and diseases are always changing. Every year, new more effective medications are developed to replace older ones that are found less effective and/or found to have dangerous long-term side effects. When daily physical activity and exercise are viewed as a potential medication, these lifestyle programs can be used by patients with almost any disease, and in many cases, physical activity and exercise have clearly been shown to achieve success in primary and secondary disease prevention (Lavie et al. 2009).

Most notable when used properly, physical activity and exercise have minimal detrimental side effects, and the accumulating scientific evidence for many different diseases provide further support for the numerous health benefits of daily physical activity and exercise (Lavie et al. 2009; Warburton, Nicol, and Brendin 2006).

From this newly founded information is the realization that a strong dose–response relationship exists between the amount or volume of daily physical activity and exercise completed and the health benefits obtained. In other words, the more daily physical activity and exercise completed or the higher the exercise intensity completed, the greater the health benefits obtained. To demonstrate this dose–response effect, Sui et al. (2007) reported cross-sectional results showing that older men and women who maintained moderate cardiorespiratory fitness levels had notably lower mortality risk than persons with low cardiorespiratory fitness. More importantly, subjects judged as having high cardiorespiratory fitness had even lower mortality risk. Furthermore, her work demonstrates that cardiorespiratory fitness is an important independent factor for lower mortality risk in older adults. Haskell (1994) reviewed the literature and reported similar findings for five large prospective studies; greater physical activity or cardiorespiratory fitness levels are associated with lower mortality risk. The work of Haskell (1994) and Sui et al. (2007) support a dose–response relationship and provide further support for daily physical activity and exercise as providing health benefits.

Medications alter how body systems function. In this regard, once physical activity and exercise programming are used as medicine, the manner in which the body systems function is changed. Not only does the body function differently, but the biologic mechanisms for functioning are changed. For example, cardiovascular exercise adaptations are numerous and consist of increasing myocardial oxygen supply as well as decreasing myocardial oxygen demand, increasing the myocardium electrical stability, and improving overall myocardial function. Daily physical activity and exercise enhance the cardiovascular functional capacity and decrease myocardial work that reduces the potential for the heart to develop an ischemic state at rest and during submaximal exercise (American College of Sports Medicine 2010). Decreased myocardial work and oxygen demand also elicit decreases in various other variables such as heart rate, systolic blood pressure, and blood catecholamine levels at rest and at any submaximal exercise work rate. Decreased blood catecholamine levels at rest and during submaximal exercise result in the likelihood of decreased ventricular fibrillation (Hull et al. 1994). Other exercise-induced cardiovascular benefits include increased myocardial function because of an increased stroke volume at rest and during submaximal or maximal exercise (American College of Sports Medicine 2010). The mechanism for increased stroke volume is associated with increased myocardium contractility and increased heart hypertrophy. All of these exercise adaptations are likely to postpone the development of a CHD event (American College of Sports Medicine 2010) and contribute to both primary and secondary prevention of CHD.

Biological changes brought on by daily physical activity and exercise are not limited to the cardiovascular system. Daily physical activity and exercise will alter the way all body systems function as well as the biologic mechanisms by which these systems function. These exercise-induced changes or adaptations include improved insulin sensitivity (Goodyear and Kahn 1998), reduced blood triglyceride levels, enhanced HDL-C levels and HDL-C/LDL-C ratio (Durstine and Thompson 2001), and decreased platelet aggregation that contributes to a lower likelihood for blood clot formation (Wang, Jen, and Chen 1995).

In addition to benefits to the cardiovascular system, daily physical activity and exercise are effectively used in the management plan for type 2 diabetes (Goodyear and Kahn 1998). Here, exercise improves glycolytic enzyme function, messenger RNA expression in the production of GLUT-4 protein (which is responsible for glucose transport into cells), and an exercise-induced pathway independent of insulin for the uptake of glucose into cells (Goodyear and Kahn 1998). These improvements can be seen with 150 min/week of moderate physical activity.

Lifestyles incorporating daily physical activity and exercise are associated with reduced weight and body fat, both of which are risk factors for cancer (You et al. 2009). Exercise is also associated with increased immune function and aids in maintaining functional capacity in persons with cancer and undergoing therapy (Stevinson, Lawlor, and Fox 2004). There is little doubt that leading a physically active lifestyle reduces the overall rate of mortality and morbidity while increasing quality of life.

The concept that a physically inactive lifestyle leads to a lower quality of life, premature morbidity, and early mortality among persons with chronic diseases has been extensively studied (Durstine et al. 2009). The results from these scientific studies have helped define the many health consequences of physical inactivity (Kesaniemi et al. 2010; U.S. Department of Health and Human Services 2008). Nonetheless, the complete economic cost of physical inactivity is very difficult to define and understand. One measure of the overall heath cost is the direct cost of medical care in treatment of chronic health conditions. Even determining this cost, because of the many different aspects of direct medical costs for caring for persons with chronic conditions, can be perplexing and difficult to carry out. One estimated cost is $1.5 trillion in 2005, which is more than 75% of the nation's medical care budget (see Table 6.1). The information in this table does not take into consideration the many

TABLE 6.1

Selected Chronic Diseases Precipitated by Physical Inactivity and Resulting Health Care Costs in the United States

Chronic Disease	Annual Cost of Condition in United States (US$)
Heart disease and stroke	448 billion
Cancer	228 billion
Diabetes	174 billion
Obesity	117 billion
Arthritis	81 billion (medical care cost)
	128 billion (medical care cost and loss of productivity)
Hypertension	76.6 billion
Cognitive and psychological disorders	Cost not known

Source: Centers for Disease Control and Prevention data 2010. With permission.

other indirect costs of chronic conditions including lost wages and decreased work productivity. Although these items are indirect costs, the losses place a heavy burden on society. For example, the estimated loss of productivity caused by arthritis alone totals more than $40 billion a year (Durstine, Peel, and LaMonte 2009). In addition to the economic burdens of physical inactivity, many personal consequences related to physical inactivity exist such as lower quality of life, loss of functional independence, depression, and mood disorders (Dudgeon et al. 2004; Kesaniemi et al. 2010; U.S. Department of Health and Human Services 2008). When all cost aspects for chronic disease are considered, the financial burden is overwhelming.

In the 1990s, a new phrase was coined: "evidence-based medicine." This phrase was developed by scientists at McMaster University and defined as "a systemic approach to analyze published research as the basis of clinical decision making" (Claridge and Fabian 2005). This phrase has been further revised and updated and has great practical value when developing a medical management plan with specific and detailed daily physical activity and exercise programming tailored to meet the needs of patients diagnosed with chronic conditions. The goal of using evidence-based guidelines is to apply the best available scientific evidence to develop an exercise plan that best fits the needs of the patient. Evidence-based guidelines seek to assess the strength of evidence for treatments benefits and risks, including lack of treatment to establish guidelines and policies. Evidence-based guidelines state how to effectively modify the standard exercise prescription to fit the specific needs of persons with chronic diseases. The use of evidence-based guidelines in the development of a management plan incorporating daily physical activity and exercise ensures the best exercise recommendations to meet the patient's personal health status. Table 6.2 shows a collection of websites in which evidence-based medicine guidelines, proper application of guidelines, current research topics, and the latest information regarding evidence-based medicine are presented. These websites will help in getting an overview of how to effectively prescribe exercise to persons with chronic diseases.

Daily physical activity and exercise programs are designed to meet individual health and fitness goals. When physical activity and exercise are part of secondary disease prevention programs, recommendations established by the American College of Sports Medicine (2010) and the U.S Department of Health and Human Services (2008) are best used. Although these two sets of recommendations differ slightly, both highlight that daily physical activity and exercise improve physical fitness and promote the concept that some physical activity and exercise is better than none. The ACSM guidelines recommend that moderate exercise intensity (40–60% VO_2R) aerobic activity should be engaged for 30 min a day, 5 days a week or that vigorous exercise intensity ($\geq$60% VO_2R) aerobic activity should be performed for 20 min each day at least 3 or more days each week. Aerobic exercises should be accompanied with 2 to 3 days each week of muscle strengthening activity where 8 to 10 strength exercises involving all major muscle groups using 8 to 12 repetitions per exercise are performed. An exercise session should incorporate both warm-up and cool-down segments as well as flexibility exercises (American College of Sports Medicine 2010). From a slightly different perspective, the U.S Department of Health and Human Services in 2008 released the *Physical Activity Guidelines for*

TABLE 6.2
Select Website Sources of Evidence-Based Medicine

Source	Description
Agency for Healthcare Research and Quality (AHRQ) www.ahrq.gov/clinic/epcix.htm	The AHRQ Web site includes links to the National Guideline Clearinghouse, Evidence Reports from the AHRQ's 12 Evidence-Based Practice Centers (EPC), and Preventative Services.
American College of Physicians Journal Club (ACPJC) www.acponline.gov/journals/acpjc/jcmenu.htm	ACP Journal Club evaluates evidence in individual articles.
Centre for Evidence Based Medicine (CEBM) www.cebm.net	The CEBM aims to promote evidence-based health care and provide support and resources to anyone who wants to make use of them. The Web site provides links to evidence-based journals and EBM-related teaching materials.
Center for Research Support, TRIP Database www.tripdatabase.com/index.html	The AHRQ began the Translating Research into Practice (TRIP) initiative in 1997 to implement evidence-based tools and information. A good place to start for EBM literature search.
Clinical Evidence, BMJ Publishing Group www.clinicalevidence.org	Searches British Medical Journal's (BMJ) Clinical Evidence Compendium for up-to-date evidence regarding effective health care. Lists available topics and describes the supporting body of evidence to date. Concludes with interventions "likely to be beneficial" vs. those with "unknown effectiveness."
Cochrane Database of Systematic Reviews www.cochrane.org	Systematic evidence reviews that are uploaded periodically by the Cochrane group. Reviewers discuss whether adequate data are available for the development of EBM guidelines for diagnosis or management.
Database of Abstracts of Reviews of Effectiveness (DARE) http://www.crd.york.ac.uk/crdweb/	Structured abstracts written by University of York CRD reviewers. Abstract summaries review articles on diagnostic or treatment interventions and discuss clinical applications.
EBM Guidelines www.ebmg.wiley.com	Evidence Based Medicine (EBM) Guidelines focuses on presenting practical and real-life information reflecting real clinical experience. EBM Guidelines is continuously updated to present the latest trends in clinical medicine.

(continued)

TABLE 6.2 (Continued)
Select Website Sources of Evidence-Based Medicine

Source	Description
Effective Health Care www.york.ac.uk/inst/crd/ehcb.htm	Bimonthly, peer reviewed bulletin for medical decision makers. Based on systematic reviews and synthesis of research on the clinical effectiveness, cost effectiveness, and acceptability of health service interventions.
Essential Evidence Plus www.essentialevidenceplus.com	Includes the InfoRetriever search system for the complete Patient-Oriented Evidence that Matters (POEMs) database and six additional evidence-based databases. Subscription is required.
Evidence-Based Medicine www.ebm.bmj.com	Bimonthly publication launched in 1995 by the BMJ Publishing Group. Article summaries include commentaries by clinical experts. Subscription is required.
Institute for Clinical Systems Improvements (ICSI) www.ICSI.org	ICSI is an independent, nonprofit collaboration of healthcare organizations, including the Mayo Clinic (Rochester, MN). Web site includes the ICSI guidelines for preventative services and disease management.
National Guideline Clearinghouse (NGC) www.guideline.gov	Comprehensive database of evidence-based clinical practice guidelines from government agencies and healthcare organizations. Describes and compares guideline statements with respect to objectives, methods, outcomes, evidence rating scheme, and major recommendations.
Open Clinical www.openclinical.org/ebm.	Open clinical aims to disseminate methods and tools for building healthcare knowledge applications that comply with the highest quality, safety, and ethical standards.
U.S. Preventative Services Task Force (USPSTF) www.ahrq.gov/clinic/uspstfix.htm	This Web site features updated recommendations for clinical preventative services based on systematic reviews by the U.S. Preventative Services Task Force.

Source: Siwek, J., et al., *Am. Fam. Phys.*, 65(2), 251–258, 2002. With permission.

Americans, and these guidelines recommend engaging in at least 150 min/week of moderate intensity aerobic activity, or 75 min/week of vigorous aerobic activity or an equivalent combination of moderate and vigorous intensity activity. Any aerobic activity can be performed in short periods or exercise bouts greater than 10 min in length. If this strategy of short physical activity and exercise bouts is used, three bouts equally spread throughout the day totaling at least 30 min is recommended. Because of the added health benefits, muscle-strengthening activities involving all major muscle groups are recommended 2 or more days each week (U.S. Department of Health and Human Services 2008).

The ACSM and U.S. Physical Activity Guidelines establish daily recommendations to meet primary disease prevention goals. In order to better meet secondary disease prevention goals, the U.S. Physical Activity Guidelines recommend that additional health benefits be achieved by increasing the time spent doing either aerobic and/or muscle-strengthening exercises. These guidelines recommend increasing weekly time spent being physically active and/or exercising to 300 min of moderate-intensity aerobic physical activity, or 150 min/week of vigorous aerobic activity or equivalent (U.S. Department of Health and Human Services 2008).

DISEASE MANIFESTATIONS AND THE ROLE OF PHYSICAL ACTIVITY IN MINIMIZING DISEASE PROCESSES

This section is concerned with several specific chronic conditions recognized as primary contributors to the world health burden and how physical activity can be used to reverse or minimize these disease manifestations. In secondary disease prevention and the care of any chronic condition, a medical management plan is developed. Such a plan includes information about the client's disease conditions, medications, exercise testing considerations, daily physical activity and exercise considerations, and special needs.

Coronary artery disease and peripheral arterial disease are the products of atherosclerosis and are the result of any one of many different factors including inflammation, lipid deposition, hypertension, and endothelial dysfunction (Libby and Ridker 2006). Atherosclerosis occurs as a progressive accumulation of lipids, calcium, platelets, macrophages, and fibrous connective tissue at a specific site on the inside wall of arteries and in time, as the accumulation grows, is termed fibrous plaque (Franklin 2009). Because of inner wall plaque buildup, the artery lumen (the area where blood flows) narrows and blood flow is reduced and eventually completely blocks blood flow through that artery, stopping the delivery of oxygen and other nutriments to surrounding tissues. When this happens in the coronary arteries of the heart, the process is referred to as a heart attack or myocardial infarction.

Of all the chronic progressive diseases, CHD has the most information regarding physical activity exercise. Thus, a great deal of information regarding evidence-based guidelines is now available for use in the development of exercise programming as part of the medical management plan to aid in achieving secondary disease prevention goals (King et al. 2009; Durstine et al. 2009). When working with CHD patients, safety is of the utmost concern. Before patients begin exercising, they must be able to define terms such as angina and identify provoking factors or symptoms of a cardiac episode, describe treatment (including the protocol for taking nitroglycerin), understand their upper limits of exercise tolerance, and know when to stop exercising (Friedman and Roberts 2009). These precautions allow for the patient to understand "how much exercise is enough," and what to do if symptoms occur. For example, if a patient develops angina during an exercise session, exercise should stop immediately and sublingual nitroglycerin administered in accordance to individual facility guidelines (Friedman and Roberts 2009). A medical management plan for CHD patients will likely include one or multiple prescribed drugs. The effects of these medications on heart rate, blood pressure, the ECG, and exercise capacity are evaluated before a supervised exercise program is initiated. During the early phase of such programming, exercise sessions are monitored by the medical staff and trained exercise personnel. Initial exercise duration is 15 to 20 min. Within this exercise session, short periods of 4 to 5 min are followed with short rest periods. The exercise session duration is slowly lengthened over time, and progression is based on the patient's functional improvement (Friedman and Roberts 2009). The exercise goal is to progress to 30 to 60 min each day, most if not all days of the week at moderate exercise intensities. Muscle-strengthening activities are recommended 2 days per week. Isometric exercises are avoided as they may cause large and sudden increases in blood pressure (Hall 2008). For more information regarding exercise programming and evidence-based medicine for CHD patients, visit the American Heart Association's website, www.americanheart.org, and the American College of Cardiology, website www.acc.org.

Hypertension is a contributing factor for atherosclerotic plaque development and is defined as a systolic blood pressure greater than or equal to 140 mm Hg and/or a diastolic blood pressure greater than or equal to 90 mm Hg (American College of Sports Medicine 2010). Generally, two factors contribute to high blood pressure: increased peripheral artery constriction and changes in inner arterial wall causing arterial narrowing. The increased peripheral narrowing is likely caused by any number of factors and includes increased renin–angiotensin system activity and increased sympathetic nervous system activity.

When developing a physical activity and exercise program for patients with hypertension, exercise training is initiated only after starting drug therapy (Gordon 2009). This procedure allows for the medications to better control blood pressure before, during, and after exercise. While exercising, blood pressure should be monitored regularly, and if systolic blood pressure exceeds 250 mm Hg and/or diastolic blood pressure exceeds 115 mm Hg, exercise should be stopped. Also, if resting systolic blood pressure is greater than 200 mm Hg and/or resting diastolic blood pressure is greater than 110 mm Hg, exercise is not recommended until blood pressure is better controlled (ACSM 2010). Hypertensive individuals should exercise aerobically most, if not all, days of the week with exercise sessions lasting longer than 30 min at an intensity of 40–60% VO_2 reserve. A muscle-strengthening regimen, 2–3 days per week, may be added as part of the exercise program, but only in combination with aerobic training. This combination is suggested because muscle-strengthening activity alone, with the exception of circuit training, has not been shown to significantly lower blood pressure. Muscle-strengthening regimens should focus on using lower resistances and higher repetitions (Gordon 2009).

Another factor associated with atherosclerosis development is an overabundance of cholesterol in the blood—a condition known as dyslipidemia or hyperlipidemia. There are several determining factors in defining dyslipidemia: a total serum cholesterol level of 200 mg dL^{-1} or higher, an LDL-C level greater than or equal to 130 mg dL^{-1} or higher, and an HDL-C level less than 40 mg dL^{-1} (American College of Sports Medicine 2010). Lipids are important for many body functions such as energy storage, components of cell membranes, insulation, and steroid hormone synthesis (Durstine, Moore, and Polk 2009). Nonetheless, lipids can only move around the body in combination with proteins. As lipids and proteins join together, the newly formed particle is termed a lipoprotein. Four distinct lipoprotein classes exist: chylomicrons, VLDL, LDL, and HDL. Chylomicrons, VLDL, and LDL are responsible for transportation of the lipids from either the intestine or the liver to all other tissues, where they are used for necessary body functions. When these blood lipid levels are too high, CHD risk is greatly increased. On the other hand, HDL is responsible for removing lipids from the body by transporting them back to the liver where they are metabolized and eliminated from the body. This action has importance because the elimination of cholesterol from the body is associated with reduced accumulation of atherosclerosis plaque (Durstine, Moore, and Polk 2009).

Dyslipidemia alone presents a chronic health condition with few exercise limitations. In most cases, daily physical activity and exercise programming for dyslipidemic patients often follow guidelines used for primary prevention. However, if a person with dyslipidemia presents with signs or symptoms for other chronic conditions such as CHD or renal disease, daily physical activity and exercise programming should follow exercise guidelines for secondary disease prevention for the diagnosed disorder (Durstine, Moore, and Polk 2009). Although muscle-strengthening and flexibility exercises are still important for persons with dyslipidemia, these forms of physical activity and exercise do not expend great amounts of energy and do not have a substantial impact on blood lipids and lipoproteins levels as compared to aerobic exercise. When using exercise in the treatment of dyslipidemia, caloric expenditure is of the utmost importance, making aerobic exercise the main focus. In order to gain optimal blood lipids and lipoproteins improvement, exercise amounts or volume larger than recommended levels are necessary to prevent chronic diseases. Reducing caloric intake and lowering dietary saturated fat consumption also are recommended (Durstine, Moore, and Polk 2009). Dyslipidemic clients should exercise at least 5 days a week and accumulate a minimum of 300 min of physical activity each week. Because of the high volume of aerobic exercise being completed, exercising several times a day is helpful. Such an arrangement allows for increased total caloric expenditure while reducing overall fatigue (Durstine, Moore, and Polk 2009).

Arthritis is a debilitating chronic condition characterized by inflammation, tissue swelling, stiffness, pain, and limited range of motion (Centers for Disease Control and Prevention 2010a). Several forms of arthritis exist, but the most common are osteoarthritis and rheumatoid arthritis. Osteoarthritis is characterized by a weakening of the cartilage in the synovial joints leading to subchondral cysts and the formation of bone spurs (Minor and Kay 2009) and is categorized as either primary or secondary. Primary osteoarthritis is due to natural wear and tear that bones experience throughout life with the greatest impact observed in menopausal women. Secondary osteoarthritis occurs as a symptom of other chronic conditions such as obesity, injury, or heredity. Rheumatoid arthritis is considered an autoimmune disease (Minor and Kay 2009) and is characterized by swelling and inflammation in the joint synovial membrane. Continued joint inflammation eventually leads to cartilage and bone deterioration around the affected joint, and is accompanied with soreness, distortion, and decreased joint functionality (Minor and Kay 2009).

The main focus of a physical activity and exercise program for clients with arthritis is the need for joint protection to reduce the chance of injury and limit pain (Minor and Kay 2009). Stretching before and after an exercise session improves range of motion and limits postexercise pain and stiffness. By limiting postexercise pain and stiffness, both duration and frequency of exercise are increased. Low-impact and functional exercises are the aerobic activities of choice and reduce stress placed on joints. Suggested activities include cycling, rowing, swimming, and walking (Minor and Kay 2009). If 30 min of exercise is too long and causes excessive joint pain, several shorter exercise bouts spread throughout the day are recommended. This procedure allows for a person to optimize the volume or amount of exercise while limiting stress placed on the joints during one exercise session.

Diabetes is a chronic metabolic disease characterized by either reduced insulin production or the body not being able to properly use insulin. Both situations result in elevated blood sugar levels or hyperglycemia (Centers for Disease Control and Prevention 2010b). Two distinct and different diabetes types exist and are caused by different factors, but result in relatively similar symptoms. Type 1 diabetes mellitus, or insulin-dependent, or juvenile diabetes is caused when insulin-secreting beta cells of the pancreas are destroyed. Type 2 diabetes is associated with hyperglycemia caused by an insulin deficiency where insulin is no longer functioning properly. In the latter case, the person is described as insulin-resistant and additional insulin is needed. The overall causes for type 2 diabetes mellitus are not well defined. Possible contributing factors include increased liver glucose production, increased fat breakdown, and insulin abnormalities that contribute to an increase insulin resistance resulting in hyperglycemia (Hornsby and Albright 2009). Hyperglycemia is a condition thought to accelerate atherosclerosis development in arteries of the brain, heart, kidneys, eyes, peripheral nerves, and lower extremities. Thus, diabetes is a leading cause of CHD, peripheral artery disease, kidney failure, blindness, and debilitating neuropathies (Goodman and Fuller 2009).

When developing physical activity and exercise programming for people with diabetes, consideration is given to severity of diabetic complications such as peripheral neuropathy, which cause loss of touch sensation in extremities, the client's medication schedule, and the current blood sugar level (Hornsby and Albright 2009). Before beginning exercise, blood sugar level is determined and if it is less than 70 mg/dL, clients should consume an adequate amount of carbohydrate to elevate blood sugar. If blood glucose level is greater than 250 mg/dL and ketones are present in the urine, blood glucose levels should be lowered before exercising. Once exercise has begun, a carbohydrate source should readily be available in the event a client's blood sugar drops severely while exercising. Persons with diabetes need to practice good foot care by wearing proper shoes and cotton socks to prevent blistering during exercise (Hornsby and Albright 2009). Because people with diabetes require longer times for sores to heal, special precautions should be taken to prevent the development of sores and blisters that may cause infections.

Although obesity is not a disease, it is associated with a host of morbid conditions. Obesity is an excessive accumulation of body fat; is linked to many chronic diseases such as CHD, hypertension, type 2 diabetes, and osteoarthritis; and leads to early morbidity and mortality (Goodman and Fuller 2009). Around the world, obesity affects 300 million people with estimates that 32% of U.S. adults are classified as obese (Centers for Disease Control and Prevention 2008a). Obesity usually occurs as an imbalance between dietary calories consumed and the amount of calories expended. When more calories are consumed than expended, the unused calories convert to energy fat stores. When associated with obesity, such an energy imbalance causes altered physiological responses including decreased growth hormone, decreased insulin sensitivity, increased fasting insulin levels, and increased cholesterol synthesis. These altered physiological responses are why obesity is linked with many other chronic diseases, and why the development of obesity has severe health consequences (Wallace and Ray 2009).

Physical activity and exercise programming for overweight and obese individuals should optimize caloric expenditure while reducing caloric intake. When weight loss is a goal, the goal for time spent in physical activity and exercise is 200 to 300 min or more with a caloric energy expenditure of 2000 kcal or greater each week (American College of Sports Medicine 2010). In order to meet time and/or caloric expenditure goals, multiple bouts of short exercise duration placed throughout the day is recommended. Use of multiple exercise bouts in 1 day is reported as an effective means of expending greater calories (National Heart Lung and Blood Institute 2010).

Persons with chronic conditions and diseases should participate in daily physical activity and exercise, but their physical activity and exercise plan should be modified and adapted to meet their specific needs and goals. In the past decade, daily physical activity and exercise recommendations for many chronic conditions have become better defined. By modifying the standard physical activity and exercise principles to ensure that patient needs are met, secondary disease prevention and health benefits are optimized while also ensuring patient safety. Persons with a chronic health condition and a medical management plan incorporating physical activity and exercise become more aware of their physical activity and exercise limitations and are better able to work within these limitations. A concise set of exercise management plans for persons with many different chronic diseases and disabilities is available (American College of Sports Medicine 2010).

MAKING LIFESTYLE CHANGES

Chronic diseases are often caused by multiple factors that fall into two categories: genetic and environmental. Although genes are not changeable, gene expression is changeable and is accomplished by altering environmental factors deemed detrimental to health through lifestyle intervention programs like daily physical activity and exercise. The opposite also is true: a physically inactive lifestyle can modify genes to promote disease and disability (Booth et al. 2002). One example of a successful improvement in a lifestyle behavior is the decline in prevalence of tobacco use from 42% to 20% of U.S. adults between 1965 and 2007 (Centers for Disease Control and Prevention 2008b). In order to achieve secondary disease prevention goals such as lessening disease severity and lessening reliance on prescription medication, incorporation of lifestyle behavior change process as part of developing a medical management or rehabilitation plan is imperative. An effective means of altering lifestyle behaviors is to make small and progressive changes that are planned and include both short-term and long-term goals with action steps for each goal. This step-by-step process is described by the Stages of Change Model (also referred to as the Transtheoretical Model) and may be a relevant process for persons with chronic diseases who are starting a behavior change program.

The first stage in the model is termed precontemplation, where patients are either not aware of a behavioral problem or denies that one exists. A person in this stage tends to defend, ignore, or deny that bad habits exist. To move to the next stage, contemplation, a person must become aware of the problem. At this point, the individual is likely indecisive as to the appropriate actions to take in order to change their behavior. In this stage, possible action steps are to do nothing and slip back to the precontemplation, or take actions steps and progress to the next stage, termed preparation. Here, a firm commitment to change is essential, and a plan for changing an undesirable behavior is developed. Once action steps for improvement are determined and a plan is prepared, the individual enters the action stage. In this stage, the person becomes actively involved in following a behavioral intervention plan, whereas in previous stages, the focus was on information gathering, decision-making, and planning for the behavior change. The final stage is maintenance, which involves keeping the behavior change a regular part of one's daily routine and avoiding relapse to previous behaviors. Ideally, the maintenance stage is the final stage. However, if an individual reverts or relapses to old behaviors, a process of relapse prevention is needed.

When formulating any intervention plan, setting reasonable and attainable goals is the best strategy to promote behavior change, because each goal achieved provides a form of positive feedback and gives encouragement toward the next goal. A popular system to encourage goal setting is referred to as the SMART system, which is an acronym for Specific, Measurable, Actionable, Realistic, and Time oriented (Moore, Marsh, and Durstine 2009). A successful plan is structured, specific, and is individualized to an individual's currents needs and wants. A structured program has attainable goals where improvement is observable and provides strong encouragement to enhance program adherence. In designing a successful intervention, simply stating "I am going to start exercising" is not enough to increase the odds of adopting a successful physical activity and exercise program. A successful exercise management plan must contain specific information such as the number of exercise days per week (frequency), the length of each exercise session (duration), and the type of exercise (mode) to be performed. Measurable goals provide the client with factual information about goal attainment and provide reinforcement to stay engaged in the program

(Moore, Marsh, and Durstine 2009). An example of engagement is someone who continues their exercise plan until a goal is reached, such as losing 10 lb or lowering blood pressure within a certain range, and then sustaining the behavior to maintain the desired outcomes.

An exercise management plan must be realistic and contain actionable goals that the client believes are attainable and truly desires to achieve. Exercise professionals can help novice exercisers choose enjoyable physical activities and exercise modes and can provide help and motivation to achieve short-term and long-term goals (Moore, Marsh, and Durstine 2009). Setting unobtainable goals leads to discouragement and decreased motivation for continued participation with a predictable dropping out of an exercise program. Finally, a goal must have a time orientation, such as having a goal to lower blood glucose levels within 4 weeks. Setting such a goal supports accountability and promotes goal achievement.

From an environmental perspective, lifestyle choices play an integral role in the development of chronic diseases. Nevertheless, human genetic makeup is an extremely important factor in the development of most chronic diseases. Human gene composition and environmental factors are involved in numerous delicate metabolic interactions that maintain balance between developing disease and not developing disease. This delicate balance may be interrupted by any number of environmental factors, such as having a physically active lifestyle. Because most modern cultures incorporate less daily time spent for physical activity, the balance between health and disease is often not maintained, and as a result, higher incident rates for chronic diseases have developed. The human body is designed for daily physical activity and exercise, and when a lifestyle includes daily physical activity and exercise, human gene expression is altered toward a reduced susceptibility for developing many different chronic diseases and their resulting disabilities (Booth et al. 2002).

SUMMARY

Chronic health conditions pose a very serious health threat to all people around the world. With the rise in prevalence of chronic diseases, great concern about proper medical management of these conditions has produced much new scientific interest and research information. Medications, diets, and surgeries have traditionally been some of the most common forms of disease treatment. However, daily physical activity and exercise are now seen as effective intervention tools in developing a management plan for many chronic diseases. While scientists continue to evaluate and determine the proper amount of physical activity and exercise for use in the medical management plan, better evidence-based guidelines are currently being developed for many chronic conditions. When a medical management plan uses scientifically proven disease-specific guidelines for physical activity and exercise, optimal health gains with safer programs are achieved. Although much work has already been completed in developing exercise evidence-based guidelines for secondary disease prevention, much work still needs to be done. Many chronic conditions and diseases have not received full scientific evaluation, and thus evidence-based guidelines for them are not yet available.

STUDY QUESTIONS

1. Define the term "evidence-based medicine." Describe at least three scenarios where using evidence-based medicine is useful in the development of an exercise prescription for the treatment of chronic conditions.
2. Compare the similarities and contrast the differences between the ACSM physical activity guidelines and the U.S. physical activity guidelines.
3. Discuss how changes in cultural norms, medical discoveries, and lifestyle behaviors led to an increased incidence of chronic conditions and decreased communicable diseases in the past century.
4. Of the numerous biologic mechanisms by which exercise may contribute to the primary or secondary prevention of coronary heart disease, in your opinion, which is the most important mechanism and why?
5. Explain how physical activity can help to reduce the risk factors associated with diabetes, arthritis, hypertension, and coronary heart disease.
6. Describe the aspects by which an exercise prescription should be modified to meet the specific needs of a specific patient.

REFERENCES

American College of Sports Medicine. 2010. *Resource Manual for Guidelines for Exercise Testing and Prescription*, 6th edition. Baltimore: Lippincott, Williams and Wilkins.

Arias, E. 2010. United States life tables, 2006. *National Vital Statistics Reports*, 58(21): 1–40. http://www.cdc.gov/nchs/data/nvsr/nvsr58/nvsr58_21.pdf (accessed July 17, 2011).

Artinian, N. T., G. F. Fletcher, D. Mozaffarian et al. 2010. American Heart Association Prevention Committee of the Council on Cardiovascular Nursing. 2010. Interventions to promote physical activity and dietary lifestyle changes for cardiovascular risk factor reduction in adults: A scientific statement from the American Heart Association. *Circulation* 122: 406–441.

Booth, F. W., M. V. Chakravarthy, S. E. Gordon et al. 2002. Waging war on physical inactivity: Using modern molecular ammunition against an ancient enemy. *J. Appl. Physiol.* 93: 3–30.

Centers for Disease Control and Prevention. 2004. The burden of chronic diseases and their risk factors: National and state perspectives 2004. http://www.cdc.gov/nccdphp/burden book2004/section01/tables.htm (accessed July 17, 2011).

Centers for Disease Control and Prevention. 2008a. Prevalence of overweight, obesity, and extreme obesity among adults: United States, trends 1976–80 through 2005–2006. http://www.cdc.gov/nchs/data/hestat/overweight/overweight_adult.pdf (accessed July 17, 2011).

Centers for Disease Control and Prevention. 2008b. Targeting Tobacco Use at a Glance 2008. http://www.cdc.gov/chronicdisease/resources/publications/AAG/osh.htm (accessed July 17, 2011).

Centers for Disease Control and Prevention. 2010a. Arthritis at a glance. http://www.cdc.gov/ chronicdisease/resources/publications/AAG/arthritis.htm (accessed July 17, 2011).

Centers for Disease Control and Prevention. 2010b. Diabetes Public Health Resource. What is diabetes? http://www.cdc.gov/diabetes/consumer/learn.htm#1 (accessed July 17, 2011).

Claridge, J. A., and T. C. Fabian. 2005. History and development of evidence-based medicine. *World J. Surg.* 29: 547–553.

Dudgeon, W. D., K. D. Phillips, C. M. Bopp et al. 2004. Physiological and psychological effects of exercise interventions in HIV disease. *AIDS Patient Care STDs* 18(2): 81–98.

Durstine, J. L., G. E. Moore, P. L. Painter et al. 2009. *ACSM's Exercise Management for Persons with Chronic Diseases and Disabilities.* Champaign, IL: Human Kinetics.

Durstine, J. L., B. Peel, and M. J. LaMonte. 2009. Exercise is medicine. In *ACSM's Exercise Management for Persons with Chronic Diseases and Disabilities*, ed. J. L. Durstine, G. E. Moore, P. L. Painter et al., 21–30. Champaign, IL: Human Kinetics.

Durstine, J. L., G. E. Moore, and D. Polk. 2009. Hyperlipidemia. In *ACSM's Exercise Management for Persons with Chronic Diseases and Disabilities*, ed. J. L. Durstine, G. E. Moore, P. L. Painter et al., 167–174. Champaign, IL: Human Kinetics.

Durstine, J. L., and P. D. Thompson. 2001. Exercise in the treatment of lipid disorders. *Cardiol. Clin.* 19: 471–488.

Franklin, B. A. 2009. Myocardial Infarction. In *ACSM's Exercise Management for Persons with Chronic Diseases and Disabilities*, ed. J. L. Durstine, G. E. Moore, P. L. Painter et al., 49–57. Champaign, IL: Human Kinetics.

Friedman, D., and S. O. Roberts. 2009. Angina and silent ischemia. In *ACSM's Exercise Management for Persons with Chronic Diseases and Disabilities*, ed. J. L. Durstine, G. E. Moore, P. L. Painter et al. 66–72. Champaign, IL: Human Kinetics.

Goodman, C. C., and K. S. Fuller. 2009. *Pathology: Implications for the Physical Therapist.* China: Saunders Elsevier.

Goodyear, L. J., and B. B. Kahn. 1998. Exercise, glucose transport and insulin sensitivity. *Annu. Rev. Med.* 49: 235–261.

Gordon, N. F. 2009. Hypertension. In *ACSM's Exercise Management for Persons with Chronic Diseases and Disabilities*, ed. J. L. Durstine, G. E. Moore, P. L. Painter et al., 107–113. Champaign, IL: Human Kinetics.

Hall, L. 2008. Disease management and discharge destinations. In *Pollock's Textbook of Cardiovascular Disease and Rehabilitation*, ed. J. L. Durstine, G. E. Moore, M. J. LaMonte et al., 131–39. Champaign, IL: Human Kinetics.

Haskell, W. L. 1994. Health consequences of physical activity: Understanding and challenges regarding dose-response. *Med. Sci. Sports Exerc.* 26: 649–660.

Hornsby Jr., W. G., and A. L. Albright. 2009. Diabetes. In *ACSM's Exercise Management for Persons with Chronic Diseases and Disabilities*, ed. J. L. Durstine, G. E. Moore, P. L. Painter et al., 182–191. Champaign, IL: Human Kinetics.

Hull Jr., S. S., E. Vanoli, P. B. Adamson et al. 1994. Exercise training confers anticipatory protection from sudden death during acute myocardial ischemia. *Circulation* 89: 548–552.

Kesaniemi, A., C. J. Riddoch, B. Reeder et al. 2010. Advancing the future of physical activity guidelines in Canada: An independent expert panel interpretation of the evidence. *Int. J. Behav. Nutr. Phys. Act.* 7: 41.

King, N. A., M. Hopkins, P. Caudwell et al. 2009. Beneficial effects of exercise: Shifting the focus from body weight to other markers of health. *Br. J. Sports Med.* 43: 924–927.

Lavie, C. J., R. J. Thomas, R. W. Squires et al. 2009. Exercise training and cardiac rehabilitation in primary and secondary prevention of coronary heart disease. *Mayo Clin. Proc.* 84: 373–383.

Libby, P., and P. Ridker. 2006. Inflammation and atherothrombosis: From population biology and bench research to clinical practice. *J. Am. Coll. Cardiol.* 48: A33–A46.

Milani, R. V., C. J. Lavie, and M. R. Mehra. 2004. Reduction in C-reactive protein through cardiac rehabilitation and exercise training. *J. Am. Coll. Cardiol.* 43: 1056–1061.

Minor, M. A., and D. R. Kay. 2009. Arthritis. In *ACSM's Exercise Management for Persons with Chronic Diseases and Disabilities*, ed. J. L. Durstine, G. E. Moore, P. L. Painter et al., 259–265. Champaign, IL: Human Kinetics.

Moore, G. E., A. P. Marsh, and J. L. Durstine. 2009. Approach to exercise and disease management. In *ACSM's Exercise Management for Persons with Chronic Diseases and*

Disabilities, ed. J. L. Durstine, G. E. Moore, P. L. Painter et al., 9–20.Champaign, IL: Human Kinetics.

Moore, G. E., P. L. Painter, G. W. Lyerly et al. 2009. Managing exercise in persons with multiple chronic conditions. In *ACSM's Exercise Management for Persons with Chronic Diseases and Disabilities*, ed. J. L. Durstine, G. E. Moore, P. L. Painter et al., 31–37. Champaign, IL: Human Kinetics.

National Heart Lung and Blood Institute. 2010. Obesity Education Initiative. http://www .nhlbi.nih.gov/about/oei/index.htm (accessed July 17, 2011).

Pescatello, L. S., B. A. Franklin, R. Fagard et al. 2004. Exercise and hypertension. *Med. Sci. Sports Exerc.* 36: 533–553.

Siwek, J., M. L. Gourlay, D. C. Slawson, and A. F. Shaughnessy. 2002. How to write an evidence-based clinical review article. *Am. Fam. Phys.* 65(2): 251–258.

Stevinson, C., D. A. Lawlor, and K. R. Fox. 2004. Exercise interventions for cancer patients: Systematic review of controlled trials. *Cancer Causes Control* 15: 1035–1056.

Sui, X., M. J. LaMonte, J. N. Laditka et al. 2007. Cardiorespiratory fitness and adiposity as mortality predictors in older adults. *JAMA* 298: 2507–2516.

Thompson, P. D., D. Buchner, D., I. L. Piña et al. 2003. Exercise and physical activity in the prevention and treatment of atherosclerotic cardiovascular disease: A statement from the council on clinical cardiology (subcommittee on exercise, rehabilitation, and prevention) and the council on nutrition, physical activity, and metabolism (subcommittee on physical activity). *Circulation* 107: 3109–3116.

U.S. Department of Health and Human Services. 2008. *Physical Activity Guidelines for Americans*. U.S. Department of Health and Human Services, 2008. ODPHP Publication No. U0036. Also available at: http://www.health.gov/paguidelines/pdf/paguide.pdf (accessed July 17, 2011).

Wallace, P. W., and S. Ray. 2009. Obesity. In *ACSM's Exercise Management for Persons with Chronic Diseases and Disabilities*, ed. J. L. Durstine, G. E. Moore, P. L. Painter et al., 192–200. Champaign, IL: Human Kinetics.

Wang, J., C. J. Jen, and H. Chen. 1995. Effects of exercise training and deconditioning on platelet function in men. *Arterioscler. Thromb. Vasc. Biol.* 15: 1668–1674.

Warburton, D. E. R., C. W. Nicol, and S. S. D. Bredin. 2006. Health benefits of physical activity: The evidence. *Can. Med. Assoc. J.* 174(6): 801–809.

World Health Organization. 2003. Diet, nutrition and the prevention of chronic diseases: Report of a joint WHO/FAO expert consultation, Geneva, 28 January–1 February 2002. http://whqlibdoc.who.int/trs/WHO_TRS_916.pdf (accessed July 17, 2011).

You, J.-F., R. Tang, C. R. Changchien et al. 2009. Effect of body mass index on the outcome of patients with rectal cancer receiving curative anterior resection. *Ann. Surg.* 249: 783–787.

7 Physical Activity in Growth and Development

Fátima Baptista and Kathleen F. Janz

CONTENTS

INTRODUCTION

Biological (growth and maturation) and behavioral development are conditioned by an interaction between genetic and environmental factors, among which physical activity, nutritional intake, diseases, and milieu stresses are of particular importance. This chapter presents evidence supporting the role of physical activity in the growth and development of school-age youth (5–17 years). Specifically, we address how physical activity contributes to childhood development with a carryover effect as healthy children become healthy adults. We also address the critical need to promote physical activity in young people because of the significant percentage of youth who are not sufficiently active enough to optimize health benefits.

Morbidity and mortality during the pediatric years mainly result from conditions that are unrelated to physical activity. But several surrogate markers of future risk for chronic diseases and behavioral outcomes, which are influenced by physical activity, are expressed during childhood and adolescence as part of a long process of pathology. The outcomes presented in this chapter refer to the most relevant outcomes for short-term well-being or for long-term health. Specifically, we discuss adiposity and fat distribution as markers of overweight and obesity, the metabolic syndrome as a marker of cardiometabolic health, bone mass and shape as markers of bone health, and emotional, behavioral, and hyperactivity disorders as markers of mental health. These outcomes, along with academic achievements, are all advantageously influenced by optimal levels of childhood physical activity. Potential adverse effects of physical activity, including injuries and menstrual disturbances, are also described. In the end, we hope to draw attention to the need for properly framing the promotion of physical activity practices for all children.

PREVALENCE OF PHYSICAL ACTIVITY

Young people are the most active group within a population (Figure 7.1). Yet, as defined by most federal health agencies, significant percentages of children and adolescents are not sufficiently active, that is, they do not acquire at least 60 min of daily physical activity of moderate or higher intensity.

Objective physical activity data from 1778 U.S. youth between 6 and 19 years and 2714 Portuguese youth between 10 and 19 years indicate that more than 50% of children younger than 11 years and more than 90% of young people between 16 and 19 years are not active enough (Figure 7.2) (Troiano et al. 2008; Baptista et al. 2011). The U.S. and Portuguese studies are particularly important for providing surveillance data and an intercultural comparison since physical activity was measured using the same brand of accelerometer-based activity monitor and the

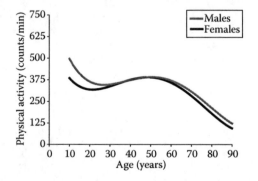

FIGURE 7.1   Cross-sectional data showing average intensity of total physical activity (PA) expressed in counts per minute by age, in a representative sample of Portuguese population (4696 participants) evaluated between 2006 and 2008. (Data from *Med. Sci. Sports Exerc.*, doi: 10.1249/MSS.0b013e318230e441, 2011.)

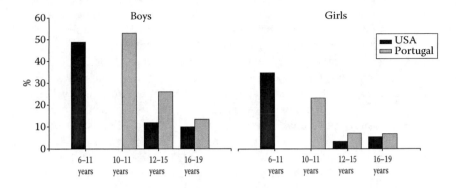

FIGURE 7.2 Prevalence of children and adolescents attaining sufficient physical activity (60 min of moderate- and vigorous-intensity physical activity per day). (Data from Troiano, R. P. et al., *Med. Sci. Sports Exerc.*, 40, 181–188, 2008; Baptista, F. et al., *Med. Sci. Sports Exerc.*, doi: 10.1249/MSS.0b013e318230e441, 2011.)

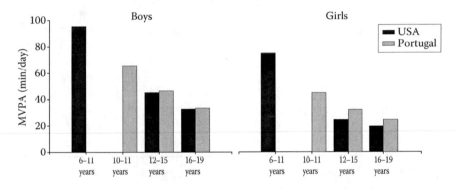

FIGURE 7.3 Moderate- and vigorous-intensity physical activity (MVPA) by age and gender in the United States and Portugal, considering every minute above this intensity threshold. (Data from Troiano, R. P. et al., *Med. Sci. Sports Exerc.*, 40, 181–188, 2008; Baptista, F. et al., *Med. Sci. Sports Exerc.*, doi: 10.1249/MSS.0b013e318230e441, 2011.)

same methodology of analysis. In both studies, boys performed, on average, more than ~20 min/day of at least moderate-intensity physical activity when compared to girls (Figure 7.3). However, both boys and girls had decreased physical activity at a similar rate throughout adolescence. Using comparable accelerometry-based methods, other investigators have reported this pattern in children and adolescents in European countries (other than Portugal).

PSYCHOSOCIAL, ENVIRONMENTAL, AND BIOLOGICAL CORRELATES OF PHYSICAL ACTIVITY

Understanding the correlates of physical activity brings to light the development of effective interventions to promote a physically active lifestyle. Variation in physical activity is explained by the independent and interactive effects of psychosocial, environmental, and biological factors. Parental/family support is one of the most influential psychosocial factors for physical activity-related behaviors in youth. A recent comprehensive review of the literature by Beets and colleagues identified four categories of parental support: instrumental (purchasing equipment, payment of fees, and transportation); conditional (doing activity with and watching/supervising); motivational (encouragement and praise); and informational (discussing benefits). These factors are often confounded by parental socioeconomic status (denoted by parental education, occupational status, and/or family income) (Beets, Cardinal, and Alderman 2010). For example, with increasing age, participation in physical activities becomes more elaborate and financially costly (e.g., sport clubs fees), which may reduce the likelihood of physical activity in adolescents from lower-income families.

Environmental influences can be especially relevant to children and adolescents because they have less autonomy in their behavioral choices (when compared to adults). One of the more important environmental correlates during childhood is school physical activity policies: the time allowed for free play, time spent outdoors, and number of field trips. These factors all show a positive association with children's physical activity levels. Potential correlates of physical activity within the proximal physical environment include availability and accessibility of physical activity programs or facilities, and neighborhood safety and neighborhood hazards (e.g., many roads, no crossings lights, heavy traffic, pollution). However, in most studies, these factors as perceived and estimated by parents are unrelated to children's physical activity levels (Ferreira et al. 2006). In adolescents, attendance of a nonvocational school and low neighborhood crime incidence have emerged as positively associated with physical activity. Other variables at school-, proximal- and macroenvironment levels are undetermined or are not possible to infer at this time from the limited number of existing studies.

Biological aspects, specifically maturity status, seem to influence physical activity only among girls who are advanced in their maturity (when compared to peers). Evidence exists that early maturing girls possess lower physical activity levels than later maturing girls (Drenowatz et al. 2010). Advanced maturation in girls is associated with greater adiposity gains and physique changes that may be less appropriate for successful engagement in sport-based physical activities. And, conversely, excessive adiposity gains predispose girls to an early puberty and a higher accumulation of body fat compared with girls who have puberty on time. Therefore, preventing excessive gains in body fat is important during and before puberty.

Physical self-concept has been advanced as a potential mediator of relations between maturity status and physical activity with positive self-concept predicting greater involvement in moderate- and vigorous-intensity physical activity. The complexity of factors and their interaction with maturity suggest the need for targeted multilevel interventions aimed at increasing, or at least maintaining, physical activity in pubescent girls.

OVERWEIGHT AND OBESITY

In most public health literature, overweight and obesity are defined as abnormal or excessive fat accumulation and expressed by body mass index (BMI), that is, the weight in kilograms divided by the square of the height in meters (kg/m^2). Children and adolescents are commonly classified as overweight and obese using age- and gender-specific BMI criteria proposed by the International Obesity Task Force (Cole et al. 2000) or by the World Health Organization (2007). Overweight and obese are equivalent to a BMI of 25 and 30 kg/m² at 19 years. The U.S. Centers for Disease Control (CDC 2000) defines overweight or obese as equivalent to a BMI at or above the 85th percentile-for-age and at or above the 95th percentile-for-age, respectively.

Therefore, comparing overweight and obesity among pediatric populations is difficult because there is no standard definition of obesity applied worldwide. However, it seems clear that the prevalence of overweight and obesity has been growing rapidly for over two decades in developed countries and also in many low- and middle-income nations. A report from the International Obesity Task Force, which was based on various surveys conducted after 1990, suggests that 10% of children and adolescents worldwide (age 5 to 17 years) are at least overweight. This is an absolute value of 155 million young people. Of these 155 million overweight youth, 30 to 45 million are classified as obese, representing about 2% to 3% of the total worldwide population of children and adolescents. Higher values of overweight/obesity prevalence have been reported in the Near and Middle East (~16%), Europe (~20%), and the Americas (~32%), whereas lower values are observed in parts of Asia/Pacific (5%) and sub-Saharan Africa (~2%).

CONSEQUENCES AND DETERMINANTS OF OVERWEIGHT AND OBESITY

Overweight and obesity in youth is a global health problem because of its high prevalence coupled with short- and long-term psychosocial and biological consequences. The short-term biological effects of overweight and obesity include an adverse impact on blood pressure, blood lipids, and blood glucose. When elevated, these factors are markers of cardiovascular disease and type 2 diabetes; specifically, they increase likelihood of these diseases in adulthood. The risk is particularly high for those who remain overweight/obese as adults. In addition to metabolic disorders, chronic diseases such as breast, colon, and kidney cancers, musculoskeletal disorders, and gall bladder disease are associated with obesity in adulthood. Other significant health problems of overweight/obesity throughout the life course include asthma, sleep disorders, and hepatic steatosis. At the psychosocial level, obesity in young people is related to poor school performance and unhealthy or risky behaviors such as alcohol and tobacco use, premature sexual behavior, inappropriate dieting practices, and physical inactivity.

Excess weight in youth tracks strongly into adulthood with approximately one-half of overweight adolescents and more than one-third of overweight children remaining obese as adults. Therefore, one of the main risk factors associated with overweight/obesity in children and adolescents is adult obesity. However, a higher BMI during adolescence, even without being overweight, predicts adverse health effects in adults, including heavier adolescents who do not become obese adults.

At this time, the complexity and multifactorial nature of childhood obesity preclude a well-defined mechanism for its cause. However, mounting evidence suggests that its antecedents appear very early during the life course. Intrauterine events and factors during the early development years predispose a child to disorders such as obesity (and the metabolic syndrome). The presence of maternal gestational diabetes, overweight and smoking, low and high birth weight, infant feeding practices, rapid infant growth, short sleep duration, and an obesogenic environment (unhealthy diet and sedentary lifestyle) are major contributors to the increasing prevalence of childhood obesity (Kumanyika et al. 2008).

OVERWEIGHT/OBESITY AND PHYSICAL ACTIVITY

The rapid change in the prevalence of obesity worldwide highlights the importance of nongenetic factors as causal determinants despite interaction between genes and lifestyle factors. The accumulation of fat is the result of a chronic positive energy balance due to a higher energy intake in relation to energy expenditure. Therefore, physical activity, which contributes significantly to total energy expenditure (and is the most modifiable component of total energy expenditure), influences adiposity levels (Figure 7.4). Indeed, associations between low levels of physical activity and high levels of obesity in children and adolescents are repeatedly observed in cross-sectional studies. It is less clear, however, if levels of physical activity are always the cause of increases in BMI or if young people with increased BMI are less likely to engage in physical activity or both (bidirectional relationship). Recently, Kwon and colleagues used a longitudinal design, an objective measure of physical activity (accelerometers), and a criterion measure of adiposity (dual-energy X-ray absorptiometry) to show the odds of being in the lowest quartile for moderate- and vigorous-intensity physical activity at age 11 were 4 times higher for children with high levels of total body fat at age 8 (when compared to age-matched children with normal or low levels of body fat) (Kwon et al. 2011). In this same cohort and using the same methods, high levels of moderate- and vigorous-intensity physical activity at age 5 was shown to predict low levels of adiposity at age 8 and at age 11 (Janz et al. 2009). Other studies have suggested that physical activity does not prevent excessive gain of fat but can reduce the rate of gain in children and adolescents (Reichert et al. 2009; Wilks et al. 2011). For example, in a 1-year randomized controlled trial, Kriemler and colleagues showed that additional moderate- or vigorous-intensity physical activity of at least 13 min/day led to a difference of −6% gains in body fat when compared to usual physical activity. The effect was seen in schoolchildren

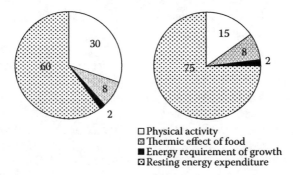

□ Physical activity
⊠ Thermic effect of food
■ Energy requirement of growth
⊡ Resting energy expenditure

FIGURE 7.4 Components (%) of total daily energy expenditure between active and inactive youth.

from grade 1 (~7 years) and grade 5 (~11 years), regardless of initial BMI (Kriemler et al. 2010). These researchers also observed a 5% improvement of cardiorespiratory fitness and a 5% reduction of cardiovascular risk, which included all the components of metabolic syndrome. In general, more longitudinal and controlled trial studies are needed to fully understand the implications of bidirectional associations between physical activity and adiposity and physical activity's effect on fat-gain trajectories.

In children and adolescents who are already overweight, physical activity at a dose of 30–60 min/day of at least moderate intensity, for 3 to 7 days/week, promotes a reduction of total body and visceral fat (Strong et al. 2005). Such programs have not yet influenced the reduction of body-fat percentages in children and adolescents with normal body weight, for which physical activity may need to be of a longer duration (>80 min/day) with a preponderance of vigorous-intensity physical activity. This suggests that the level of intensity needed to shift adiposity population curves in youth is higher than what is needed for reduction of obesity in children.

In infant and preschool children, interventions to promote healthy eating and/ or increase in energy expenditure through physical activity (reduction in television watching/sedentary behaviors or exercise/play interventions) have been limited in their effectiveness for preventing overweight and obesity or in limiting weight gain. These results suggest the difficulty of modifying these behaviors at an early age (Monasta et al. 2011). Nevertheless, the preschool years have been regarded as a critical period for the programming of energy balance, via the concept of early "adiposity rebound." That is, children who undergo early adiposity rebound are at increased risk of later obesity.

EARLY ADIPOSITY REBOUND

Among the various periods of life for the development of obesity, the period at which the adiposity rebound occurs is considered one of the most critical. The adiposity rebound corresponds to the minimum or nadir of BMI, which occurs at ages 5 to 7 years, and precedes the second rise in the BMI curve during the growing years (Figure 7.5) (Rolland-Cachera et al. 2006). The adiposity rebound is classified as

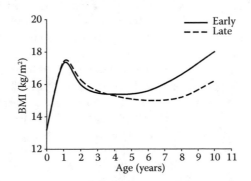

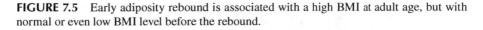

FIGURE 7.5   Early adiposity rebound is associated with a high BMI at adult age, but with normal or even low BMI level before the rebound.

"early" when it occurs before age 5. Early timing of the adiposity rebound has been associated with advanced biological maturity during adolescence and with a high BMI during adolescence and young adulthood.

The period of life in which the adiposity rebound occurs should be considered important for the control of energy balance. Some studies observed that in more physically active children, adiposity rebound occurs later and fat mass gains are ~4% to 7% lower than in less active children (Deheeger, Rolland-Cachera, and Fontvielle 1996; Janz et al. 2002). This suggests physical activity's potential for the control of energy balance in young children and the possibility of preventing early adiposity rebound. Recent evidence reviewed by Reilly (2008) suggests that associations between timing of adiposity rebound and later obesity may not reflect genetic programming, but potentially denote "obesogenic" growth trajectories established during the preschool period.

INTERACTION BETWEEN OBESITY-RELATED GENES AND PHYSICAL ACTIVITY

Among the various genes related to obesity, the FTO (fat mass and obesity-associated) gene variant, particularly the rs9939609 homozygous AA allele, is strongly associated with BMI, risk of obesity, and obesity-related traits in populations of different ethnicities and ages (7 years and older). The prevalence of this risk allele in the white population is approximately 40%. Even though genetic factors play a role in obesity, an elevated BMI should not be viewed as an inevitable product of genetics since health-related behaviors, such as regular physical activity and dietary habits, are likely to be equally important. In fact, the effect of the FTO rs9939609 polymorphism on body-fat parameters (BMI, fat percentage, and waist circumference) seems to be much lower in adolescents who meet physical activity recommendations (i.e., ≥60 min/day of moderate- and vigorous-intensity physical activity) compared with those who do not (Ruiz et al. 2010).

METABOLIC SYNDROME

The metabolic syndrome consists of the clustering of the most dangerous risk factors for cardiovascular disease and type 2 diabetes, including abdominal obesity, elevated triglycerides, elevated blood pressure, impaired fasting glucose, and reduced high-density lipoprotein cholesterol level. Although the metabolic syndrome is traditionally reported in adults, it has recently been observed in young people and is likely related to the rapid rise in obesity in this population. At this time, the clustering of cardiometabolic risk factors appears to be a better measure of metabolic health in children and adolescents than single risk factors. Therefore, the metabolic syndrome in young people should be viewed as contributing to a high risk of health complications and should be distinguished from simpler cases of uncomplicated obesity. Since fat distribution, lipid levels, blood pressure, insulin sensitivity, and insulin secretion change normally with growth and maturation, the development of the definition of the metabolic syndrome is differentiated by age groups: age 6 years to younger than 10 years; age 10 years to younger than 16 years; and 16 years or older (Zimmet et al. 2007). In children younger than 10 years, the metabolic syndrome is not diagnosed;

TABLE 7.1

Definition of Metabolic Syndrome in Children and Adolescents, According to the International Diabetes Federation

Age Group (years)	Obesity[a] (WC)	Triglycerides	HDL-C	Blood Pressure	Glucose
6–<10	≥90th percentile	N/A	N/A	N/A	N/A
10–<16	≥90th percentile or adult cutoff if lower	≥1.7 mmol/L (≥150 mg/dL)	<1.03 mmol/L (<40 mg/dL)	systolic ≥130 or diastolic ≥85 mm Hg	≥5.6 mmol/L (100 mg/dL) or known T2DM

≥16 (adult criteria)	Central obesity (defined as waist circumference ≥94 cm for Europid men and ≥80 cm for Europid women, with ethnicity-specific values for other groups) plus any two of the following four factors:

✓ Triglycerides: ≥1.7 mmol/L (≥150 mg/dL) or treatment for high triglycerides

✓ HDL-C: <1.03 mmol/L (<40 mg/dL) in males and <1.29 mmol/L (<50 mg/dL) in females, or treatment for low HDL

✓ Systolic BP ≥130 mm Hg or diastolic BP ≥85 mm Hg, or treatment for hypertension

✓ Fasting plasma glucose ≥5.6 mmol/L (≥100 mg/dL) or known T2DM

Note: WC, waist circumference; HDL-C, high-density lipoprotein cholesterol; T2DM, type 2 diabetes mellitus.

[a] Risk factors and cutoff values by age groups used to diagnose Metabolic Syndrome.

however, weight reduction is recommended for those with abdominal obesity, that is, a waist circumference ≥90th percentile (Table 7.1).

For older children and adolescents 10 to 16 years old, the metabolic syndrome is diagnosed with abdominal obesity (waist circumference ≥90th percentile) and the presence of two or more of the other clinical features. Waist circumference percentile regression values in nationally representative samples of African–American, European–American, and Mexican–American children and adolescents can be obtained from tables produced by Fernandez et al. (2004). For young people older than 16 years, the criteria are the same as used for adults. As in adults, waist measurement is the main component of the metabolic syndrome because it is an independent predictor of insulin resistance, lipid levels, and blood pressure.

Using the definition of the International Diabetes Foundation, the prevalence of the metabolic syndrome in youth ranges from ~0.2% at 10 years in European countries (Ekelund et al. 2009) to ~7.1% at 16 to 17 years in U.S. adolescents (Ford et al. 2008). The prevalence increases with age and is higher in boys than in girls. However, the prevalence for youth is significantly lower than the ~25% prevalence observed in the adult population worldwide. However, about 15–20% of adolescents in some European countries are obese or have at least two metabolic risk factors without being obese.

According to data from the European Youth Heart Study, the results of which are extensively documented in peer-reviewed journals, inactivity, physical activity, and cardiorespiratory fitness seem to contribute separately to metabolic risk. The association between television viewing (a surrogate marker of inactivity) and clustered metabolic risk may be mediated by adiposity, whereas physical activity and cardiorespiratory fitness are associated with individual and clustered metabolic-risk indicators independent of obesity. Physical activity and cardiorespiratory fitness were 20% and 25% lower, respectively, in children categorized as having the metabolic syndrome when compared to those children categorized without it. An increase in physical activity by 30–40 min/day (0.5 SD increase) of at least moderate-intensity activity is associated with a risk reduction of 33%. At an absolute level, 116 min/day of moderate- and vigorous-intensity physical activity at 9 years and 88 min/day at 15 years decreased the risk of cardiometabolic risk-factor clustering. The risk reduction associated with a 1-SD increase in physical activity or cardiorespiratory fitness was similar (60% and 67%, respectively) (Andersen et al. 2006). This suggests significant health benefits associated with increasing levels of either physical activity or physical fitness in youth. However, from a public health perspective, it is more feasible to increase daily moderate-intensity physical activity rather than increase cardiorespiratory fitness, which requires more demanding vigorous-intensity exercise. These European Youth Heart Study findings support that the health guidelines of at least 60 min/day of physical activity of at least moderate intensity (e.g., U.S. Health and Human Services and World Health Organization Physical Activity Guidelines) may be insufficient to prevent metabolic risk in youth. The benefits of higher duration of physical activity appear to be equally extended to children at lower metabolic risk.

BONE HEALTH

Healthy bone development is one of the more important reasons for promoting physical activity during the growing years, since approximately 50% of the variability in bone mass in older adults is attributable to their degree of earlier bone mineralization. In addition, bone mineral mass and distribution appear to track through childhood, adolescence, and young adulthood (Baxter-Jones et al. 2008). Thus, to achieve maximal effects, intervention strategies aimed at reducing the incidence of osteoporosis (bone fragility) must begin in childhood. The effect of physical activity on the skeleton appears to be higher during early and mid-puberty (pubertal stage P2 and P3) when compared to late puberty and postpuberty (pubertal stage P4 and P5) (Hind and Burrows 2007), again suggesting the need for early interventions (see Table 7.2 for criteria of Tanner for pubertal development).

Physical activity affects not only material bone properties (i.e., bone mass) but also structural bone properties that are related to bone mass distribution (i.e., size, shape, and internal architecture). These latter properties are indicators of axial, bending, and torsional strength, and consequently indicators of the bone's resistance to mechanical loads. Boys and girls who are more physically active have more favorable characteristics of bone mass distribution and, therefore, bone strength. These physical activity-related structural changes, which appear to be unique to the growing years, are derived mainly from increased bone apposition in the outer surface of bone.

TABLE 7.2

Stages of Puberty According to Criteria of Tanner for Genital and Breast Development

Genitals (male)

1. Prepubertal (I)—prepubertal (testicular volume less than 1.5 mL; small penis of 3 cm or less)
2. Early puberty (II)—testicular volume between 1.6 mL and 6 mL; skin on scrotum thins, reddens and enlarges; penis length unchanged
3. Mid-puberty (III)—testicular volume between 6 mL and 12 mL; scrotum enlarges further; penis begins to lengthen to about 6 cm
4. Late puberty (IV)—testicular volume between 12 mL and 20 mL; scrotum enlarges further and darkens; penis increases in length to 10 cm and circumference
5. Postpuberty (V)—testicular volume greater than 20 mL; adult scrotum and penis of 15 cm in length

Breasts (female)

1. Prepubertal (I)—no glandular tissue; areola follows the skin contours of the chest (prepubertal)
2. Early puberty (II)—breast bud forms, with small area of surrounding glandular tissue; areola begins to widen
3. Mid-puberty (III)—breast begins to become more elevated, and extends beyond the borders of the areola, which continues to widen but remains in contour with surrounding breast
4. Late puberty (IV)—increased breast size and elevation; areola and papilla form a secondary mound projecting from the contour of the surrounding breast
5. Post puberty (V)—breast reaches final adult size; areola returns to contour of the surrounding breast, with a projecting central papilla

Although at least 60% of peak bone mass is genetically determined, an adequate dietary intake of calcium and proteins, vitamin D, and regular weight-bearing physical activity contribute significantly to bone mass acquisition. Among these factors, physical activity is the most critical to the peak bone mass. Physical activity maximizes the deposition of bone mineral particularly in bone regions where the mechanical demands are greatest (Figure 7.6). Moderate- to high-impact weight-bearing physical activity with ground impact greater than 2 times body weight, such as jogging, running, or jumping, have a higher osteogenic potential compared to nonweight-bearing physical activity (activities in the water or in the seated position) or reduced weight-bearing physical activities such as walking and dancing. The greater the osteogenic potential of an activity, which is dependent on the intensity of the mechanical load, the shorter the duration of physical activity that will be needed to achieve desirable results. For example, the accumulation of ~30 min/day of vigorous-intensity physical activity, such as jogging or running, would be expected to lead to bone results equivalent to those produced by the accumulation of 10–15 min/day, 2–3 times/week of vigorous-intensity activities with greater mechanical demands, such as jumping (Janz et al. 2001; Sardinha, Baptista, and Ekelund 2008; Weeks, Young, and Beck 2008). This is because each cell in the bone matrix, in particular osteocytes, is sensitive to stimuli induced by components of mechanical loading (matrix deformation, fluid flow, and streaming potentials), generating

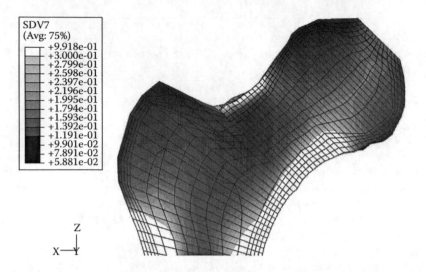

FIGURE 7.6 Heterogeneous bone mass distribution in a proximal femur. Finite element analysis was used to analyze distribution of bone mass according to location of applied loads during weight-bearing physical activity: femoral head and great trochanter. Figure shows increase in bone mineral content in some areas (first colors of the scale) compared with others (last colors of the scale). (Data from Cardadeiro, G. et al., *J. Bone Miner. Res.*, 25, 2304–2312, 2010. With permission. Courtesy of Joana Silva and Paulo Fernandes, IDMEC-IST, TU Lisbon.)

intra- and intercellular signals (mechanotransduction) to regulate the behavior of neighboring cells. The end result is the recruitment of osteoblasts to form new bone, or lining cells to recruit new osteoblasts.

The mineralization of the skeleton is most rapid (peak bone mass accrual) between ~11.5 and 13.5 years in girls and between ~13 and 15 years in boys. During these 2-year periods, about 26% of the total bone mineral content is acquired and 100% is reached between 20 and 30 years, that is, peak bone mass is achieved. The percentage of bone mineral content acquired during the 2 years around puberty is similar to what is lost in 30 years between ages 50 and 80 years. Since boys' peak velocity of linear growth occurs later than girls (11.8 vs. 13.4 years), boys have more time to grow and also more time for bone mineral acquisition. In addition, boys have a higher peak bone mass accrual (322 vs. 407 g/years). Even after peak bone mass accrual, males have an advantage over females since bone mass gains persist in males after puberty. During postpuberty (P5), when growth is less than 1 cm/ year, significant increases in bone mass occur through their 20s. Continued bone mineralization is not significant in postpubertal females. Gender-specific growth and maturation patterns explain the differences of 10% in height and of 25% in peak bone mass between males and females. They also contribute to making women more vulnerable to fracture than men, particularly after the menopause.

The large volume or intensity of physical activity, which occurs in sports training, leads to favorable differences in bone mass of up to 30% between athletes and nonathletes. Baxter-Jones and colleagues (2008) have reported a difference of up to

10% in bone mass between nonathlete young adult's who were physically active during adolescence (when compared to those adults who were inactive as adolescents). Bone mass differences between those who are habitually physically active and those who are not is a contributing factor to the prevention of bone fractures, not only among adolescents but also in the elderly. In postmenopausal women, an increase in peak bone mass of 10% during adolescence can delay the onset of osteoporosis by 13 years and prevent the risk of fracture by 50%. The importance of peak bone mass to the prevention of osteoporosis and fractures supports early interventions to ensure all children and adolescents engage in adequate levels of bone-enhancing physical activity.

MENTAL HEALTH

Mental health is defined as a state of well-being in which every individual realizes his or her own potential, can cope with the normal stresses of life, can work productively, and is able to make a contribution to her or his community (World Health Organization 2005). The most common mental health disorders and difficulties during childhood and the teenage years include emotional disorders (anxiety and depression), conduct or behavioral disorders (substance abuse, bullying and fighting, eating disorders including anorexia nervosa and bulimia), and attention deficit hyperactivity disorders. In youth, the worldwide average prevalence of these disorders is 12% (Costello, Egger, and Angold 2005), which is comparable to diabetes, asthma, and other diseases of youth. In some developed countries, the overall prevalence of these disorders in young people can reach ~22%. There is a need for early intervention of these disorders, since mental health disorders have a significant impact on how children develop and mature into adulthood. Without effective prevention/treatment, children and adolescents with mental health difficulties are at increased risk of academic underachievement, substance abuse, isolation, and suicide.

In a nationally representative sample of U.S. adolescents, emotional disorders were the most common mental health condition, followed by behavioral disorders, and substance use disorders. The median age for the onset of this array of disorders varies considerably, ranging from the earliest median age of onset of 6 years for anxiety, followed by 11 years for behavioral, 13 years for mood, and 15 years for substance use (Merikangas et al. 2010). Boys seem to have a greater prevalence of attention-deficit/hyperactivity disorders than girls, whereas girls have 2-fold higher rates of mood disorders than boys. No gender differences have been noted in the rates of anxiety or behavioral disorders.

The majority of studies investigating associations between physical activity and mental health problems have focused on adults, but studies in youth also indicate that physical activity is important to reduce mental health disorders. Physically active boys and girls show fewer symptoms of mental health disorders than their inactive peers. For example, an increase in physical activity of about 1 h/week has been associated with an 8% decrease in the odds of depressive symptoms in both boys and girls (Rothon et al. 2010). The authors of this study suggest that the association may be independent of physical activity intensity, since the intensity of the activity appeared to have very little influence on the mental health level of the participants.

Sedentary behaviors have been linked to mental health problems in children, including attention and behavioral conduct disorders. However, Griffiths and colleagues (2010) recently reported that young children (age 5 years) who used screen entertainment for any duration but also participated in sport demonstrated fewer total difficulties—emotional, behavioral, hyperactivity–inattention, and peer relationship problems and more prosocial behaviors—than children who used screen entertainment for ≥2 h/day and did not participate in sport. Physiologic (e.g., monoamine and endorphin hypotheses) and psychological (e.g., distraction, "mastery," social support, and self-esteem hypotheses) mechanisms are proposed to underlie the mental health benefits resulting from physical activity involvement. Additionally, persistent physical inactivity, primarily during adolescence, may increase the risk of later problems due to excess alcohol and illicit drug use.

ACADEMIC ACHIEVEMENT

Direct indicators of academic achievement include grade-point averages, scores on standardized tests, and grades in specific courses. Indirect measures of academic achievement include concentration, memory, and classroom behavior. Positive correlations between academic performance and several forms of physical activity (i.e., participation in sports, physical education, exercise, and nonorganized physical activity) suggest that high amounts of physical activity are associated with academic benefits (Trudeau and Shephard 2010). Physiological influences such as greater arousal and an increased secretion of neurotrophins and psychosocial influences such as increased self-esteem and connectedness to the school culture are proposed as potential mediating variables in this relationship. The influence of physical activity on academic achievement may even occur before and beyond school age, since early stimulation of brain structures seems to increase the reserves of brain function, as characterized by both the number of neurons and the extent of their interconnections.

Studies have shown that introducing up to an additional hour per school day of curricular time dedicated to physical education does not negatively affect academic achievement in other subjects in elementary school. Cardiorespiratory fitness, however, is not significantly associated with cognitive performance. This finding suggests that the benefits derived from physical activity to academic achievement are acute and likely transient. Therefore, in order to optimize the relationship between physical activity and academic achievement, children and adolescents should engage in daily activity.

INJURIES

Engaging in physical activity has numerous health benefits, but also carries the risk of injury. Injuries can counter the beneficial effects of physical activity at a young age, particularly if the child or adolescent is unable to continue to be active because of the residual effects of injury or if he or she loses enthusiasm for physical activity because of negative associations with injuries. Consequently, the prevention of physical activity injuries in youth is an important component of ensuring physically active children and adolescents.

Most injuries resolve with conservative management and rest, but some may result in long-term growth disturbance or joint degeneration (Maffulli et al. 2010). Follow-up of young athletes with meniscus surgery indicates that more than 50% of individuals will eventually have knee osteoarthritis and associated pain and functional impairment. Injuries are most common among athletes, but the incidence of injuries among nonathletes inside and outside of the school environment is also significant. Injury rates per hourly exposure to various sports range from 0.04 to 127.3 per 1000 h of participation. In general, the highest injury risk is for ice hockey and the lowest for soccer (Spinks and McClure 2007). For school activities, Verhagen and colleagues (2009) reported an overall injury-incidence density of 0.48 per 1000 h of exposure to physical education, sports, and leisure-time physical activity for children (age 10–12 years). The lowest incidence density was for leisure-time physical activity, followed by physical education, and sports (Verhagen et al. 2009). Of these injuries, 40% required medical treatment and 14% resulted in one or more days of absence from regular school activities. Outside of the school environment, those youth (grades 6 to 10) who reported high levels of physical activity had a 2-fold higher risk of injury than those reporting lower levels of physical activity (Warsh, Pickett, and Janssen 2010). Injury incidence increased with age and with augmented exposure to new activities and risks. Gender differences were often nonsignificant, but girls are injured at a higher rate than boys in most studies reporting gender differences. Gender differences in injury risks may become significant particularly during the growth spurt, which occurs earlier in girls than in boys. Disproportionate growth and a decline in physical fitness may be the culprit in girls' increased risk of injury during this time.

MENSTRUAL DISTURBANCES

One of the most frequent reasons for gynecological consultation by girls who perform intensive and/or extensive physical activity is for the diagnosis and treatment of severe menstrual disturbances: oligomenorrhea (irregularities in menstrual cycle length) and amenorrhea (absence of regular periods). In fact, the prevalence of severe menstrual disturbances in athletes is 5 to 10 times higher than the general population. In addition, subtle menstrual disturbances, such as anovulation (absence of ovulation) and a short luteal phase (phase after ovulation) are also present in competitive athletes or recreationally active women with regular menstrual cycles (De Souza et al. 2010). Among athletes, the prevalence of menstrual disturbances appears to be highest for those who are young, have high training loads, and participate in sports where leanness may enable competitive advantages. The latter category includes sports with a strong aesthetic component (e.g., diving), sports of long distances, and sports with weight categories. The estimated prevalence of menstrual disturbances among females who train under these conditions is 50%. Girls who begin extensive training programs before the occurrence of menarche, that is, before the complete maturation function of hypothalamic–pituitary–gonadal axis, may delay the onset of menstruation and also increase their risk for secondary amenorrhea. The reduction in body weight below limits compatible with the energy availability for the regulation of major metabolic activities is one of the strongest explanations for the occurrence of these hormonal dysfunctions. During long periods of insufficient energy, the body maintains the metabolic activities necessary for survival by providing energy for cellular maintenance of essential functions such as thermoregulation and loco-motion, whereas less critical processes such as reproductive function, deposition of adipose tissue, and growth are compromised. Observations that athletes with amen-orrhea consume fewer calories (1250 to 2150 kcal/day) than eumenorrheic athletes (normal menstrual cycles) (1700 to 2500 kcal/day) with a similar level of training, confirmed that unhealthy eating behaviors are present. Beyond fertility problems, menstrual disturbances have been associated with decreased bone density, increased prevalence of stress fractures, and vascular dysfunction.

PHYSICAL FITNESS

Physical fitness is a set of attributes that people have or achieve that relates to the ability to perform physical activity. Good physical fitness enhances the practice of more demanding physical activities, quantitatively (duration) and qualitatively (inten-sity and complexity). For most children and adolescents, optimal physical activity programs for promoting physical fitness are of longer duration and intensity than typically recommended. However, in preschool children, physical activity programs should focus on the development and improvement of motor skills, namely, loco-motor skill (i.e., running, galloping, skipping, hopping, sliding, leaping) and object control skill (throwing, catching, bouncing, kicking, striking, rolling), which are pre-requisites to safely and enjoyably engaging in fitness-promoting activities (Figure 7.7). Children with lower motor competency (or perceived lower motor competence) are likely to have poor physical fitness, decreased participation in physical activity, and increased cardiovascular risk factors later in life.

The greatest benefits of high levels of physical fitness are expected in the preven-tion of obesity and the metabolic syndrome and in the promotion of bone health. Low levels of cardiorespiratory fitness have been associated with the increased prevalence of cardiovascular and metabolic risk factors in children. Longitudinal data support a high level of cardiorespiratory fitness during adolescence as positively associated to a healthy cardiovascular profile for later in life (Twisk, Kemper, and van Mechelen 2002). Cardiorespiratory fitness is quantified as VO_{2max} or VO_{2peak} with units that describe the oxygen uptake in milliliters per kilogram of body weight per minutes ($mL\ kg^{-1}\ min^{-1}$). Data from the European Youth Heart Study reported that children (9-year-old) and adolescents (15-year-old) who have a VO_{2max} below

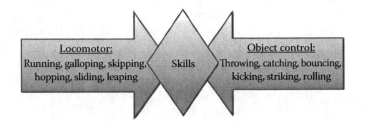

FIGURE 7.7 Prerequisite motor skills to be active that should be developed during early childhood (preschool years).

37.4 and 33.0 mL kg^{-1} min^{-1} for girls, respectively, and 43.6 and 46.0 mL kg^{-1} min^{-1} for boys, respectively, may be at risk for metabolic syndrome (Adegboye et al. 2011).

Mean values of VO$_{2peak}$ during adolescence usually range from 45 to 60 mL kg^{-1} min^{-1}. Boys have higher values than girls at ages of 5 years and beyond; however, cardiorespiratory fitness tends to increase at the same rate in both genders until the end of puberty. After puberty, cardiorespiratory fitness values accelerate in boys and decrease in girls. This is mainly due to the increase of adipose tissue that accompanies puberty in girls but may also be associated with a general decline in vigorous-intensity activity by girls.

Physical activity and physical fitness are reciprocally related but have independent effects on health during the growing years and therefore should be considered separately. Different strategies should be used based on the goals of an intervention program, for example, behavioral modification for improving physical activity and a period of exercise training for increasing physical fitness. In addition to aerobic exercise, resistance training has a positive impact on the development of lean body mass and muscular strength, both of which provide health benefits and assist in the long-term participation of regular physical activity.

TRACKING OF PHYSICAL ACTIVITY

Physical activity tracking studies quantify how well individuals maintain their activity rank within a cohort over time. The major aims of these studies are to address the stability of an individual's physical activity level over time and whether physical activity at an earlier time can be used to predict future physical activity behavior. Tracking studies are valuable because they provide insight as to when initial precursors and factors that determine physical activity occur and if specific population subgroups should receive targeted high-risk intervention early in life. Pediatric tracking studies measuring physical activity via survey methods generally indicate low to moderate ($r \sim 0.30$) tracking and a decline in interage associations with longer intervals between measures. Most of these studies find some predictability of later physical activity levels based on initial levels and minimal gender differences. Interage stability coefficients and predictability are generally greater for sport participation than "everyday" physical activity. This may be real or an artifact of the difficulty of measuring usual physical activity (when compared to sport). When objective monitors (usually accelerometry-based activity monitors) are used to assess physical activity, unadjusted associations tend to be similar to questionnaire results (Janz, Burns, and Levy 2005; Kelly et al. 2007). However, Kristensen and colleagues (2008) have shown that more sophisticated modeling of objective data, which includes adjustment for sources of physical activity variation (e.g., seasonal effects, within-week variation, instrumental measurement error), significantly increases tracking coefficients ($\sim$0.50) and predictability odds ratios. When coupled with previous studies, these findings would suggest that physical activity habits are established early and continue with the individual. However, given that, at best, tracking is moderate, some children initially categorized as active will become inactive (and vice versa). Therefore, population approaches, where all children are the focus of the intervention, should be used in conjunction with more targeted strategies.

INTERVENTIONS TO KEEP KIDS ACTIVE

Surveillance data clearly indicate that children and adolescents need to become more physically active. Interventions that target physical activity (rather than using physical activity as a strategy to improve health outcomes) are becoming increasingly more sophisticated and comprehensive. For example, early physical activity interventions used psychosocial theories to inform strategies that focused almost exclusively on changing an individual's perception or motivation to become active. Although determinants were theoretically defined, they were seldom tested as mediators of changes in physical activity, so little was learned about the pathway for change. Current intervention studies are primarily informed by socioecologic models that include integrated approaches to support physical activity behaviors at multiple levels (e.g., individual, peer, community, policy). In addition, more sophisticated statistical models and larger sample sizes are allowing researchers to construct pathway analyses to more clearly identify exactly what factors were affected during the intervention to change physical activity levels (Naylor et al. 2006). These newer interventions typically take place at schools or within communities with schools playing a dominant role. In children, school-based interventions have generally been successful in modestly (2 to 6 min) increasing physical activity via increasing children's physical activity levels during physical education classes. In adolescents, school-based interventions show positive and significant outcomes particularly when family and/or community involvement is included as a component of the intervention. However, family-based or community-based interventions that do not include schools have not shown promising results, and in a systematic review of the literature of controlled trials, van Sluijs and colleagues (2008) have concluded that as an intervention, education alone is ineffective.

CONCLUSION

Physical activity practiced in sufficient quantities (at least 60 min/day of moderate or higher intensity) has beneficial effects on health and the attenuation of genetic predispositions to certain conditions such as obesity. In the short term, physical activity prevents gains in adiposity and the occurrence of risk factors/behaviors for cardiometabolic health (independent of adiposity). Physical activity also improves bone and mental health and is associated with academic benefits. In the long term, physical activity during childhood and adolescence promotes the acquisition of good physical-activity habits later in life; prevents the incidence of diseases related to cardiovascular, bone, and mental health risk factors/behaviors; and improves brain function. The intensity of activity does not appear to be decisive for the effects on mental health and academic achievement, but vigorous-intensity activity can produce better results in optimizing bone and cardiometabolic health. The practice of vigorous-intensity physical activity is conditioned by the level of fitness, so it is important to develop physical fitness during the pediatric years.

Available data indicate that the prevalence of surrogate markers for future chronic diseases in young people can reach 7% for the metabolic syndrome, 22% for mental health disorders, and 30% for overweight, whereas the prevalence of insufficient physical activity in youth can reach 90%. It is therefore imperative to understand the determinants of physical activity and sedentary behaviors in youth and to develop interventions to promote a safe, physically active lifestyle for both boys and girls. Targeted and innovative strategies may be needed for girls, who show reduced physical activity levels when compared to boys and are more prone to obesity, osteoporosis, and depression in adulthood.

STUDY QUESTIONS

1. Identify three biological and psychosocial consequences in the short-term of overweight/obesity in young people.
2. Explain the importance of weight-bearing physical activity for bone health during puberty. List three types of physical activities considered to be weight bearing.
3. How can injuries counter the beneficial effects of physical activity at a young age?
4. Explain one of the main reasons for the occurrence of menstrual disturbances in physically active girls.
5. What is the value of developing motor skill competence during growing years on physical activity and health during adulthood?
6. Do you feel that physical fitness or physical activity should be the main outcome of public health programs? Why?
7. How do the current results from tracking studies support early targeted interventions to increase physical activity levels in subgroups of children?
8. Use a socioecologic model to propose a novel intervention to improve physical activity levels in youth.

REFERENCES

Adegboye, A. R., S. A. Anderssen, K. Froberg et al. 2011. Recommended aerobic fitness level for metabolic health in children and adolescents: A study of diagnostic accuracy. *Br. J. Sports Med.* 45: 722–728.

Andersen, L. B., M. Harro, L. B. Sardinha et al. 2006. Physical activity and clustered cardiovascular risk in children: A cross-sectional study (The European Youth Heart Study). *Lancet* 368: 299–304.

Baxter-Jones, A. D., S. A. Kontulainen, R. A. Faulkner et al. 2008. A longitudinal study of the relationship of physical activity to bone mineral accrual from adolescence to young adulthood. *Bone* 43: 1101–1107.

Baptista, F., D. A. Santos, A. M. Silva et al. 2011. Prevalence of the Portuguese population attaining sufficient physical activity. *Med. Sci. Sports Exerc.*, doi: 10.1249/MSS.0b013e318230e441.

Beets, M. W., B. J. Cardinal, and B. L. Alderman. 2010. Parental social support and the physical activity-related behaviors of youth: A review. *Health Educ. Behav.* 37: 621–644, doi: 10.1177/1090198110363884.

Cardadeiro, G., F. Baptista, V. Zymbal, L. A. Rodrigues, and L. B. Sardinha. 2010. Ward's area location, physical activity, and body composition in 8- and 9-year-old boys and girls. *J. Bone Miner. Res.* 25: 2304–2312.

Centers for Disease Control and Prevention. 2000. Clinical growth charts. http://www.cdc
.gov/growthcharts/clinical_charts.htm (accessed 7/17/2011).

Cole, T. J., M. C. Bellizzi, K. M. Flegal et al. 2000. Establishing a standard definition for child
overweight and obesity worldwide: International survey. *BMJ* 320: 1240–1243.

Costello, E., H. Egger, and A. Angold. 2005. 10-year research update review: The epidemiology of child and adolescent psychiatric disorders: I. Methods and public health burden.
J. Am. Acad. Child Adolesc. Psychiatry 44: 972–986.

Deheeger, M., M. F. Rolland-Cachera, and A. M. Fontvielle. 1996. Physical activity and body
composition in 10 year old French children: Linkages with nutritional intake? *Int. J.
Obes.* 21: 372–379.

De Souza, M. J., R. J. Toombs, J. L. Scheid et al. 2010. High prevalence of subtle and severe
menstrual disturbances in exercising women: Confirmation using daily hormone measures. *Hum. Reprod.* 25: 491–503.

Drenowatz, D., J. C. Eisenmann, K. A. Pfeiffer et al. 2010. Maturity-related differences in
physical activity among 10- to 12-year-old girls. *Am. J. Hum. Biol.* 22: 18–22.

Ekelund, U., S. Anderssen, L. B. Andersen et al. 2009. Prevalence and correlates of the metabolic
syndrome in a population-based sample of European youth. *Am. J. Clin. Nutr.* 89: 90–96.

Fernandez, J. R., D. T. Redden, A. Pietrobelli et al. 2004. Waist circumference percentiles
in nationally representative samples of African–American, European–American, and
Mexican–American children and adolescents. *J. Pediatr.* 145: 439–444.

Ferreira, I., K. van der Horst, W. Wendel-Vos et al. 2006. Environmental correlates of physical
activity in youth—a review and update. *Obes. Rev.* 8: 129–154.

Ford, E. S., C. Li, G. Zhao et al. 2008. Prevalence of the metabolic syndrome among U.S.
adolescents using the definition from the International Diabetes Federation. *Diabetes
Care* 31: 587–589.

Griffiths, L. J., M. Dowda, C. Dezateux et al. 2010. Associations between sport and screen-
entertainment with mental health problems in 5-year-old children. *Int. J. Behav. Nutr.
Phys. Act* 7: 30.

Hind, K., and M. Burrows. 2007. Weight-bearing exercise and bone mineral accrual in children and adolescents: A review of controlled trials. *Bone* 40: 14–27.

Janz, K. F., T. L. Burns, and S. M. Levy. 2005 Tracking of activity and sedentary behaviors in
childhood: The Iowa Bone Development Study. *Am. J. Prev. Med.* 29: 171–178.

Janz, K. F., T. L. Burns, J. C. Torner et al. 2001. Physical activity and bone measures in young
children: The Iowa bone development study. *Pediatrics* 107: 1387–1393.

Janz, K. F., S. Kwon, E. M. Letuchy et al. 2009. Sustained effect of early physical activity on
fat mass in older children. *Am. J. Prev. Med.* 37: 35–40.

Janz, K. F., S. M. Levy, T. L. Burns et al. 2002. Fatness, physical activity, and television viewing in children during the adiposity rebound period: The Iowa bone development study.
Prev. Med. 35: 563–71.

Kelly, L. A., J. J. Reilly, D. M. Jackson et al. 2007. Tracking physical activity and sedentary
behavior in young children. *Pediatr. Exerc. Sci.* 19: 51–60.

Kriemler, S., L. Zahner, C. Schindler et al. 2010. Effect of school based physical activity programme (KISS) on fitness and adiposity in primary schoolchildren: Cluster randomized
controlled trial. *BMJ* 340: c785.

Kristensen, P. L., N. C. Møller, L. Korsholm et al. 2008. Tracking of objectively measured
physical activity from childhood to adolescence: The European Youth Heart Study.
Scand. J. Med. Sci. Sports 18: 171–78.

Kumanyika, S. K., E. Obarzanke, N. Stettler et al. 2008. Scientific statement from American
Heart Association Council on Epidemiology: Promotion of healthful eating, physical
activity, and energy balance. *Circulation* 118: 428–464.

Kwon, S., K. F. Janz, T. L. Burns et al. 2011. Effects of adiposity on physical activity in childhood: Iowa Bone Development Study. *Med. Sci. Sports Exerc.* 43: 443–448.

Maffulli, N., U. G. Longo, N. Gougoulias et al. 2010. Long-term health outcomes of youth sports injuries. *Br. J. Sports Med.* 44: 21–25.

Merikangas, K. R., J. P. He, M. Burstein et al. 2010. Lifetime prevalence of mental disorders in U.S. adolescents: Results from the National Co-morbidity Survey Replication—Adolescent Supplement (NCS-A). *J. Am. Acad. Child Adolesc. Psychiatry* 49: 980–989.

Monasta, L., G. D. Batty, A. Macaluso et al. 2011. Interventions for the prevention of overweight and obesity in preschool children: A systematic review of randomized controlled trials. *Obes. Rev.* 12: e107–e118.

Naylor, P., H. M. Macdonald, J. A. Zebedeea et al. 2006. Lessons learned from Action Schools! BC. *J. Sci. Med. Sport* 9: 413–423.

Reichert, F. F., A. M. Batista Menezes, J. C. Wells et al. 2009. Physical activity as predictor of adolescent body fatness—a systematic review. *Sports Med.* 39: 279–294.

Reilly, J. J. 2008. Physical activity, sedentary behaviour and energy balance in the preschool child: Opportunities for early obesity prevention. *Proc. Nutr. Soc.* 67: 317–325.

Rolland-Cachera, M. F., M. Deheeger, M. Maillot et al. 2006. Early adiposity rebound: Causes and consequences for obesity in children and adults. *Int. J. Obesity* 30: S11–S17.

Rothon, C., P. Edwards, K. Bhui et al. 2010. Physical activity and depressive symptoms in adolescents: A prospective study. *BMC Med.* 8: 32.

Ruiz, J. R., I. Labayen, F. B. Ortega et al. 2010. Attenuation of the effect of the FTO rs9939609 polymorphism on total and central body fat by physical activity in adolescents: The HELENA study. *Arch. Pediatr. Adolesc. Med.* 164: 328–333.

Sardinha, L. B., F. Baptista, and U. Ekelund. 2008. Objectively measured physical activity and bone strength in 9 year old boys and girls. *Pediatrics* 122: e728–e736.

Spinks, A. B., and R. J. McClure. 2007. Quantifying the risk of sports injury: A systematic review of activity-specific rates for children less than 16 years of age. *Br. J. Sports Med.* 41: 548–557.

Strong, W. B., R. M. Malina, C. R. J. Blimkie et al. 2005. Evidenced based physical activity for school-age youth. *J. Pediatr.* 146: 732–737.

Troiano, R. P., D. Berrigan, K. W. Dodd et al. 2008. Physical activity in the United States measured by accelerometer. *Med. Sci. Sports Exerc.* 40: 181–188.

Trudeau, F., and R. J. Shephard. 2010. Relationships of physical activity to brain health and the academic performance of schoolchildren. *Am. J. Lifestyle Med.* 4: 138–150.

Twisk, J. W., H. C. Kemper, and W. van Mechelen. 2002. The relationship between physical fitness and physical activity during adolescence and cardiovascular disease risk factors at adult age. The Amsterdam Growth and Health Longitudinal Study. *Int. J. Sports Med.* 23: S8–S14.

van Sluijs, E. M., A. M. McMinn, and S. J. Griffin. 2008. Effectiveness of interventions to promote physical activity in children and adolescents: Systematic review of controlled trials. *BJM* 42: 653–657.

Verhagen, E., D. Collard, M. C. A. Paw et al. 2009. A prospective cohort study on physical activity and sports-related injuries in 10–12-year-old children. *Br. J. Sports Med.* 43: 1031–1035.

Warsh, J., W. Pickett, and I. Janssen. 2010. Are overweight and obese youth at increased risk for physical activity injuries? *Obes. Facts* 3: 225–230.

Weeks, B. K., C. M. Young, and B. R. Beck. 2008. Eight months of regular in-school jumping improves indices of bone strength in adolescent boys and girls: The POWER PE study. *J. Bone Miner. Res.* 23: 1002–1011.

World Health Organization. 2005. *Promoting Mental Health: Concepts, Emerging Evidence, Practice: A Report of the World Health Organization, Department of Mental Health and Substance Abuse in Collaboration with the Victorian Health Promotion Foundation and the University of Melbourne.* Geneva: World Health Organization.

World Health Organization. 2007. Growth Reference Data for 5–19 years. http://www.who
.int/growthref/who2007_bmi_for_age/en/.
Wilks, D. C., H. Besson, A. K. Lindroos et al. 2011. Objectively measured physical activity
and obesity prevention in children, adolescents and adults: A systematic review of prospective studies. *Obes. Rev.* 12: e119–e129.
Zimmet, P., K. G. Alberti, F. Kaufman et al. 2007. The metabolic syndrome in children and
adolescents—An IDF consensus report. *Pediatr. Diabetes* 8: 299–306.

8 Physical Activity and Healthy Adulthood

Kelley K. Pettee Gabriel and Jennifer L. Gay

CONTENTS

INTRODUCTION

Physical activity has been shown to reduce the risk of premature death and chronic conditions and improve health risk factors, physical fitness, and functional capacity (Haskell et al. 2007; U.S. Department of Health and Human Services 2008). Accordingly, physical activity has been identified as a critical element of *healthy aging* (Kesaniemi et al. 2001), a term used to characterize optimal physical, mental, and social well-being in older adults. To achieve optimal health, it is recommended that all healthy adults participate in both aerobic and muscle-strengthening activity (Haskell et al. 2007) and avoid excessive time in discretionary sedentary pursuits. Engaging in activities that result in improvement in other facets of physical fitness (e.g., flexibility and balance/coordination) is also important. However, in 2007, less than half (49.3%) of U.S. adults met the guidelines for physical activity (Centers for Disease Control and Prevention 2008).

Given the importance of physical activity to health and aging, it is important to expand the definition of "healthy aging" to adults younger than 65 years. Changing our scientific lens to view adults aged 18–64 years as potentially vulnerable to— rather than protected from—the development of chronic disease will lead to a better understanding of the correlates and determinants of age-related declines in physical activity. Unfortunately, very little is currently known regarding the factors that are most related to the reduction in physical activity levels over the life course, particularly during the adult years. However, it is important as improved knowledge in this area could potentially lead to the development of more effective and sustainable physical activity interventions that foster health and well-being across the span of adulthood.

This chapter will briefly explore the importance of physical activity in adults including the health-enhancing benefits of specific activity types or domains relevant to adults. Next, current recommendations for physical activity will be summarized and at-risk population subgroups will be identified. Then, transitional periods across adulthood that could potentially influence physical activity levels will be discussed and strategies for promoting physical activity will be provided, particularly for at-risk populations.

CURRENT ACTIVITY GUIDELINES FOR ADULTS

The most recent physical activity recommendations, the *2008 Physical Activity Guidelines for Americans* (U.S. Department of Health and Human Services 2008), suggest that for substantial health benefits, adults should accumulate at least 150 min of moderate-intensity aerobic physical activity, 75 min of vigorous-intensity, or the equivalent combination of moderate- to vigorous-intensity physical activity (MVPA) per week. Furthermore, it is recommended that aerobic activity is accumulated in bouts lasting at least 10 min. In addition, the guidelines specify that adults can achieve more extensive health benefits by participating in a higher volume of aerobic physical activity (i.e., at least 300 min of moderate-intensity, 150 min of vigorous-intensity physical activity or the comparable combination of MVPA). The *2008 Physical Activity Guidelines for Americans* (U.S. Department of Health and Human

Services 2008) also recommend that adults participate in moderate- to vigorous-intensity muscle strengthening activities that encompass all major muscle groups on at least 2 (preferably nonconsecutive) days per week. Although not specifically recommended for adults aged 18–64 years, participation in additional facets of physical fitness (e.g., flexibility and balance/coordination exercises) are also beneficial to health.

BRIEF OVERVIEW OF PHYSICAL ACTIVITY EPIDEMIOLOGY APPLIED TO ADULTS

Early research beginning in the 1950s focused on the associations between aerobic activity and all-cause mortality and coronary heart disease (Morris et al. 1953). Since then, substantial evidence-based research has emerged to show benefit with a multitude of additional health outcomes (U.S. Department of Health and Human Services 1996, 2008) and risk factors in adults (U.S. Department of Health and Human Services 1996). In addition, aerobic activity can reduce overall adiposity, which is another important modifiable risk factor for chronic disease development (U.S. Department of Health and Human Services 1996). Muscle-strengthening activities provide health benefits beyond those gained from aerobic activity and can help adults maintain their independence as they grow older. However, the improvements to muscular strength and endurance are limited to the muscles doing the work; thus, it is important for adults to strengthen all the major muscle groups recommended in the *2008 Physical Activity Guidelines for Americans* (U.S. Department of Health and Human Services 2008). Muscle-strengthening activities promote the development and maintenance of metabolically active lean muscle mass, which improves glucose metabolism (Ishii et al. 1998) and reduces the risk of metabolic disorders including type 2 diabetes mellitus (Eves and Plotnikoff 2006). Furthermore, mechanical loading on skeletal tissue enhances bone formation in young adults and slows bone loss in middle age (Vuori 2001), which likely results in reduced risk of bone-related health outcomes, such as osteoporosis (Courneya and Friedenreich 1997). In addition to improved body and bone composition, muscle-strengthening activities may also reduce risk of all-cause mortality (FitzGerald et al. 2004; Katzmarzyk and Craig 2002).

In summary, there is substantial evidence to support the health-enhancing effects of physical activity in adults. Given that the development of chronic diseases typically do not occur until later in life (e.g., after age 50), maintaining the recommended levels of aerobic and muscle-strengthening activity combined with avoiding prolonged exposure to sedentary activities in adulthood will set the stage for a healthy aging process by reducing risk of debilitating chronic disease while maximizing functional and cognitive ability.

PHYSICAL ACTIVITY LEVELS IN ADULTS

Age-related decreases in physical activity levels are well documented in public health literature; however, little is known about the underlying cause(s) or characteristics of this decline. In addition to the age-related declines, there can also be differences in physical activity levels and features of this age-related decline by gender and racial/ethnic representation.

WOMEN VERSUS MEN

Figure 8.1 shows the prevalence of U.S. women and men that met the 1995 U.S. Centers for Disease Control and Prevention–American College of Sports Medicine (CDC–ACSM) physical activity recommendations across five age categories using data collected from the 2007 CDC Behavioral Risk Factor Surveillance System (BRFSS) (Centers for Disease Control and Prevention 2008). Adults were classified as meeting the physical activity recommendations if s/he reported engaging in at least 30 min of moderate-intensity physical activity for five or more days per week or at least 20 min of vigorous-intensity physical activity for three or more days per week (Pate et al. 1995). Across all age categories, men were more likely to meet recommendations for physical activity when compared with women (Centers for Disease Control and Prevention 2008). More specifically, among women aged 18–24 years, the proportion of women reporting at least 30 min of moderate-intensity activity at least five times per week or at least 20 min of vigorous-intensity physical activity on at least three days of the week was 54.1%. In similarly aged men, the prevalence that met physical activity recommendations was 63.3%. Among 25- to 34-year-olds, the percentage of those meeting current recommendations decreased in both women and men (i.e., 51.4% vs. 55.0%, respectively). In the 35–44 years age group, prevalence estimates were similar (i.e., 49.4% vs. 49.7%); however, men tended to be slightly more active. These gender-based differences became more disparate among 45–64 and 65+-year-old women and men (i.e., 46.0% vs. 47.3% and 35.9% vs. 44.0%) (Centers for Disease Control and Prevention 2008).

CONSIDERATIONS FOR PHYSICAL ACTIVITY PROMOTION IN WOMEN

Given the gender-related differences in physical activity, some interventions focus solely on promoting physical activity in women. Social support and behavioral strategies such as goal setting, diaries or logs, and feedback from intervention staff are strategies frequently used in interventions for women. Interventions are now targeting specific subpopulations of women, including pregnant women and those transitioning through menopause. Given the time constraints for most new parents or

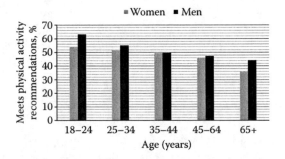

FIGURE 8.1 Prevalence of U.S. adults who meet recommendations for physical activity by gender and age group. (Data from CDC BRFSS, 2007; Centers for Disease Control and Prevention, 2008. With permission.)

those part of the "sandwich generation" (i.e., responsible for taking care of children and parents), some interventions are now turning to technology, such as use of telephones, the Internet, electronic gaming, and/or video exercise routines, to deliver programs to enhance participant flexibility. For example, one Australian program contacted postpartum women using text messages that reinforced goal-setting, self-monitoring, and social support for exercise (Fjeldsoe, Miller, and Marshall 2010). This is only one example of a physical activity promotion strategy pertaining to women that will be discussed within the context of life-course transitions.

UNDERSERVED POPULATIONS

Adults representing racial/ethnic minorities tend to be less active than whites (Centers for Disease Control and Prevention 2008). Differences in leisure-time physical activity may be attributable to historical disparities in educational attainment, household income level, and family and work responsibilities. Furthermore, according to data from the BRFSS in 2007 (Centers for Disease Control and Prevention 2008), physical activity participation decreases in all race/ethnicity groups (i.e., white, Black, Hispanic, and other) across successive age groups (Figure 8.2). Among 18- to 24-year-olds, the percentage of those meeting recommendations was 62.5% for white, 49.2% for Black, 55.1% for Hispanic, and 57.1% for those representing other racial/ethnic groups. The prevalence decreased among adults aged 25–34 years (56.8% for white, 49.0% for Black, 45.8% for Hispanic, and 51.5% for adults representing other racial/ethnic groups). Then the prevalence decreased in each successive age group (34–44 years: white, 52.8%; Black, 44.3%; Hispanic, 42.2%; other, 43.2%; 45–64 years: white, 49.3; Black, 36.8%; Hispanic, 38.6%; other, 41.9%; and 65+ years: white, 41.1%; Black, 26.2%; Hispanic, 34.1%; other, 38.7%) across all race/ethnicity groups. These data show that across all age categories, Blacks are the least active race/ethnicity population subgroup in nonoccupational physical activities (Centers for Disease Control and Prevention 2008) and whites are the most active. Although the data are not shown, men report more physical activity than women in all race/ethnic groups and across all age levels. These observations highlight the importance of providing evidence-based physical activity interventions for women

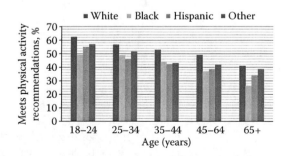

FIGURE 8.2 Prevalence of U.S. adults who meet recommendations for physical activity by race/ethnicity and age group. (Data from CDC BRFSS, 2007; Centers for Disease Control and Prevention, 2008. With permission.)

across all race/ethnic and age groups to prevent mobility disabilities associated with aging and early mortality.

In 2003–2004, another U.S. Surveillance System, the National Health and Nutrition Examination Survey (NHANES), collected accelerometer data in 7176 individuals aged ≥6 years (Troiano et al. 2008). This was the first time that a U.S. national surveillance system incorporated a direct measure of physical activity into their data collection procedures. According to the 2003–2004 NHANES data, the average minutes of accelerometer-derived MVPA among non-Hispanic Black and Mexican-American women, ages 20 to 59 years, was 20.0 and 22.1 min/day, respectively. In similarly aged non-Hispanic Black and Mexican–American men, the average MVPA was higher (i.e., 37.9 and 45.7 min/day, respectively). It is likely that occupational physical activity contributed to the amounts of movement recorded. Therefore, based on these data, it appears as if non-Hispanic Black and Mexican–American adult men were meeting the 1995 CDC–ACSM physical activity recommendations and women were close. In adult men, the percentage meeting the 1995 CDC–ACSM physical activity recommendations was 39.1% and 41.8%, respectively. These data suggest two things: first, self-report instruments such as the ones used in the BRFSS may not be adequately quantifying physical activity levels in these population subgroups. For example, BRFSS questions focus largely on leisure-time physical activity, whereas individuals representing racial/ethnic minorities may accumulate physical activity in other domains, such as during work, domestic activities, or childcare (Kriska 2000). Second, the self-report and accelerometer are measuring two related, but not entirely equivalent, constructs of physical activity. Activity monitors, such as the accelerometer used in the NHANES accelerometer module, predominantly assess ambulatory activities (e.g., walking or jogging), whereas self-report tools measures might also query about time spent in other nonambulatory activities (e.g., bicycling, swimming, or weight training). Thus, the accelerometer may not be measuring exactly the same types of activities as a self-report measure. Similar to differences by gender seen in the BRFSS self-report data for nonoccupational physical activity, 2003–2004 NHANES also demonstrated an age-related decline in accelerometer-derived MVPA among both Black and Hispanic adults (Troiano et al. 2008).

CONSIDERATIONS FOR PHYSICAL ACTIVITY PROMOTION IN UNDERSERVED ADULTS

Since the mid-1990s, there has been an emphasis by the U.S. federal government on eliminating racial/ethnic disparities in health. This emphasis has been realized in studies and programs tailored for underserved populations. Marcus and colleagues (2006) define underserved populations as those of low socioeconomic status or racial and/or ethnic minorities. When working with any population the intervention materials should be tailored not only to the level of readiness for physical activity, but programs should also be tailored to cultural and linguistic norms.

Several examples exist of interventions being administered through faith-based organizations such as churches as one strategy to reach underserved adult populations. The informational materials may reference biblical passages to motivate intervention participants or link physical activity to spirituality. For example in the Faith, Activity and Nutrition and Health-E-AME Internet-based intervention targeting

African–American adults attending African Methodist Episcopal churches in South Carolina, faith-based messages promoted physical activity and healthy lifestyles among church members. Physical activity breaks were also incorporated into church services and activities so attendees could stand and move around to break up continuous sitting often experienced in traditional church services and/or to attend organized sessions held in the church (Wilcox et al. 2007). While the Health-E-AME program targeted African–American adults, faith-based physical activity interventions have been tested in Hispanic communities as well (Bopp, Fallon, and Marquez 2008). In the Faithful Footsteps intervention, held in Hispanic Catholic church settings in Kansas, priests or other church officials spoke to churchgoers about healthy lifestyles, including physical activity. Intervention sessions included such topics as (1) the benefits of physical activity to health, (2) the importance of physical activity to prevent/manage heart disease and diabetes and enhance mental health, and (3) strategies to becoming more active using pedometer step counters.

Another strategy to increase adult participation in physical activity is the use of community health outreach workers to deliver information and lead physical activity groups among inactive adults. Although community health workers have traditionally been employed in cardiovascular disease and/or diabetes interventions, they are now delivering information that specifically target ways in which to increase physical activity. In the United States, community health workers referred to as *promotoras* often provide intervention support with Hispanic communities as they are seen as a credible source of information (Reininger et al. 2010). International interventions in Guatemala (Bailey and Coombs 1996) and India (Van Rompay et al. 2008) have also used community health workers to disseminate interventions to adults in the community.

PERIODS OF TRANSITION THROUGH ADULTHOOD

Although an age-related decline in physical activity levels has been well documented in both genders and across all racial/ethnic population subgroups, very little is known about the factors that may cause this decline (Corder, Ogilvie, and van Sluijs 2009). Some hypothesize that the reduction in physical activity levels is gradual and attributable to the aging process, whereas other researchers postulate that changes in physical activity behavior are a result of key events, defined as *life-course transitions*, that occur over the lifespan (Corder, Ogilvie, and van Sluijs 2009). The inability to conclusively identify the underlying factors that relate to variable physical activity levels over time in adults is likely because a small number of longitudinal studies have been specifically designed to explore the determinants of physical activity behavior change across the lifespan using high-quality physical activity measures (Corder, Ogilvie, and van Sluijs 2009). The majority of what is currently known in this area is derived from cross-sectional studies, which are limited in that they can only uncover and document correlates of behavior change; therefore, causality is unknown. In the relatively few studies that have been conducted, the correlates of physical activity behavior change have been examined in specific population subgroups (e.g., women within a particular age group) and, therefore, have not been concurrently examined across different genders, age, or race/ethnicity groups.

The concept of life-course transitions and their role on physical activity levels was repopularized when Allender, Cowburn, and Foster (2006) noted that life circumstances seemed to influence participation when synthesizing the literature related to barriers and motives to physical activity. In a follow-up review article, Allender, Hutchinson, and Foster (2008) summarized the findings of previous studies that included a life event as the exposure and physical activity as the outcome and characterized five general transitional periods during adulthood that could influence physical activity levels. These periods included a change in (1) employment status, (2) residence, including moving away for school, (3) health or physical status, (4) relationships, and (5) family structure. It is important to note that these periods of flux may only be applicable to, or differentially affect, specific population subgroups. Although there is little supportive literature regarding specific health promotion theories and interventions that have been evaluated within the context of life-course transitions, these key life-course events could be used as targets for promoting physical activity. Each of the five transitional periods, with applicable health promotion strategies, will be described in more detail in following sections.

CHANGE IN EMPLOYMENT STATUS

Changes in employment status including transitioning from high school or higher education (e.g., college, university, or graduate training) to the workforce, moving from employment to unemployment and vice versa, and retirement may influence physical activity participation. Given that work and related demands encompass a substantial proportion of an individual's waking hours, it seems intuitive that shifting from no or little (i.e., part-time) work to a full-time job would negatively impact physical activity levels. This is shown in data from the youngest age cohort (i.e., aged 18–23 years in 1996) enrolled in the Australian Longitudinal Study of Women's Health (i.e., Women's Health Australia). A study by Brown and Trost (2003), examining data collected on the baseline (i.e., collected in 1996) and second (i.e., collected in 2000) survey showed a reduction in physical activity levels among women who had initiated paid work during the 4-year observational period. This finding was adjusted for important factors such as age, income, educational attainment, primary language, and body mass index. The role of employment status was later verified in a study by Bell and Lee (2006), using data from a subsample of the same age cohort in Women's Health Australia that also completed a targeted survey in 2002 that focused on the timing of key life-course transitions. They found that women with no reported physical activity had a younger mean age (i.e., 18.9 ± 2.4 years) at the initiation of her first full-time job, when compared with women in the low, moderate, and high active group (i.e., 20.1 ± 2.5, 20.5 ± 2.5, and 20.7 ± 2.5 years, respectively). In another study by Bell and Lee (2005), baseline data (i.e., collected in 1996) showed a direct relationship between physical inactivity and unemployment status. However, the association was not confirmed in the longitudinal analysis, also included in this paper that likewise used data collected 4 years later (i.e., collected in 2000). A longitudinal study by Evenson et al. (2002) compared the physical activity levels of Atherosclerosis Risk in Communities study participants who reported working at baseline, but had retired by the 6-year follow-up, with participants who reported working at both time points (i.e., baseline and 6-year follow-up). Results showed that retirement was associated with a significant increase in sport and exercise participation, as well as television watching (Evenson et al. 2002). Thus, this life transition was associated with both an increase in physical activity and sedentary behavior.

POTENTIAL STRATEGIES TO INCREASE PHYSICAL ACTIVITY DURING EMPLOYMENT TRANSITIONS

Interventions that promote physical activity in adults that transition from unemployment to employment or change positions might consider goal-setting and time management strategies and/or identify ways to promote access to places or opportunities to engage in physical activity. An employment transition can result in changes to work schedule, insurance benefits that incentivize participants to make healthy lifestyle choices (e.g., wellness programs), and access to on-site workout facilities. Goal-setting strategies (Locke and Latham 1990) can help adults identify barriers to being physically active and propose possible solutions to those barriers within the constraints of their new responsibilities. Using the goal-setting theory of Locke and Latham (1990), an individual would identify a goal, determine possible, realistic solutions for reaching the goal, self-monitor his/her progress, and then once the goal is attained, reward him- or herself for reaching the goal. Rewards for goal attainment should be linked to the goal or behavior, for example, with physical activity, a new pair of sneakers or workout clothes would be appropriate, rather than rewards that are unrelated to the goal (e.g., money).

To assist employees in reaching physical activity and health/wellness goals, some employers have implemented worksite wellness policies and programs. These policies and programs can be useful strategies to enhance time management and access to places to be physically active. For example, Blue Cross Blue Shield, a health insurance company, offers a worksite walking program to employees to encourage physical activity participation during the workday and long-term weight loss. Some Blue Cross Blue Shield locations and other corporations/companies have onsite gym facilities with cardiorespiratory equipment, weight training, and group fitness classes, which provide flexibility related to potential time-related barriers and an established place to be active. Although not all companies offer these benefits, many companies offer educational wellness materials that link insurance discounts to the amount of employee physical activity participation.

CHANGE IN RESIDENCE OR CIRCUMSTANCE

Changes in residence may include shifts in both geographical location and life circumstance. Examples of these types of transitions include relocating from one geographical location to another, downsizing from a single-family residence to an apartment, moving from a parent's home to college/university, moving to another part of town, or moving in with a significant other. Although not studied in this context, moving from one geographical location to another, particularly if the move included a stark climate change, may also influence physical activity levels. For example, adults who move from a geographical location with four distinct seasons to a desert climate may have higher physical activity levels during the winter than if they had not moved (Matthews et al. 2001; Newman et al. 2009). In a 5-month follow-up study by Butler et al. (2004), there was no change in physical activity levels among a small sample of U.S. female freshmen who relocated from home to university. In addition to a change in physical location, adapting to a new circumstance at home can also affect physical activity levels. Using longitudinal data from the youngest cohort enrolled in Women's Health Australia, Bell and Lee (2005) found that moving in with a significant other was also associated with lower physical activity levels. However, when interpreting these results, it is important to note that the physical activity levels of college roommate(s) and significant others were not ascertained, so it is difficult to know the role of social support and modeling on physical activity levels.

POTENTIAL STRATEGIES TO PROMOTE PHYSICAL ACTIVITY FOLLOWING GEOGRAPHICAL CHANGES

Potential health promotion strategies to increase physical activity levels among adults who move to a new geographic location include identifying convenient and accessible facilities for physical activity as well as increasing awareness of opportunities for physical activity within the community such as group fitness classes, hiking and biking trails, and events such as 5K races. The current evidence suggests that the built environment, especially within neighborhoods, is associated with both increased and reduced physical activity levels (Humpel et al. 2002). Neighborhoods that provide safe, supportive, and interesting places to walk show increased levels of walking physical activity. Neighborhoods that lack sidewalks, perceptions of safety, and low engagement in physical activity by residents often show lower levels of physical activity (Brownson et al. 2001). The Social Ecological Model (McLeroy et al. 1988) describes how multiple levels of environment and interpersonal interactions influence individual behavior. Related to a change in residence, institutional/organizational-, community-, and policy- level factors contribute to establishing an environment supportive of physical activity. Institutional factors may provide residents free access to neighborhood recreational facilities or identify school campuses that can be used by adults during after-school hours. Community factors are defined by networks of organizations and institutions, as well as informal relationships across groups. Community parks and recreation departments could collaborate with neighborhood associations to build parks and playgrounds to enhance access to places to be physically active in certain neighborhoods. Finally, the policy level includes any policies or practices at the local, state, or national level that can influence physical activity participation. Adults transitioning to new neighborhoods might experience improved sidewalks, curb cutouts, and street lighting when compared to their previous neighborhood—characteristics that could potentially augment opportunities to be physically active. It is also important to note that changing one's residence might also negatively impact physical activity levels. Therefore, municipalities, communities, and local organizations should continuously work toward promoting available facilities, equipment, events, and other opportunities for physical activity participation to individuals moving into their community.

Change in Physical Status

Changes in physical or health status can include events such as pregnancy, acute illness, or development of chronic disease or disability. Results from two longitudinal studies (Devine, Bove, and Olson 2000; Grace et al. 2006) suggested that pregnancy had little impact on a woman's physical activity levels. In the study by Devine Bove, and Olson (2000), the relationship between lifestyle factors (i.e., diet and exercise) and weight fluctuations during pregnancy and postpartum were examined. In-depth interviews were conducted at mid-pregnancy, 6 weeks, and 12 months postpartum. Results showed that the new role of motherhood did little to influence lifestyle factors that were developed before pregnancy (Devine, Bove, and Olson 2000). The study by Grace et al. (2006) explored changes in health-promoting behaviors (e.g., consuming a healthy diet and engaging in physical activity) across the transition of motherhood and return to work (i.e., maternity group) versus a comparison group of slightly older nonpregnant women (i.e., 32.6 ± 4.2 vs. 41.0 ± 7.8 years). Participants in the maternity group completed study surveys while pregnant (range 17–39 weeks gestation), during maternity leave (average age of babies: 10.0 ± 3.7 months), and when they returned to work (average age of babies 13.9 ± 4.3 months), whereas the comparison group completed surveys at baseline and then, again, at a time that corresponded to when the maternity group returned to work. Study findings showed that physical activity levels were not different between the maternity and comparison group, nor did physical activity change over the postpartum period among maternity group participants. It is important to note that study participants in the Devine, Bove, and Olson (2000) and Grace et al. (2006) studies were recruited while pregnant; therefore, estimates of prepregnancy physical activity levels were historically recalled and could be subject to bias. In addition to limited information regarding prepregnancy health behaviors, data collection for the Devine et al. (2000) and Grace et al. (2006) studies ended during postpartum, which limits interpretation of the long-term impacts of pregnancy and physical activity.

The development, diagnosis, and subsequent management of a chronic disease or condition may also impact physical activity levels. In two retrospective studies (Blanchard et al. 2003; Courneya and Friedenreich 1997), cancer survivors self-reported a decrease in exercise levels from pre- to postdiagnosis. However, a 2002 longitudinal study by Pinto et al. (2002) showed no changes in exercise participation over a 12-month period among women undergoing breast cancer treatment. It is, again, important to be cautious when interpreting these results. Many chronic diseases are transient in nature, meaning that there will likely be periods from prediagnosis to diagnosis to management where physical activity levels will fluctuate. For example, an individual undergoing rigorous chemotherapy treatment or rehabilitating from a heart attack and bypass surgery will likely be less active than they were at prediagnosis or during the management phase of the disease course. Or, they may be more active if they are engaged in a rehabilitation exercise program. Research that examines the distribution of physical activity over the entire disease control continuum is greatly needed, both in the general population and specific population subgroups, alike.

Finally, the impact of childhood illness and physical activity levels in adulthood were explored in a study by Kuh and Cooper (1992). In this study, they found reduced adult physical activity levels in (1) all individuals who suffered a physical disability by age 13, and (2) women who suffered a serious illness during childhood or adolescence. Additional research studies examining the role of timing of disease or disability during the life course on subsequent physical activity levels are greatly needed.

POTENTIAL STRATEGIES TO PROMOTE PHYSICAL ACTIVITY FOLLOWING CHANGES IN PHYSICAL STATUS

For both pregnant women and patients recovering from chronic diseases, such as cardiovascular disease or cancer, attitudes and beliefs about what dose of physical activity is healthful can vary. For example, women may believe that physical activity is not allowed during pregnancy or individuals recovering from a chronic condition (e.g., myocardial infarction) may not be aware of the health benefits of physical activity to manage risk factors or prevent subsequent events. The theory of planned behavior (Ajzen 1991) is commonly used in health promotion-related research with a central tenet that specifies the intention to engage in a behavior is the best predictor of future participation in that behavior. Within this theory, three specific constructs influence intention to engage in a given behavior: (1) attitudes toward the behavior, (2) influence of important others, and (3) perceived behavioral control. When these constructs are applied to physical activity, the theory of planned behavior asserts that adults will engage in physical activity when they have a positive attitude about participating, they think that family or friends will approve, and they feel they have control over how they engage in physical activity.

In pregnant women, several studies (Hausenblas and Downs 2004) indicate that theory of planned behavior is useful to promote physical activity behaviors during this important life-course transition. They showed that attitudes and perceived control of physical activity participation related to one's intention to be physically active—an important predictor to long-term behavior change. Interestingly, the influence of others was not predictive of intention in study participants. Similarly, interventions targeted at cardiac rehabilitation and cancer survivors have used theory of planned behavior to increase physical activity participation. In a study of 377 breast cancer survivors randomized into a theory-based intervention versus a control group, the participants receiving the intervention reported improved attitudes toward exercise, increased intentions to engage in physical activity, and greater physical activity participation (Vallance et al. 2008).

CHANGE IN RELATIONSHIPS

Changes in relationship status can include a transition from being single to married or from being married to single due to divorce, separation, or widowhood. In general, studies examining the relationship between physical activity and marital status have garnered mixed results (Trost et al. 2002). In the study of Booth et al. (2000), individuals who reported of having an active partner were more likely to also be physically active. Yet, among the youngest age cohort of the Women's Health Australia, marriage led to a reduction in physical activity levels (Bell and Lee 2005; Brown and Trost 2003). Similar findings were shown in a cross-sectional study by Salmon et al. (2000). In this study, unmarried males were 34% more likely to participate in any form of leisure-time physical activity when compared to married males. Findings were similar in women (i.e., unmarried women were 35% more likely to be physically active than married women). Several other investigations have shown no significant association between marital status and physical activity. In a study by Sternfeld, Ainsworth, and Quesenberry (1999), marital status was not related to sport/exercise among women aged 20–65 years that were members of the Northern California Kaiser Permanente Medical Care Program. This lack of association between physical activity and marital status was also shown in women aged ≥40 years enrolled in the U.S. Women's Determinants Study (Brownson et al. 2000; King et al. 2000). Furthermore, in a 10-year follow-up of participants aged 25–75 years, marriage did not impact physical activity participation. King et al. (1998) showed a decline in physical activity levels during the premarital period that leveled off after marriage. Transitioning from marriage to being single has been largely understudied. A 3-year study by Umberson (1992) found a reduction in physical activity levels after divorce in men, but no change in women. This study also found that widowhood and low physical activity levels were correlated in men.

POTENTIAL STRATEGIES TO PROMOTE PHYSICAL ACTIVITY FOLLOWING RELATIONSHIP CHANGES

The *Guide to Community Preventive Services* (Task Force on Community Preventive Services 2002) published by the CDC, supports the importance of social support strategies to enhance physical activity participation. Social support can be enhanced by strengthening existing interpersonal bonds or by creating new supportive relationships or networks and can be effective regardless of whether an individual is newly married or recently divorced or widowed. There are four types of social support: emotional, appraisal, informational, and instrumental (House 1981). Emotional support is what people typically think of as social support and includes concern and caring about whether a friend is engaging in activity. Appraisal support can come from a variety of sources (e.g., family, coworkers) and is oftentimes evaluative, such as when a friend provides positive feedback about physical activity participation. Informational support includes other persons sharing opportunities for physical activity participation such as location or time information. Finally, instrumental support, also known as tangible support, generally consists of monetary support, providing equipment or clothing for physical activity, and transportation to facilities or events. Intervention strategies can include establishing a buddy system among study participants or community members, walking groups, or creating contracts to increase accountability with other participants.

CHANGE IN FAMILY STRUCTURE

The role of changes to family structure on physical activity levels in adults has largely focused on the addition of children. Data from the Women's Health Australia showed that becoming a mother for the first time lead to decreased physical activity for the following 4 years (Bell and Lee 2005; Brown and Trost 2003). Results from an 18-year follow-up study of Swedish students aged 16 years at baseline found that having a first child before 34 years was associated with subsequent inactivity (Barnekow-Bergkvist et al. 1996), particularly among female participants. However, it is possible that total number of pregnancies, child-care dynamics (e.g., stay-at-home mom vs. daycare), and the mother going back to work soon after having a child, all contribute to a woman's change in physical activity status after childbirth. Other changes to family dynamics, such as divorce or death of a spouse or significant other, are covered in previous sections, whereas others factors such as an elderly parent moving in to live with their adult children or the impact of children leaving home on physical activity levels have not been well studied. The lack of conclusive information related to family dynamic changes, supports the work of future research in this area.

POTENTIAL STRATEGIES TO PROMOTE PHYSICAL ACTIVITY FOLLOWING CHANGES IN FAMILY STRUCTURE

Little is known about how to engage adults with new family structures in physical activity. Recent pilot studies suggest that the use of self-regulation may be important in increasing and maintaining physical activity levels in adults. Self-regulation is similar to the goal-setting strategies (Locke and Latham 1990) discussed in the "Potential Strategies to Increase Physical Activity during Employment Transitions section Health Promotion Strategies" section of this chapter, but also adds the element of personal control. Individuals who participate in physical activity for enjoyment or self-satisfaction, rather than because a doctor, spouse, or employer told them to become more active, exhibit internal control that enhances one's physical activity participation. Furthermore, adults who perceive that they are in control of their physical activity participation (i.e., perceived locus of causality), including the type(s) of activity and setting, are more likely to maintain activity over time (Chatzisarantis et al. 2003). Although research in this area is new, one intervention study compared families with young children who received planning and self-regulation information with families who received general physical activity information. The families who received the planning and self-regulation in addition to general physical activity information reported greater physical activity, particularly activities done with the family (Rhodes, Naylor, and McKay 2010). These results are encouraging since children who are active and who have active parents are more likely to become active adults.

CONSIDERATIONS FOR FUTURE RESEARCH

Although results to date regarding the role of life-course transitions on physical activity levels are promising, much work in this area is still needed—particularly in relation to evaluating the effectiveness of health promotion strategies to optimize physical activity levels during key life-course events/transitions. As mentioned previously, much of what we know has been gleaned from results from a select number of cross-sectional and longitudinal studies that examined these issues in specific population subgroups (i.e., young women). In an invited commentary, Corder, Ogilvie, and van Sluijs (2009) proposed several answered questions about the age-related decline in physical activity levels that have yet to be explored in the literature. For example, does physical activity decrease across all four domains of physical activity (i.e., leisure time, occupational, transportation, or domestic/self-care), or does it target only a few domains? What are the individual-, intrapersonal-, or environmental characteristics that predominately cause physical activity to decrease across the lifespan? Finally, given that much of what we know has been derived via self-report assessments of physical activity, will the use of more sophisticated measures of physical activity and sedentary behavior result in more informative findings? Uncovering the correlates or determinants of the decline will help health promotion experts better target these characteristics to ultimately attenuate the well-documented reduction in physical activity levels across the lifespan.

CONCLUSION

The beneficial role of a physically active lifestyle among adults cannot be disputed. Regardless of how physical activity is accumulated within a given day, be it during leisure time, work, or active commute, maintaining adequate levels has been shown to decrease the risk of premature death and development of a multitude of chronic diseases and improve mental health and physical function. As the population of older adults in the United States and around the world grows, the role of health lifestyle behaviors, including increased physical activity and reduced periods in sedentary pursuits, is critical to reduce the burden and high costs associated with chronic disease. There are many factors that influence an adult's choice to be physically active. Some of these are related to personal choices, such as moving to new locations, and others are beyond one's control, such as the death of a spouse. Therefore, it is important for health promotion efforts to encourage the adoption of healthy lifestyle behaviors in early adulthood, with continued messaging for physical activity maintenance, in order to provide the foundation for healthy aging across the lifespan.

STUDY QUESTIONS

1. Characterize the difference in physical activity patterns obtained from national surveillance systems across the adult lifespan in these population subgroups. What are the limitations of these studies?
2. Explain the differences that women and minority groups face in meeting the physical activity recommendations, as well as in maintaining physical activity levels across a lifespan.
3. How are physical activity levels influenced by changes in employment status, residence, health, and relationships? Why is it important to identify the role of life-course transitions on physical activity levels? What are the limitations of these studies?
4. Why should strategies to encourage physical activity in adults fit the needs of the target population? Discuss in detail the potential individual-, intra-personal-, or environmental-level characteristics that should be considered

when designing interventions to increase/maintain optimal physical activity levels during key life-course events.

5. Explain the value of "healthy aging" in older adults to reduce overall burden from chronic disease conditions? Discuss the importance of extending this concept to adult men and women between the ages of 18 and 65 years.

ACKNOWLEDGMENT

The authors thank Amy E. Pettee, BS, MSEd, for her thoughtful review of the chapter and expertise in the area of literacy and question development.

REFERENCES

Ajzen, I. 1991. The theory of planned behavior. *Organ. Behav. Hum. Decis.* 50: 179–211.

Allender, S., G. Cowburn, and C. Foster. 2006. Understanding participation in sport and physical activity among children and adults: A review of qualitative studies. *Health Educ. Res.* 21: 826–835.

Allender, S., L. Hutchinson, and C. Foster. 2008. Life-change events and participation in physical activity: A systematic review. *Health Promot. Int.* 23: 160–172.

Bailey, J. E., and D. W. Coombs. 1996. Effectiveness of an Indonesian model for rapid training of Guatemalan health workers in diarrhea case management. *J. Community Health* 21: 269–276.

Barnekow-Bergkvist, M., G. Hedberg, U. Janlert et al. 1996. Physical activity pattern in men and women at the ages of 16 and 34 and development of physical activity from adolescence to adulthood. *Scand. J. Med. Sci. Sports* 6: 359–370.

Bell, S., and C. Lee. 2006. Does timing and sequencing of transitions to adulthood make a difference? Stress, smoking, and physical activity among young Australian women. *Int. J. Behav. Med.* 13: 265–274.

Bell, S., and C. Lee. 2005. Emerging adulthood and patterns of physical activity among young Australian women. *Int. J. Behav. Med.* 12: 227–235.

Blanchard, C. M., M. M. Denniston, F. Baker et al. 2003. Do adults change their lifestyle behaviors after a cancer diagnosis? *Am. J. Health Behav.* 27: 246–256.

Booth, M. L., N. Owen, A. Bauman et al. 2000. Social–cognitive and perceived environment influences associated with physical activity in older Australians. *Prev. Med.* 31: 15–22.

Bopp, M., E. A. Fallon, and D. X. Marquez. 2008. Faithful footsteps: A faith-based physical activity intervention for Hispanics. Paper presented at the Public Health without Borders: Proceedings of the American Public Health Association 136th Annual Meeting and Expo, San Diego, CA.

Brown, W. J., and S. G. Trost. 2003. Life transitions and changing physical activity patterns in young women. *Am. J. Prev. Med.* 25: 140–143.

Brownson, R. C., A. A. Eyler, A. C. King et al. 2000. Patterns and correlates of physical activity among U.S. women 40 years and older. *Am. J. Public Health* 90: 264–270.

Brownson, R. C., E. A. Baker, R. A. Housemann et al. 2001. Environmental and policy determinants of physical activity in the United States. *Am. J. Public Health* 91: 1995–2003.

Butler, S. M., D. R. Black, C. L. Blue et al. 2004. Change in diet, physical activity, and body weight in female college freshman. *Am. J. Health Behav.* 28: 24–32.

Centers for Disease Control and Prevention. 2008. *2007 Behavioral Risk Factor Surveillance System Survey Data.* Atlanta, GA: Department of Health and Human Services, Centers for Disease Control and Prevention.

Chatzisarantis, N. L. D., M. S. Hagger, S. J. H. Biddle et al. 2003. A meta-analysis of perceived locus of causality in exercise, sport, and physical education contexts. *J. Sport Exerc. Psychol.* 25: 284–306.

Corder, K., D. Ogilvie, and E. M. van Sluijs. 2009. Invited commentary: Physical activity over the life course—Whose behavior changes, when, and why? *Am. J. Epidemiol.* 170: 1078–1081.

Courneya, K. S., and C. M. Friedenreich. 1997. Relationship between exercise pattern across the cancer experience and current quality of life in colorectal cancer survivors. *J. Altern. Complement. Med.* 3: 215–226.

Devine, C. M., C. F. Bove, and C. M. Olson. 2000. Continuity and change in women's weight orientations and lifestyle practices through pregnancy and the postpartum period: The influence of life course trajectories and transitional events. *Soc. Sci. Med.* 50: 567–582.

Evenson, K. R., W. D. Rosamond, J. Cai et al. 2002. Influence of retirement on leisure-time physical activity: The atherosclerosis risk in communities study. *Am. J. Epidemiol.* 155: 692–699.

Eves, N. D., and R. C. Plotnikoff. 2006. Resistance training and type 2 diabetes: Considerations for implementation at the population level. *Diabetes Care* 29: 1933–1941.

Fitzgerald, S., C. Barlow, J. B. Kampert et al. 2004. Muscular fitness and all-cause mortality: Prospective observations. *J. Phys. Act. Health* 1: 7–18.

Fjeldsoe, B. S., Y. D. Miller, and A. L. Marshall. 2010. Mobilemums: A randomized controlled trial of an SMS-based physical activity intervention. *Ann. Behav. Med.* 39: 101–111.

Grace, S. L., A. Williams, D. E. Stewart et al. 2006. Health-promoting behaviors through pregnancy, maternity leave, and return to work: Effects of role spillover and other correlates. *Women Health* 43: 51–72.

Haskell, W. L., I. M. Lee, R. R. Pate et al. 2007. Physical activity and public health: Updated recommendation for adults from the American College of Sports Medicine and the American Heart Association. *Med. Sci. Sports Exerc.* 39: 1423–1434.

Hausenblas, H. A., and D. S. Downs. 2004. Prospective examination of the theory of planned behavior applied to exercise behavior during women's first trimester of pregnancy. *J. Reprod. Infant Psychol.* 22: 199–210.

House, J. S. 1981. *Work Stress and Social Support*. Reading, MA: Addison-Wesley.

Humpel, N., N. Owen, E. Leslie et al. 2002. Environmental factors associated with adults' participation in physical activity: A review. *Am. J. Prev. Med.* 22: 188–199.

Ishii, T., T. Yamakita, T. Sato et al. 1998. Resistance training improves insulin sensitivity in Niddm subjects without altering maximal oxygen uptake. *Diabetes Care* 21: 1353–1355.

Katzmarzyk, P. T., and C. L. Craig. 2002. Musculoskeletal fitness and risk of mortality. *Med. Sci. Sports Exerc.* 34: 740–744.

Kesaniemi, Y. K., E. Danforth Jr., M. D. Jensen et al. 2001. Dose-response issues concerning physical activity and health: An evidence-based symposium. *Med. Sci. Sports Exerc.* 33: S351–S358.

King, A. C., C. Castro, S. Wilcox, A. A. Eyler, J. F. Sallis, and R. C. Brownson. 2000. Personal and environmental factors associated with physical inactivity among different racial-ethnic groups of U.S. middle-aged and older-aged women. *Health Psychol.* 19: 354–364.

King, A. C., M. Kiernan, D. K. Ahn et al. 1998. The effects of marital transitions on changes in physical activity: Results from a 10-year community study. *Ann. Behav. Med.* 20: 64–69.

Kriska, A. 2000. Ethnic and cultural issues in assessing physical activity. *Res. Q. Exerc. Sport* 71: S47–S53.

Kuh, D. J., and C. Cooper. 1992. Physical activity at 36 years: Patterns and childhood predictors in a longitudinal study. *J. Epidemiol. Community Health* 46: 114–119.

Locke, E. A., and G. P. Latham. 1990. *A Theory of Goal Setting and Task Performance*. Englewood Cliffs, NJ: Prentice-Hall.

Marcus, B. H., D. M. Williams, P. M. Dubbert et al. 2006. Physical activity intervention studies: What we know and what we need to know: A scientific statement from the American Heart Association Council on Nutrition, Physical Activity, and Metabolism (Subcommittee on Physical Activity); Council on Cardiovascular Disease in the Young; and the Interdisciplinary Working Group on Quality of Care and Outcomes Research. *Circulation* 114: 2739–2752.

Matthews, C. E., P. S. Freedson, J. R. Hebert et al. 2001. Seasonal variation in household, occupational, and leisure time physical activity: Longitudinal analyses from the seasonal variation of blood cholesterol study. *Am. J. Epidemiol.* 153: 172–183.

McLeroy, K. R., D. Bibeau, A. Steckler et al. 1988. An ecological perspective on health promotion programs. *Health Educ. Q.* 15: 351–377.

Morris, J. N., J. A. Heady, P. A. Raffle et al. 1953. Coronary heart-disease and physical activity of work. *Lancet* 265: 1111–1120.

Newman, M. A., K. K. Pettee, K. L. Storti et al. 2009. Monthly variation in physical activity levels in postmenopausal women. *Med. Sci. Sports Exerc.* 41: 322–327.

Pate, R. R., M. Pratt, S. N. Blair et al. 1995. Physical activity and public health. A recommendation from the Centers for Disease Control and Prevention and the American College of Sports Medicine. *JAMA* 273: 402–407.

Pinto, B. M., J. J. Trunzo, P. Reiss et al. 2002. Exercise participation after diagnosis of breast cancer: Trends and effects on mood and quality of life. *Psychooncology* 11: 389–400.

Reininger, B. M., C. S. Barroso, L. Mitchell-Bennett et al. 2010. Process evaluation and participatory methods in an obesity-prevention media campaign for Mexican Americans. *Health Promot. Pract.* 11: 347–357.

Rhodes, R. E., P. J. Naylor, and H. A. McKay. 2010. Pilot study of a family physical activity planning intervention among parents and their children. *J. Behav. Med.* 33: 91–100.

Salmon, J., N. Owen, A. Bauman et al. 2000. Leisure-time, occupational, and household physical activity among professional, skilled, and less-skilled workers and homemakers. *Prev. Med.* 30: 191–199.

Sternfeld, B., B. E. Ainsworth, and C. P. Quesenberry. 1999. Physical activity patterns in a diverse population of women. *Prev. Med.* 28: 313–323.

Task Force on Community Preventive Services. 2002. Recommendations to increase physical activity in communities. *Am. J. Prev. Med.* 22: 67–72.

Troiano, R. P., D. Berrigan, K. W. Dodd et al. 2008. Physical activity in the United States measured by accelerometer. *Med. Sci. Sports Exerc.* 40: 181–188.

Trost, S. G., N. Owen, A. E. Bauman et al. 2002. Correlates of adults' participation in physical activity: Review and update. *Med. Sci. Sports Exerc.* 34: 1996–2001.

U.S. Department of Health and Human Services. 1996. *Physical Activity and Health: A Report of the Surgeon General.* Atlanta, GA: U.S. Government Printing Office.

U.S. Department of Health and Human Services. 2008. Physical Activity Guidelines Advisory Committee Report.

Umberson, D. 1992. Gender, marital status and the social control of health behavior. *Soc. Sci. Med.* 34: 907–917.

Vallance, J. K., K. S. Courneya, R. C. Plotnikoff et al. 2008. Analyzing theoretical mechanisms of physical activity behavior change in breast cancer survivors: Results from the Activity Promotion (Action) trial. *Ann. Behav. Med.* 35: 150–158.

Van Rompay, K. K., P. Madhivanan, M. Rafiq et al. 2008. Empowering the people: Development of an HIB peer education model for low literacy rural communities in India. *Hum. Resour. Health* 6: 6.

Vuori, I. M. 2001. Dose-response of physical activity and low back pain, osteoarthritis, and osteoporosis. *Med. Sci. Sports Exerc.* 33: S551–S586; discussion 609–610.

Wilcox, S., M. Laken, M. Bopp et al. 2007. Increasing physical activity among church members: Community-based participatory research. *Am. J. Prev. Med.* 32: 131–138.

9 Physical Activity and Healthy Aging

David M. Buchner

CONTENTS

INTRODUCTION

The focus of this chapter—physical activity and healthy aging—is part of a large topic in gerontology dealing with determinants of healthy aging. People often assume (incorrectly) that genes are the key determinant of healthy aging. We hear people say they expect to live a long healthy life because their parents did. In fact, public health science shows lifestyle choices are stronger determinants of healthy aging. For example, one study estimated that 82% of cardiovascular disease in women could be prevented or delayed by adopting a healthy lifestyle (no use of tobacco, a healthy diet and body weight, regular physical activity, alcohol in moderation) (Stampfer et al. 2000). People with healthy lifestyles may live 10 or more years longer than those without such behaviors (Fraser and Shavlik 2001).

This chapter emphasizes issues in physical activity of primary importance to older adults: (1) the potential public health impact of promoting physical activity in older adults; (2) the effect of physical activity on physical and mental functional limitations, falls, and disability; (3) the promotion of physical activity in clinical settings; and (4) the translation of research findings into evidence-based, community programs to promote physical activity in older adults. The chapter introduces these topics with a brief history of public health research and practice in promoting physical activity in older adults.

Of course, topics covered in other chapters are highly relevant to older adults. These topics include sedentary behavior, chronic disease prevention, therapeutic physical activity, injury prevention, and the chapters dealing with promotion of physical activity.

BACKGROUND AND TERMINOLOGY

Following the usage of the *2008 Physical Activity Guidelines for Americans*, this chapter regards older adults at age 65 and older. In older adults, *active life expectancy* refers to the number of years an individual can expect to live without a major disability. A major disability is often regarded as inability to perform a basic activity of daily living (ADL) (e.g., ability to eat, transfer, or use the toilet) or sometimes inability to perform an instrumental ADL (IADL) (e.g., ability to shop, do laundry, and do housekeeping). A feature of healthy aging is compression of morbidity (Vita et al. 1998). The compression-of-morbidity hypothesis holds that (1) humans have a maximum lifespan, (2) interventions can increase active life expectancy, and (3) therefore morbidity and major disability can be compressed into a few years at the end of life. Note that physical activity does not increase the maximal lifespan, but decreases the risk of morbidity and premature mortality.

Public health practice related to physical activity in older adults has changed dramatically over the past 40 years. Historically, there were concerns that it was "too late" for physical activity to make a difference, that older adults had too high an injury risk, and that older adults were not capable of much physical activity because of low fitness. By the 1980s, it was proven that older adults experienced improvements in fitness from both aerobic training and resistance training. By the 1990s, there was consensus that older adults experienced major health benefits from regular physical activity, could do activity safely, and it was never "too late" to benefit (U.S. Department of Health and Human Services 1996). The past decade has witnessed steady growth in evidence-based approaches to promoting physical activity in older adults.

Over the past 20 years, research has addressed the effects of physical activity on the disablement process. This chapter discusses this research using terminology of the Nagi framework (Pope and Tarlov 1991, pp. 76–108), which recognized effects can be measured at four different levels:

1. *Pathology*—at the level of cells and tissue (e.g., effect of physical activity on growth of new neurons in the brain)
2. *Physiologic impairment*—at the level of organs and organ systems (e.g., effect of physical activity on VO_2max)
3. *Functional limitations*—at the level of behavioral ability and performance in neutral environments (e.g., effect of physical activity on walking speed)
4. *Disability*—at the level of ability to do tasks of life in actual environments (e.g., effect of physical activity on ability to shop for groceries)

PUBLIC HEALTH IMPORTANCE

A strong case can be made for the importance and feasibility of promoting physical activity in older adults. The case rests on several observations:

(1) Older adults have been the most rapidly growing segment of the U.S. population. The percentage of the U.S. population over age 65 will continue to grow steadily from about 13% in 2010 to about 20% in 2040 (U.S. Census Bureau 2008).

(2) U.S. older adults are the least physical active age group. Results from the National Health and Nutrition Examination Survey (NHANES) raise the possibility that older adults are much less active than indicated by self-report questions on surveys. When NHANES measured the level of activity using an accelerometer, less than 5% of older adults met the 1995 U.S. Centers for Disease Control and Prevention–American College of Sports Medicine (CDC–ACSM) public health recommendation for physical activity (Troiano et al. 2008).

(3) There is strong evidence that regular physical activity provides major health benefits in older adults. The first major conclusion of the 1996 Surgeon General's report, *Physical Activity and Health*, is "People of all ages, both male and female, benefit from regular physical activity" (U.S. Department of Health and Human Services 1996). Consider a study of more than 2700 older adults enrolled in a home care program, who typically have high rates of disability and a short life expectancy. Older adults who obtained more than 2 h/week of physical activity had roughly a 50% lower risk of mortality (Landi et al. 2004). A study in nursing home residents reported that resistance training improved the resident's mobility and gait speed (Fiatarone et al. 1994).

The beneficial effects of physical activity can be stronger, more immediate, and or more easily demonstrated in older adults, because older adults are at highest risk for most chronic conditions prevented by physical activity. For example, the Diabetes Prevention Project conducted a randomized trial of a combined physical activity and weight loss intervention in adults with impaired glucose tolerance (prediabetes). Overall, the intervention reduced risk of diabetes by 58% (Diabetes Prevention Program Research Group 2004). The benefits of the intervention were strongest in adults age 60 and older, where risk of diabetes was reduced by 71%.

(4) Major benefits of physical activity occur at levels of physical activity that are feasible in older adults. The majority of older adults are capable (at least after some training) of walking 150 min/week. Because the dose–response relationship between physical activity and health benefit is curvilinear (greater benefits at lower levels of activity, and relatively less benefit from increasing activity to very high levels), this level of activity provides major health benefits. Consider the results of the Women's Health Initiative Observational Study (WHI) in Figure 9.1 (Manson et al. 2002). A woman who does a brisk walk (at 3.4 METs [metabolic equivalent]) for 150 min/week does 8.5 MET-h of activity, and ranks in the third WHI quintile of physical activity. Depending on her age, she would experience a reduction in risk of cardiovascular disease of 14–37%. Even women in the second quintile, who are insufficiently active, experience meaningful reductions in risk.

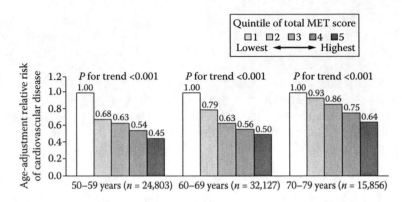

FIGURE 9.1 Age-adjusted relative risk of cardiovascular disease by age and by quintile of total MET-hours per week of physical activity, in 73,743 women in Women's Health Initiative Observational Study. Numbers above the bars and height of bars indicate relative risk. Range of MET-hours is by quintile (Q) is: Q1, 0–2.4; Q2, 2.5–7.2; Q3, 7.3–13.4; Q4, 13.5–23.3; Q5, 23.4 and higher. (From Manson, J. E. et al., *New Engl. J. Med.*, 347, 716–725, 2002. With permission.)

(5) Older adults prefer walking, which is the most feasible type of physical activity. Walking requires no special equipment or special facilities; opportunities to walk are widely available. Walking has low risk of injury—about 1 injury for every 1000 h of walking (Physical Activity Guidelines Advisory Panel 2008, pp. G10-1 to G10-58). It is remarkable that something as mundane as walking 30–60 min each day can cause a large improvement in the health of older adults (Lee and Buchner 2008).

(6) U.S. surveillance data shows encouraging trends in levels of physical activity of older adults. Between 1988 and 2002, the percentage of older adults inactive in leisure time has declined; for example, women age 70+ showed a decline from about 50% inactive to about 40% inactive (Centers for Disease Control and Prevention 2004).

(7) Medical expenditures are lower in active older adults. A longitudinal study reported that inactive older adults at baseline, who increase activity to three or more days per week, have annual medical expenditures that are $2202 less than older adults who remain inactive (Martinson et al. 2003). A study of EnhanceFitness participants reported a dose–response relationship between exercise participation and reduction in medical care expenditures. Participants overall had medical care expenditures of 94% of nonparticipants, whereas participants who attended at least twice per week had expenditures of 79% of nonparticipants (Ackermann et al. 2003). This study also reported that one hospitalization was prevented for every 20 older adults who exercised.

(8) Longer life expectancy due to physical activity may not increase medical expenditures, because of compression of morbidity. A recent study used Medicare data to simulate the effect of disability status at age 70 on life expectancy, active life expectancy, and expected cumulative medical

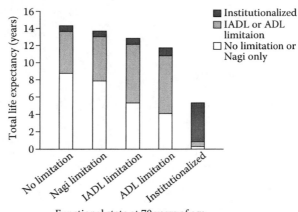

FIGURE 9.2   Life expectancy at age 70 years by functional status at age 70, based on data from 1992–1998 Medicare Current Beneficiary Survey. Height of each bar indicates total life expectancy. Shading in bars indicates expected number of years of life without a functional limitation ("no limitation or Nagi limitation"), with IADL or ADL limitations, or in an institution. For example, an older adult with no limitations at age 70 has a life expectancy of an additional 14.3 years. On average, the older adult will spend 0.7 years in an institution, 4.9 years with a limitation in ADLs or IADLs, and 8.7 years without a major limitation. (Lubitz, J. et al., *New Engl. J. Med.*, 349, 1048–1055, 2003. With permission.)

expenditures (Figure 9.2) (Lubitz et al. 2003). Several results in Figure 9.2 are worth noting. (a) As expected, life expectancy is longest for people with no functional limitations at baseline. (b) Older adults commonly experience transitions between better and worse health as they age. Even older adults with baseline ADL limitations at age 70 have (on average) several remaining years of life with no major limitations. (c) The figure shows compression of morbidity. Adults with no limitations at baseline had the fewest absolute years of disability (disability defined as institutionalization, or an ADL/IADL impairment).

But the most remarkable finding of this study was that expected cumulative (lifetime) medical expenditures did not differ by baseline functional status (Figure 9.3) (Lubitz et al. 2003). That is, keeping older adults healthy did not place an extra burden on the medical care system. It appears we have a best-case scenario: regular physical activity such as walking reduces risk of premature mortality (Lee and Buchner 2008), extends active life expectancy (Ferrucci et al. 1999), compresses morbidity (Vita et al. 1998), yet does not increase medical care expenditures.

PHYSICAL ACTIVITY AND FUNCTIONAL HEALTH

One of the most important health benefits of physical activity in older adults is the prevention of functional limitations and disability. There is moderate to strong

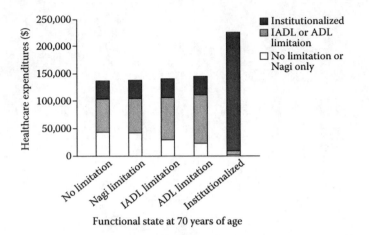

Functional state at 70 years of age

FIGURE 9.3 Cumulative expected medical expenditures from age 70 years of age until death, according to functional status at age 70, based on data from 1992–1998 Medicare Current Beneficiary Survey. For example, a person with no limitations at age 70 is expected to have cumulative expenditures of $136,000: about $32,000 during the time an older adult is institutionalized, about $60,000 during the time a person has an ADL or IADL dependency, and about $44,000 during the time an older adult has no major limitations. (From Lubitz J. et al., *New Engl. J. Med.*, 349, 1048–1055, 2003. With permission.)

evidence for preventive effects involving physical function, cognitive function, and falls (Physical Activity Guidelines Advisory Panel 2008).

PHYSICAL FUNCTIONAL HEALTH

Table 9.1 provides a framework for considering the benefits of physical activity on physical function in older adults.

- Physical activity has a fitness benefit that enhances physical performance, such as ability to run a 5K race or compete in a triathlon. Naturally, this effect occurs in all age groups and has been thoroughly studied in exercise physiology.
- Physical activity has a primary prevention benefit—reducing risk of future moderate-to-severe functional limitations and disability in relatively healthy adults.
- Some older adults have substantial functional limitations, but are not yet severely impaired. In this group, physical activity has a secondary prevention benefit—preventing or delaying the onset of severe impairment and major disability.
- Physical activity is used in rehabilitation to restore physical function in people with functional limitations and disability.

TABLE 9.1

Framework for Considering the Health Benefits of Physical Activity on Physical and Cognitive Function in Older Adults

Benefit	Group of Older Adults	Physical Function	Cognitive Function
Fitness	Relatively healthy	Enhanced physical performance	Enhanced cognitive performance
Primary prevention	Relatively healthy	Prevention of moderate to severe physical functional limitations	Prevention of moderate to severe cognitive impairment
Secondary prevention	Moderate-age related decline with some functional limitations	Prevention of severe physical functional limitations	Prevention of severe cognitive impairment
Treatment and rehabilitation	With a specific disease	Restore loss of physical function due to disease(s)	Restore loss of cognitive function due to disease(s)

These benefits are not mutually exclusive, as high levels of physical activity in relatively healthy older adults both improve performance and reduce risk of future functional limitations.

Prospective cohort studies demonstrate the value of physical activity for primary prevention of functional limitations. In a recent review, every cohort study reported that active older adults were at lower risk of mobility limitations (Figure 9.4) (Physical Activity Guidelines Advisory Committee 2008, pp. G6-1 to G6-31). Furthermore, there was a dose–response effect. Similarly, Figure 9.5 summarizes

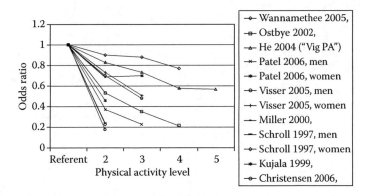

FIGURE 9.4 Prospective cohort studies assessing association between level of physical activity and risk of mobility limitations, from the evidence review of Physical Activity Guidelines Advisory Committee. Figure shows reported odds ratio of mortality for each level of physical activity in a study, with lowest level of activity assigned to the referent category. Data demonstrate a dose–response effect: generally, the higher the level of activity, the lower the odds ratio for morbidity limitations. (Physical Activity Guidelines Advisory Committee, *Physical Activity Guidelines Advisory Committee Report*, Washington, DC: U.S. Department of Health and Human Services, pp. G6-1–G6-31, 2008.)

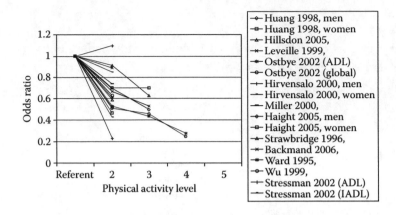

FIGURE 9.5 Prospective cohort studies assessing association between level of physical activity and risk of ADL dependency, IADL dependency, or major disability, from the evidence review of Physical Activity Guidelines Advisory Committee. Figure shows reported odds ratio for each level of physical activity in a study, with lowest level of activity assigned to the referent category. Data demonstrate a dose–response effect: generally, the higher the level of activity, the lower the odds for ADL, IADL, dependency, or major disability. (Physical Activity Guidelines Advisory Committee, *Physical Activity Guidelines Advisory Committee Report*, Washington, DC: U.S. Department of Health and Human Services, pp. G6-1–G6-31, 2008.)

cohort studies of the effect of physical activity on risk of ADL, IADL, and global outcomes related to disability. All but one study reported physical activity reduced risk. Again, there was a dose–response effect.

There are no randomized trials showing physical activity reduces risk of future functional limitations. However, there are many randomized trials of the immediate effect of physical activity on measures of functional limitations and/or disability. Several of these trials provide moderate evidence for a secondary prevention effect (Physical Activity Guidelines Advisory Committee 2008, pp. G6-1 to G6-31). For example, the LIFE-P (Lifestyle Interventions and Independence for Elders Pilot) study enrolled 424 older adults with moderate functional limitations (The LIFE Study Investigators 2006) in a randomized trial of an exercise. The study reported that older adults assigned to exercise maintained the same gait speed over a year of follow-up, whereas gait speed in control participants declined. A trial in women aged 45–75 years reported a dose–response effect between physical activity and improvement in functional limitations (SF-36 physical functioning subscale) and disability (SF-36 role physical subscale) (Martin et al. 2009).

Adverse events and injuries are a concern with exercise in older adults in general, and particularly in those with chronic diseases as in LIFE-P. However, the LIFE-P study reported that rates of adverse health events were virtually identical between the exercise and control participants (The LIFE Study Investigators 2006).

Excess body fat increases risk of functional limitations, because the more a person weighs, the more difficult it is to move. If the goal is to improve functional limitations by weight loss, does it matter whether older adults lose weight by caloric restriction or by physical activity? The answer is probably yes. One study reported that weight loss due to physical activity significantly improved 6-min walk distance, but similar weight loss due only to caloric restriction did not (Messier et al. 2004). Also, physical activity was essential to improving performance in stair climbing.

COGNITIVE FUNCTIONAL HEALTH

Table 9.1 provides a framework for considering the types of benefits of physical activity on brain health and cognitive function. The cognitive benefits are analogous to the physical function benefits described above.

The fitness benefit involves whether regular physical activity improves cognitive performance, for example, as measured by IQ tests. (This issue in older adults is analogous to the issue in children of whether activity improves academic performance.) There is strong evidence that physical activity improves mental "fitness" and cognitive function in older adults. A meta-analysis of 18 randomized trials reported a moderate effect size (0.48) of physical activity on a variety of cognitive tests (Colcombe and Kramer 2003).

Research has identified mechanisms by which exercise affects cognitive function (Kramer, Erickson, and Colcombe 2006). In animal studies, exercise causes growth of neurons in areas of the brain affected by dementia. Exercise affects the levels of neurotransmitters and hence brain activity. A feature of cognitive impairment is decreased blood flow to the brain, and physical activity increases brain blood flow.

There is strong evidence from observational studies that physical activity reduces risk of cognitive impairment due to dementia, including Alzheimer-type dementia. One meta-analysis of 16 studies found a 37% reduction in risk of dementia (Physical Activity Guidelines Advisory Committee 2008, pp. G8-1 to G8-58). There is also solid evidence from randomized trials that physical activity improves cognitive function in older adults with cognitive impairment. A meta-analysis of 30 studies reported a moderate effect size (0.57) of exercise on cognitive function in adults with dementia (Heyn, Abreu, and Ottenbacher 2004).

FALLS

Fall-related injuries are a major public health problem in older adults. Falls can lead to major injuries such as head injuries and fractures, particularly hip fracture. In 2001, about 10,300 fatal and 2.6 million nonfatal fall-related injuries occurred in the United States (Stevens et al. 2006). Direct medical costs of falls were about $19 billion.

Physical activity reduces risk of falls in older adults. Most evidence supports an exercise program that involves balance training at least three days each week and resistance training, along with walking on a few days each week (Physical Activity Guidelines Advisory Committee 2008, pp. E-1 to E-35). The Otago Exercise Program for falls causes about a 40% reduction in risk of falls, injurious falls, hospitalization for falls, and medical care expenditures for falls (Robertson et al. 2002). The CDC has identified evidence-based programs to prevent falls (Stevens and Sogolow 2008). At present, all evidence-based programs are exercise programs. But some research indicates that activities such as dancing can reduce fall risk (Keogh et al. 2009).

Balance training and resistance training are the most important component of fall prevention exercise programs (Physical Activity Guidelines Advisory Committee 2008, pp. E-1 to E-35). For example, tai chi exercise improves both balance and strength, and reduces risk of falls. Balance training involves exercises over a fixed base of support, such as standing with feet together or on one leg. It also involves dynamic exercises, such as walking backward and walking heel to toe.

CLINIC-BASED PROMOTION OF PHYSICAL ACTIVITY IN OLDER ADULTS

As discussed in the "Public Health Importance" section, public health uses a variety of approaches to promote physical activity across the lifespan. One approach that is more essential for older adults is clinic-based promotion of physical activity. Older adults are more likely than younger adults and children to have regular clinic visits that provide an opportunity for counseling. Older adults commonly view their primary care provider as the most important source of information about physical activity. Primary care providers and other clinicians must advise older adults with chronic conditions on whether the condition limits their choice or amount of physical activity. Clinicians also prescribe physical activity as treatment for chronic conditions.

The five "A"s are appropriate for promoting physical activity in clinical settings: ask, advise, assess, assist, and arrange. (1) Ask about the amount and types of physical activity in a typical week. (2) Advise older adults to participate in regular physical activity that is appropriate for their abilities and chronic conditions. (3) Assess the next step or steps for increasing physical activity in insufficiently active older adults. (4) Assist the older adult in taking these steps. (5) Arrange a follow-up appointment to monitor progress, and address problems related to increasing physical activity.

The U.S. Preventive Services Task Force issues recommendations on the effectiveness of various types of clinical counseling. The Task Force found insufficient evidence to recommend for or against clinical counseling (U.S. Preventive Services Task Force 2002). However, counseling protocols vary among research studies; some are reported to be effective and some are not. Hence, a reasonable approach in a clinic is to use an approach shown to be effective, and evaluate it. The New Zealand Green prescription is an example of a protocol for promoting physical activity that has been shown to be effective in middle-age and older adults (Elley et al. 2003). In this protocol, the medical system assesses the level of physical activity, the primary care provider provides a prescription, and the patient is referred to the community-based support and counseling for increasing physical activity.

A framework developed by Frieden (2010), "The Health Impact Pyramid," is useful in understanding the public health role of clinical interventions. The pyramid involves five tiers, with interventions in the first tier having the most effect, and those in the fifth tier having the least. The tiers are (1) socioeconomic factors, (2) changing the context to make individuals' default decisions healthy decisions, (3) long-lasting protective interventions, (4) clinical interventions, and (5) counseling and education.

Despite traditional emphasis on clinical interventions and patient education, these interventions likely have the least impact. However, a comprehensive approach to a health issue involves interventions at all tiers of the model. Clinical interventions have a role to play in older adults as necessary, but not sufficient, components of physical activity promotion.

Clinical interventions can be driven by policy interventions, such as a clinic policy requiring measuring the quality of clinic-based promotion of physical activity. The National Committee on Quality Assurance has developed a physical activity quality of care measure for older adults. It assesses if clinicians ask and advise about physical activity at least once a year (Agency for Healthcare Research and Quality 2010).

Some experts recommend that inactive older adults have a medical screening before initiating physical activity. However, there is no evidence that medical consultation in healthy people of any age can reduce risk of adverse events from physical activity (Physical Activity Guidelines Advisory Committee 2008, pp. E-1 to E-35). The U.S. Preventive Services Task Force recommends against routine screening for coronary artery disease in adults at low risk (U.S. Preventive Services Task Force 2004). In adults at high risk for coronary heart disease, the Task Force concluded that there was insufficient evidence to recommend for or against screening with existing screening tests.

TRANSLATIONAL RESEARCH AND EVIDENCE-BASED PHYSICAL ACTIVITY PROGRAMS

Exercise programs for older adults have proliferated in community settings, including both center-based and home-based programs. The quality of many programs is unknown. Hence, health organizations have begun to systematically identify evidence-based programs. For example, the National Council on Aging (2010) and the Administration on Aging (AoA) collaborated to identify evidence-based programs whose implementation would be funded by AoA. To be an evidence-based program, the health benefits of the program must be demonstrated by scientifically valid research studies or evaluations. EnhanceFitness (Project Enhance 2010) is an example of an evidence-based exercise program. The program includes strength training, balance training, aerobic training, and stretching in a 1-hour class. The health benefits of the program, such as improvements on the Functional Fitness test, are documented in research studies (Belza et al. 2006). The implementation of the program is routinely evaluated and program instructors must be certified.

Programs that help older adults increase physical activity are also increasingly common. These programs do not involve exercise classes, but involve activities such as telephone counseling or workshops. The programs seek to assist older adults in adhering to their own individualized plan for regular physical activity. An example of such an evidence-based program is Active Living Every Day, which is provided by the Cooper Institute (2010). This program emphasizes moderate-intensity physical activity, such as a brisk walking. It teaches people skills related to sustaining an active lifestyle, such as skills in identifying and overcoming barriers to activity. It emphasizes fitting activity into life in realistic ways, and individualizing the goals and activities of a physical activity program. Originally designed as a 20-session program, it is now available as a 12-session program supported by a participant workbook, online materials, a facilitator's guide, and training for facilitators.

Evidence-based programs have been developed for older adults to assist them in managing a chronic disease such as diabetes or arthritis. Such programs typically help older adults understand the role of physical activity in managing a chronic condition. An example of such a program is the Chronic Disease Self-Management Program (CDSMP) (Stanford Patient Education Research Center 2010). This program involves six workshops lasting 2½ h delivered in community settings. Workshops are facilitated by trained leaders—at least one of whom is a nonhealth professional. Participation in CDSMP often results in increased physical activity.

It is challenging to disseminate evidence-based physical activity programs in the community. To address the challenge of translation, the Robert Wood Johnson Foundation funded "Active for Life" to demonstrate that programs (e.g., Active Living Every Day) could be successfully implemented in diverse community settings. In Active for Life, two physical activity interventions tested in research studies were translated into nine community settings, including a church, a YMCA, a public health department, a nonprofit health plan, and an aging services network. The nine settings successfully delivered the physical activity interventions to more than 8,000 older adults; the health and behavior effects observed in community sites were quite similar to the health and behavior effects reported in the original research studies (Wilcox et al. 2008). However, programs did require some modifications. For example, because programs were commonly viewed as "too long" by participants, Active Living Every Day was shortened to a 12-week version as discussed above.

SUMMARY

Regular physical activity is essential for healthy aging. Physical activity reduces risk of many age-related chronic diseases and of premature mortality. Physical activity improves quality of life in older adults by improving physical and cognitive performance, and by reducing risk of physical and cognitive limitations and disability. Physical activity reduces risk of fall injuries. Active older adults are more likely to "age in place" and live independently.

Promoting physical activity in older adults is of high public health importance: older adults are the most rapidly growing age group, yet are the least active; there is strong evidence of major health benefits from moderate levels of physical activity that are realistic and achievable by older adults; active older adults have substantially lower medical expenditures; and promoting physical activity may not increase a person's cumulative (lifetime) medical expenditures in old age. There are effective approaches to promoting physical activity in older adults, including protocols for clinic-based counseling and evidence-based community programs. Programs such as Active for Life demonstrate that we can translate programs from research settings into effective community programs that reach diverse and less advantaged subgroups of older adults.

STUDY QUESTIONS

1. Describe the four different levels of measurement of the disablement process in the Nagi framework.
2. What are the three components of the compression-of-morbidity hypothesis and how does physical activity relate to the hypothesis?
3. Why is the dose–response relationship between physical activity and health benefits important in older adults? What four specific examples of a dose–response relationship are mentioned in the chapter?
4. How would you describe the evidence that physical activity provides the benefits to brain health and cognitive function described in the framework of Table 9.1?
5. What two types of physical activity are most important to fall prevention in older adults, and how could you design a program for older adults to perform these activities?
6. What are the five "A"'s of physical activity promotion in clinical settings and how can these be incorporated into a physical activity program for older adults?
7. How would you describe that evidence supporting the importance of medical screening of inactive older adults who seek to increase their physical activity?
8. Describe how the five tiers of the Health Impact Pyramid can be incorporated into a broad-based program to promote physical activity in older adults.
9. Identify how three different genres of evidence-based programs in older adults have influenced current practices for promoting physical activity in older adults.

REFERENCES

Ackermann, R. T., A. Cheadle, N. Sandhu et al. 2003. Community exercise program use and changes in healthcare costs for older adults. *Am. J. Prev. Med.* 25: 232–237.

Agency for Healthcare Research and Quality. 2010. National qualify measures clearinghouse. http://www.qualitymeasures.ahrq.gov/content.aspx?id=14987 (Accessed January 14, 2011).

Belza, B., A. S. Shumway-Cook, E. A. Phelan et al. 2006. The effects of a community-based exercise program on function and health in older adults: the EnhanceFitness program. *J. Appl. Gerontol.* 25: 291–306.

Centers for Disease Control and Prevention. 2004. Prevalence of no leisure-time physical activity—35 states and the District of Columbia, 1988–2002. *MMWR* 53: 82–86.

Colcombe, S., and A. F. Kramer. 2003. Fitness effects on cognitive function of older adults: A meta-analytic study. *Psychol. Sci.* 14: 125–130.

Diabetes Prevention Program Research Group. 2004. Reduction in the incidence of type 2 diabetes with lifestyle intervention or metformin. *New Engl. J. Med.* 346: 393–403.

Elley, D. R., N. Kerse, B. Arroll et al. 2003. Effectiveness of counseling patients on physical activity in general practice: Cluster randomized controlled trial. *BMJ* 326: 793–798.

Ferrucci, L., G. Izmirlian, S. Leveille et al. 1999. Smoking, physical activity, and active life expectancy. *Am. J. Epidemiol.* 149: 645–653.

Fiatarone, M. A., E. F. O'Neill, N. D. Ryan et al. 1994. Exercise training and nutritional supplementation for physical frailty in very elderly people. *New Engl. J. Med.* 330: 1769–1775.

Fraser, G. E., and D. J. Shavlik. 2001. Ten years of life. Is it a matter of choice? *Arch. Intern. Med.* 151: 1645–1652.

Frieden, T. R. 2010. A framework for public health action: The Health Impact Pyramid. *Am. J. Public Health* 100: 590–595.

Heyn, P., B. C. Abreu, and K. J. Ottenbacher. 2004. The effects of exercise training on elderly persons with cognitive impairment and dementia: A meta-analysis. *Arch. Phys. Med. Rehabil.* 85: 1694–1704.

Keogh, J. W. L., A. Kilding, P. Pidgeon et al. 2009. Physical benefits of dancing for healthy older adults: A review. *J. Aging Phys. Activity* 17: 479–500.

Kramer, A. F., K. I. Erickson, and S. J. Colcombe. 2006. Exercise, cognition, and the aging brain. *J. Appl. Physiol.* 101: 1237–1242.

Landi, F., M. Cesari, G. Onder et al. 2004. Physical activity and mortality in frail, community-living elderly patients. *J. Gerontol. Med. Sci.* 59A: 833–837.

Lee, I., and D. M. Buchner. 2008. The importance of walking to public health. *Med. Sci. Sports Exerc.* 40: S512–S518.

Lubitz, J., L. Cai, E. Kramarow et al. 2003. Health, life expectancy, and health care spending among the elderly. *New Engl. J. Med.* 349: 1048–1055.

Manson, J. E., P. Greenland, A. Z. LaCroix et al. 2002. Walking compared with vigorous exercise for the prevention of cardiovascular events in women. *New Engl. J. Med.* 347: 716–725.

Martin, C. K., T. S. Church, A. M. Thompson et al. 2009. Exercise dose and quality of life. *Arch. Intern. Med.* 169: 269–278.

Martinson, B. C., A. L. Crain, N. P. Pronk et al. 2003. Changes in physical activity and short-term changes in health care charges: A prospective cohort study of older adults. *Prev. Med.* 37: 319–326.

Messier, S. P., R. F. Loeser, G. D. Miller et al. 2004. Exercise and dietary weight loss in overweight and obese older adults with knee osteoarthritis. The Arthritis, Diet, and Activity Promotion Trial. *Arthritis Rheum.* 50: 1501–1510.

National Council on Aging. 2010. Evidence-based Programs. http://www.healthyagingprograms.org/content.asp?sectionid=32 (accessed January 14, 2011).

Physical Activity Guidelines Advisory Committee. 2008. *Physical Activity Guidelines Advisory Committee Report, 2008.* Washington, DC: U.S. Department of Health and Human Services.

Pope, A. M., and A. R. Tarlov. 1991. *Disability in America. Toward a National Agenda for Prevention.* Washington, D.C.: National Academy Press.

Project Enhance. 2010. About EnhanceFitness. http://www.projectenhance.org/ind_ef_aboutclass.html (access January 14, 2011).

Robertson, M. C., A. J. Campbell, M. M. Gardner et al. 2002. Preventing injuries in older people by preventing falls: A meta-analysis of individual-level data. *J. Am. Geriatr. Soc.* 50: 905–911.

Stampfer, M. J., F. B. Hu, J. E. Manson et al. 2000. Primary prevention of coronary heart disease in women through diet and lifestyle. *New Engl. J. Med.* 343: 16–22.

Stanford Patient Education Research Center. 2010. Chronic disease self-management program. http://patienteducation.stanford.edu/programs/cdsmp.html (accessed January 14, 2011).

Stevens, J. A., and E. D. Sogolow. 2008. *Preventing Falls: What Works. A CDC Compendium of Effective Community-Based Interventions from Around the World.* Atlanta, GA: Centers for Disease Control and Prevention, National Center for Injury Prevention and Control.

Stevens, J. A., P. S. Corso, E. A. Finkelstein et al. 2006. The costs of fatal and nonfatal falls among older adults. *Injury Prev.* 12: 290–295.

The Cooper Institute. 2010. Curricula/programs. Active Living Every Day (ALED). http://www.cooperinstitute.org/personal-training-education/health-fitness-consulting/curricula.cfm (access January 14, 2011).

The LIFE Study Investigators. 2006. Effects of a physical activity intervention on measures of physical performance: Results of the Lifestyle Interventions and Independence for Elders Pilot (LIFE-P) study. *J. Gerontol. Med. Sci.* 61A: 1157–1165.

Troiano, R. P., D. Berrigan, K. W. Dodd et al. 2008. Physical activity in the United States measured by accelerometer. *Med. Sci. Sports Exerc.* 40: 181–188.

U.S. Census Bureau. 2008. Percent distribution of the projected population by selected age groups and sex for the United States: 2010 to 2050. http://www.census.gov/population/www/projections/summarytables.html (accessed January 14, 2011).

U.S. Department of Health and Human Services. 1996. *Physical Activity and Health: A Report of the Surgeon General.* Atlanta, GA: U.S. Department of Health and Human Services, Centers for Disease Control and Prevention, National Center for Chronic Disease Prevention and Health Promotion.

U.S. Preventive Services Task Force. 2002. Behavioral counseling in primary care to promote physical activity. http://www.uspreventiveservicestaskforce.org/uspstf/uspsphys.htm (accessed January 14, 2011).

U.S. Preventive Services Task Force. 2004. Screening for coronary heart disease. http://www.uspreventiveservicestaskforce.org/uspstf/uspsacad.htm (accessed January 14, 2011).

Vita, A. J., R. B. Terry, H. B. Hubert et al. 1998. Aging, health risks, and cumulative disability. *New Engl. J. Med.* 338: 1035–1041.

Wilcox, S., M. Dowda, L. C. Leviton et al. 2008. Active for life. Final results from the translation of two physical activity programs. *Am. J. Prev. Med.* 35: 340–351.

10 Physical Activity and Obesity

Catrine Tudor-Locke

CONTENTS

INTRODUCTION

It is difficult to overlook the fact that there is a worldwide obesity epidemic. Various media bombard us regularly with messages about this condition and its widespread effects. We are first-hand witnesses to the phenomenon, and quite possibly are also among those who are now (or will be) counted as overweight or obese. The relationship between physical activity and obesity is complex; however, the purpose of this chapter is to define important terms and provide an introduction to select relevant current topics: an overview of the obesity epidemic; an introduction to the notion of creeping obesity; a review of the role of physical activity in preventing weight gain, promoting weight loss, and preventing weight regain; a discussion of the relationships between sedentary behavior and obesity, and also walking and obesity; and an introduction to the fitness-versus-fatness debate.

DEFINITIONS

It is necessary to provide clear definitions of the concepts used repeatedly in this chapter. *Physical activity* is "any bodily movement produced by skeletal muscles that results in energy expenditure," whereas *exercise* is "a subcategory of physical activity defined as planned, structured movement undertaken to improve or maintain one or more aspects of physical fitness" (Caspersen, Powell, and Christenson 1985). Physical activity dimensions have been described in terms of frequency (typically expressed as the number of sessions per week or bouts per day), intensity (expressed as METs [metabolic equivalent], or as a rate, e.g., kilocalories/hour), duration (minutes/day, minutes/week, hours/week), or an aggregated estimate of volume typically derived from these elements (MET-min or MET level of an activity multiplied by its duration in minutes, MET-hours or MET level multiplied by hours, PALs or physical activity level defined as total energy expenditure divided by resting energy expenditure, or total kilocalories expended). Subcategories of leisure-time, occupational, transportation, and domestic physical activity have been studied. *Walking* is bipedal locomotion undertaken for any purpose (e.g., for transport, exercise, in the course of occupation or domestic duties). *Sedentary behavior* refers to any activity, characterized by minimal body movement, that does not substantially increase energy expenditure (Pate, O'Neill, and Lobelo 2008). Examples include sleeping, eating, standing still (e.g., waiting in line), sitting, television viewing, reading, working on a computer, talking on a phone, and passive commuting (e.g., riding on a train or in a car). *Sedentarism* attempts to capture a lifestyle pattern lacking in physical activity and is primarily characterized by sedentary behaviors (Tudor-Locke and Myers 2001). Sedentarism has been inferred according to comparatively low levels of total energy expenditure, time or distance walked, or stairs climbed, through lack of self-reported participation in vigorous leisure activities (including sports and exercise), failing to achieve minimal public health guidelines, taking less than 5000 pedometer-determined steps/day (Tudor-Locke and Bassett 2004), and most recently generating less than 100 activity/counts per minute as monitored by an accelerometer (Matthews et al. 2008). *Energy expenditure* is not synonymous with physical activity. It is the metabolic cost of living and reflects the thermic effect of feeding as well as sex, age, and body mass effects on resting metabolic rate, physical activity, and posture (Lamonte and Ainsworth 2001).

Body mass index (BMI) is a density measure (computed as weight in kilograms divided by height in square meters) used to make inferences about body composition. An overweight adult is typically defined as having a BMI ≥ 25 kg/m^2 but less than 30 kg/m^2, and obesity is ≥ 30 kg/m^2 (National Institutes of Health 1998). The limitations of BMI as an indicator of body fatness/obesity include the fact that it underestimates body fat in individuals who have lost muscle mass and overestimates body fat in athletes (because of their increased muscularity) (National Institutes of Health 1998). Despite this individual-level caveat, BMI continues to be used as an important measure of overweight and obesity in population-level studies of relative risk of disease (National Institutes of Health 1998).

Overweight and obesity are distinctly different conditions. Obviously, they differ in body composition indicators such as body weight, circumference measures, and percentage of body fat. Fundamentally, however, obesity requires a pronounced positive energy balance (i.e., an energy imbalance favoring energy intake over energy expenditure) that has been sustained for a prolonged period (Bouchard and Katzmarzyk 2010). Obese individuals have a much higher resting metabolic rate (and also overall energy expenditure rate) than normal-weight or overweight individuals (Elbelt et al. 2010), attributed primarily to the energy requirements of their much larger mass. Overweight can theoretically be achieved with a reduction in energy expenditure without any change in energy intake. However, the sustained and pronounced positive energy balance underlying obesity is believed to require both hyperphagia (i.e., overeating) and relatively reduced energy expenditure caused by both a lack of physical activity and increased time spent in sedentary behaviors (Bouchard and Katzmarzyk 2010).

Cardiometabolic risk communicates a composite risk profile reflective of both cardiovascular disease and diabetes. It includes traditional risk factors such as genetic susceptibility, sex, age, smoking, blood pressure, and cholesterol, as well as emerging risk factors that include visceral adiposity, insulin resistance, dsylipidemia, and the metabolic syndrome (itself a combination of abdominal obesity, dysfunctional glucose metabolism, dyslipidemia, and elevated blood pressure) (Janiszewski and Ross 2009).

OBESITY EPIDEMIC

The prevalence of adult obesity based on response to the Behavioral Risk Factor Surveillance System (BRFSS) increased from 12.0% in 1991 (Mokdad et al. 1999) to 19.8% in 2000 (Mokdad et al. 2001). In 2001, the U.S. Surgeon General issued a report advocating a focus on *preventing and decreasing* the growing epidemic of overweight and obesity that threatens the health and welfare of our nation (U.S. Department of Health and Human Services 2001). Despite the urgency of this call to action, the 2007 BRFSS indicated that overall obesity had risen to 25.6% (Centers for Disease Control and Prevention 2008), providing continuing evidence of an epidemic trend. All of these preceding estimates were based on self-reported data. Flegal et al. (2010) recently reported that although prevalence of obesity was 32.2% and 35.5% among adult men and women, respectively, the prevalence does not seem to be continuing at the same rate over the past 10 years. Regardless of whether the increasing prevalence has slowed down, it is still high and the lifetime medical and financial burden of overweight and obesity underscore the need to continue to invest in prevention efforts (Wang et al. 2008). The best approach to the continuing problem is to prevent it by strategies aimed at prevention and attenuation of weight gain (U.S. Department of Health and Human Services 2001).

CREEPING OBESITY

Creeping obesity is a colloquial phrase that attempts to capture the insidious and incremental weight gain that accumulates over time and results in overweight or obesity. Annual average weight gains (resulting from small chronic excesses of energy intake over energy expenditure) of 0.5–1.0 kg can be expected (Burke et al. 1996). In a study of the prevalence of weight fluctuations in a community sample (age 20–45 years), more than half (53.7%) gained weight within 12 months (Crawford, Jeffery, and French 2000). In a related study, 9.3% of this population experienced large weight gains (≥5% of initial body weight) in 1 year of observation (Jeffery, McGuire, and French 2002). A study that combined three observational cohorts (Coronary Artery Risk Development in Young Adults, Atherosclerosis Risk in Communities Study and Cardiovascular Health Study) to study BMI change between 1989 and 1996 in adults reported that the mean change was approximately 0.1 unit/year greater than that from previous representative, longitudinal measurements collected in the United States between 1971 and 1984 (Kahn and Cheng 2008), suggesting that the rate of weight gain has also increased over time. It is logical to pursue prevention and attenuation of this type of weight gain if we are to implement strategies aimed at preempting and/or reversing the obesity epidemic.

ROLE OF PHYSICAL ACTIVITY IN PREVENTING WEIGHT GAIN

At its simplest level, energy balance is achieved when energy intake (i.e., diet) and energy expenditure are in equilibrium. The National Health and Nutrition Examination Survey (NHANES) indicates that dietary energy intakes have increased over the past 30 years; exact values of change in kilocalories are hampered by survey method changes (Kant, Graubard, and Kumanyika 2007). However, at least some of this increase can be explained by the fact that collectively Americans are also larger people. Mean BMI has increased 2–4 units over the same period (Wang, Colditz, and Kuntz 2007), and increased dietary intake is necessary to maintain energy balance (i.e., basal requirements are greater) in this altered state. Modest decreases in energy intake (on the order of 100 kcal/day, roughly equivalent to a single slice of bread) have been recommended as part of a program designed to prevent weight gain (Hill et al. 2003). It is important to emphasize that this magnitude of energy decrease is not likely to produce significant weight loss; rather, its prescription is implicitly aimed at prevention and attenuation of weight gain.

Another potential culprit that contributes to creeping obesity is reduced physical activity. However, self-reported participation in leisure-time physical activity has remained relatively stable over time (Centers for Disease Control and Prevention 2001) and actually appears to have increased slightly as recently as between 2001 and 2005 (Centers for Disease Control and Prevention 2007), even amid evidence of increasing trends for overweight and obesity of epidemic proportions. Although this apparent paradox would seem to point exclusively toward dietary indiscretion as the principal cause of the obesity epidemic (McCrory, Suen, and Roberts 2002), it remains possible that relatively small population gains in leisure-time physical activity may insufficiently compensate for diminished alternative sources of energy expenditure. For example, there have been obvious societal shifts in work-related energy demands (shifting over time from heavy labor to sedentary occupations), mechanization of domestic tasks with widespread adoption of labor-saving devices, short-distance transportation mode choices and patterns (replacing walking and bicycling with motorized travel), and an almost universal preference for passive leisure time pursuits, including television watching and engaging in other technology-based sedentary behaviors.

One strategy in the battle against the obesity epidemic is to prevent primary weight gain (U.S. Department of Health and Human Services 2001). Since weight gain over time is the normative trend, and body weight itself is not stable from day to day, healthy weight changes can be observed as (1) no change over time (i.e., weight stability defined generally as a change of 3.2 kg or less, or less than 3% change in body weight; Physical Activity Guidelines Advisory Committee 2008); (2) modest weight loss, which then must be defined as at least 3% decrease in body weight), or (3) even modest gain if attenuated compared to a control group. The U.S. Physical Activity Guidelines Committee recently issued a report (2008) that included a review of studies of weight stability and weight loss. Based on short-term clinical trials, a dose of physical activity in the range of 13–26 MET-h/week produced a modest 1–3% weight loss, consistent with strategies aimed at preventing weight gain. The committee identified 13 MET-h/week as equivalent to walking at a 4 mile/h pace for 150 min/week or jogging at a 6 mile/h pace for 75 min/week. The American College of Sports Medicine (ACSM) recently issued a position stand that included a statement that between 150 and 250 min/week of moderate intensity physical activity is effective in preventing weight gain (i.e., a weight gain greater than 3%) (Donnelly et al. 2009).

The current evidence of efficacy of weight gain prevention interventions is based on a very small number of studies (Lemmens et al. 2008). These have not necessarily considered other healthy weight change outcomes including modest weight loss and weight gain attenuation. Furthermore, those that have included a physical activity component have focused primarily on structured exercise undertaken as leisure-time physical activity (Lemmens et al. 2008). The continued limited focus on leisure-time physical activity as the sole intervenable opportunity confines a relatively large requisite energy expenditure (e.g., 1200 to 2000 kcal/week) (Donnelly et al. 2009) to a limited amount of personal time, conjuring questions about sustainability. An alternative, or perhaps an adjunctive, prevention strategy is to focus on nonexercise activity thermogenesis (or NEAT) that represents energy expenditures of all physical activities *excluding* volitional sports or exercise (Levine 2007). A "whole day" approach, which includes leisure-time physical activity, but also extends to other everyday activities (i.e., work, chores, transportation) offers a logically optimal strategy. The ACSM position stand (Donnelly et al. 2009) focused on appropriate physical activity weight management interventions indicated that "it is reasonable to conclude that increasing lifestyle physical activity should be a strategy included in weight management efforts."

ROLE OF PHYSICAL ACTIVITY IN WEIGHT LOSS

Compared to studying prevention of weight gain, there is much more research examining the role of physical activity in weight loss. Overall, weight loss achieved from physical activity alone has been modest when compared to that produced from dietary intervention alone.

A reasonable weight loss goal is 10% of body weight over a 6-month period (National Institutes of Health 1998). This can be achieved from a negative energy balance produced by eliciting an energy deficit of 300–500 kcal/day (or 0.5 to 1 lb/week if BMI is between 27 and 35 kg/m^2 at baseline) or 500–1000 kcal/day (or 1–2 lb/week if BMI is >35 kg/m^2 at baseline) through manipulations of energy intake and energy expenditure (National Institutes of Health 1998). The magnitude of this energy deficit has also been called the "energy gap" (Hill et al. 2003), and the greater the gap, the greater the weight loss. The personal time, attention, and work required to achieve this magnitude of energy deficit differs greatly between physical activity and dietary intervention strategies. For example, choosing not to indulge in a

200-kcal donut may be comparatively less personally challenging than choosing to go for a brisk walk for $\cong$40 min (150 lb individual, 3.5 miles/h pace). The amount of physical activity required to achieve an energy deficit of 500–1000 kcal/day may be difficult for most people to sustain in the long term. That being said, physical activity can potentiate weight loss effects of moderate dietary intervention (e.g., dietary restrictions of 500–700 kcal) strategies, and therefore both strategies are commonly recommended (Donnelly et al. 2009). The ACSM position statement (Donnelly et al. 2009) concluded that <150 min/week of physical activity produces minimal weight loss, >150 min/week produces a modest weight loss of approximately 2–3 kg, and 225–420 min/week can produce a 5–7.5 kg weight loss, clearly illustrating a dose–response effect for physical activity and weight loss. Furthermore, physical activity provides additional health effects, including preservation of fat-free mass, and enhanced cardiometabolic risk profile.

ROLE OF PHYSICAL ACTIVITY IN PREVENTING WEIGHT REGAIN

Unfortunately, weight regain is a normative occurrence after weight loss. Physical activity remains a premiere strategy to combat weight regain; however, the exact amount required is not clear and may vary widely for individuals. That being said, it is commonly held that "more is better," and the ACSM-issued recommendation for weight maintenance (allowing <3% fluctuation) following weight loss is approximately 60 min (or 4 miles) of walking per day at a moderate intensity (Donnelly et al. 2009).

SEDENTARY BEHAVIOR AND OBESITY

Data from the American Time Use Survey shows that the most frequently reported nonwork, nonsleep sedentary ($1.0 \leq MET < 1.6$) activity is watching television/movies (80.1%), second only to eating and drinking (95.6%) (Tudor-Locke, Johnson, and Katzmarzyk 2010). Furthermore, almost 60% of U.S. adults appear to watch more than 2 h of television a day (Bowman 2006). In fact, time spent watching television has often been used as a proxy indicator of sedentary behaviors in research just because it is so ubiquitous (Pate, O'Neill, and Lobelo 2008). In a study of more than 14,000 men and women stratified according to self-reported hours spent watching television or engaging in vigorous physical activity, those who watched comparatively more television and were the least active had higher BMI and blood pressure values compared to those who watched little television and were the most active (Jakes et al. 2003). Interestingly, the apparently protective effects of vigorous activity participation observed in this study were reduced with increasing time spent watching television.

Television watching has also been associated with weight gain in longitudinal studies. For example, male health professionals who reported watching 21 h or more of television per week in 1988 were more than 40% more likely to become overweight 2 years later than those who watched 1 h or less per week (Ching et al. 1996). In more than 50,000 women followed up for 6 years, a dose–response relationship between television watching and development of obesity was observed such that each

2 h/day increment in television watching was associated with an additional 23% increase in risk of obesity (Hu et al. 2003).

Weight regain following a weight loss can also been impacted by television watching. Based on data from adults who had reported weight loss the previous year in the 1999–2002 NHANES, those who averaged 4 h or more of television watching a day were twice as likely to report subsequent weight regain compared to those who averaged less than 1 h/day (Weiss et al. 2007). The National Weight Control Registry has also shown that high baseline levels of television watching and also increases in television watching are independently associated with weight regain over 1 year (Raynor et al. 2006).

WALKING AND OBESITY

Simply walking, undertaken during the course of the day in transportation, occupation, shopping, chores, walking a dog, and during leisure-time (for nonexercise purposes) is a clear example of the "whole day" approach to physical activity accumulation described above. To emphasize, walking for exercise is a purposefully undertaken physical activity behavior typically performed in a single, somewhat lengthy (30 to 70 min representing 25th and 75th percentiles for time) bout (Tudor-Locke et al. 2005). As such, its saliency makes it more easily detected using traditional physical activity assessment approaches that focus on leisure-time activities. Unfortunately, incidental, intermittent, and irregular accumulation of walking as part of day-to-day living is more difficult to distinguish using these same approaches. However, analysis of the American Time Use data has shown that, on any given day in 2003–2004, only 4.8% of Americans walked for exercise, but 31.6% walked for shopping purposes, 12% walked for transportation, 4.4% engaged in other transportation-related walking, and 2.5% walked the dog (Tudor-Locke and Ham 2008). Walking, in all its forms and purposes, provides ample opportunity for cumulative energy expenditure unshackled by intensity or bout duration requirements. At least in terms of energy balance, it is logical that every step counts.

There is an inverse cross-sectional relationship between steps/day and both BMI and waist circumference (Dwyer et al. 2007). Modeling the relationship showed that, for men habitually taking only 2000 steps/day, an extra 2000 steps/day was associated with a 2.8-cm reduction in waist circumference compared with a 0.7-cm reduction for men already walking 10,000 steps/day. For women, the potential differences in waist circumference were 2.2 cm and 0.6 cm, respectively, for a 2000-step addition to either 2000 steps/day or 10,000 steps/day. For each habitual level of steps/day, additional steps were associated with incrementally improved waist circumference and BMI measures. However, the greatest relative benefits (in terms of both waist circumference and BMI) were still apparent with relatively small increases at the lowest habitual levels of steps/day. A separate cross-sectional analysis of adult data combined from Australia, Canada, France, Sweden, and the United States showed that a normal BMI in adults was associated with at least 11,000 to 12,000 steps/day in men and 8000 to 12,000 steps/day in women, and was consistently higher for younger people (Tudor-Locke et al. 2008).

A meta-analysis of 24 randomized and controlled walking (no dietary change) trials (mean duration, 34.9 weeks; mean total volume of walking, 188.8 min/week) produced estimated reductions in body weight (1.1%; on the order of 0.2 kg to 2.0 kg) and BMI (1.9%) (Murphy et al. 2007). In all but one of the studies reviewed, control groups increased body weight by 0.1 kg to 4.2 kg. In a separate meta-analysis focused on pedometer-based programs, Richardson et al. (2008) reported that participants engaged in nine randomized and controlled programs increased their activity by 1800–4500 steps/day (from baseline values between ≅4700 and 7000 steps/day) and lost a modest amount of weight (on the order of approximately 0.05 kg/week). Most pedometer-based interventions to date have focused on relatively short-term changes over 4–16 weeks; however, there is a strong negative relationship between study duration and resulting weight loss, indicating that benefits are potentiated with prolonged adherence (Richardson et al. 2008). Miyatake et al. (2002) followed 31 Japanese males who were instructed to increase their daily steps. Visceral adipose tissue was reduced and daily walking expressed as steps/day was found to be a greater predictor of its reduction compared to changes in exercise capacity at a 1-year examination. McTiernan et al. (2007) conducted a yearlong exercise trial and reported that both male and female participants who achieved the greatest incremental steps/day changes assessed at 12 months from baseline also realized the greatest improvements in weight, hip circumference, BMI, body fat, and intraabdominal fat.

Although these change magnitudes may appear minor in comparison to results from weight loss studies that have included low calorie and very low calorie diets as well as surgical interventions (American Dietetic Association 2009), they are vitally important to preventing, maintaining, reversing (through modest weight loss), or attenuating the insidious weight gain that leads to the problem in the first place. To be clear, interventions focused on walking produce a modest weight change that accumulates over time and prevents the weight gain typical of unintervened populations (Slentz et al. 2004).

FITNESS AND FATNESS

Evidence supports the independent effects of physical activity on health outcomes that extend beyond the effects of body weight, or even weight loss. For example, fitness has been linked inversely with mortality regardless of BMI-defined weight status (Lee, Blair, and Jackson 1999). It is likely that fitness and fatness have related but also different effects on health. In a large study of more than 5,000 overweight and obese individuals with type 2 diabetes (Wing et al. 2007), BMI categories and fitness quintiles were related. However, when considered together (adjusted for age, race, smoking, and diabetes duration), HbA1c (an indicator of diabetes control), ankle-brachial index (an indicator of cardiovascular health), and a cardiovascular risk score were more strongly associated with fitness. However, systolic blood pressure was more strongly related to fatness.

Although physical activity alone can elicit modest weight loss, and can also amplify weight loss when combined with dietary intervention, physical activity can also improve cardiometabolic risk profiles in the absence of weight change. For example, it is apparent that 3 months of regular physical activity (approximately

40–60 min/day) can produce 10–19% reductions in visceral fat despite no significant changes in body weight (Janiszewski and Ross 2009). In addition, improvements in insulin sensitivity, blood pressure, HbA1c, HDL cholesterol, and triglycerides can occur with chronic exercise even without significant weight change.

CONCLUSION

Physical activity encompasses the full range of human movement, including but not limited to exercise, and results in energy expenditure. A positive energy balance (favoring energy intake over energy balance) leads to weight gain. Physical activity plays an important role in preventing weight gain, facilitating weight loss, and preventing weight regain after weight loss. Sedentary behavior (e.g., television watching) produces minimal energy expenditure and thus is a concern in terms of weight gain, weight loss, and weight regain prevention. Walking (in all its forms) represents an accessible, feasible, acceptable, and sustainable physical activity. The benefits of a physically active lifestyle extend far beyond simple manipulations of energy balance.

STUDY QUESTIONS

1. Explain the meaning of the concept, "It is better to be fit and fat than lean and not fit," to an adult who has had trouble maintaining weight loss.
2. Compare and contrast the energy expenditure of obese and normal weight individuals during sedentary and active conditions.
3. Distinguish the differences in light, moderate, and vigorous intensity physical activity in inducing an energy deficit.
4. How is it possible to engage in recommended amounts of moderate-to vigorous-intensity leisure-time physical activity but still gain weight?
5. Why is the physical activity recommendation for preventing weight gain more than the recommendation for weight loss?
6. Why is walking an effective physical activity choice for preventing weight gain, promoting weight loss, and preventing weight regain after weight loss?

REFERENCES

American Dietetic Association. 2009. Position of the American Dietetic Association: Weight management. *J. Am. Diet Assoc.* 109: 330–346.

Bouchard, C., and P. T. Katzmarzyk. 2010. Defintion and assessement of physical activity and obesity: Introduction. In *Physical Activity and Obesity*, ed. C. Bouchard and P. T. Katzmarzyk. Champaign, IL: Human Kinetics.

Bowman, S. A. 2006. Television-viewing characteristics of adults: Correlations to eating practices and overweight and health status. *Prev. Chronic Dis.* 3: A38.

Burke, G. L., D. E. Bild, J. E. Hilner et al. 1996. Differences in weight gain in relation to race, gender, age and education in young adults: The CARDIA Study. Coronary Artery Risk Development in Young Adults. *Ethnicity Health* 1: 327–335.

Caspersen, C. J., K. E. Powell, and G. M. Christenson. 1985. Physical activity, exercise, and physical fitness: Definitions and distinctions for health-related research. *Public Health Rep.* 100: 126–131.

Centers for Disease Control and Prevention. 2001. Physical activity trends—United States, 1990–1998. *Morb. Mortal. Wkly. Rep.* 50: 166–169.

Centers for Disease Control and Prevention. 2007. Prevalence of regular physical activity among adults—United States, 2001 and 2005. *Morb. Mortal. Wkly. Rep.* 56: 1209–1212.

Centers for Disease Control and Prevention. 2008. State-specific prevalence of obesity among adults—United States, 2007. *MMWR Morb. Mortal. Wkly. Rep.* 57: 765–768.

Ching, P. L., W. C. Willett, E. B. Rimm et al. 1996. Activity level and risk of overweight in male health professionals. *Am. J. Public Health* 86: 25–30.

Crawford, D., R. W. Jeffery, and S. A. French. 2000. Can anyone successfully control their weight? Findings of a three year community-based study of men and women. *Int. J. Obes. Relat. Metab. Disord.* 24: 1107–1110.

Donnelly, J. E., S. N. Blair, J. M. Jakicic et al. 2009. American College of Sports Medicine position stand. Appropriate physical activity intervention strategies for weight loss and prevention of weight regain for adults. *Med. Sci. Sports Exerc.* 41: 459–471.

Dwyer, T., D. Hosmer, T. Hosmer et al. 2007. The inverse relationship between number of steps per day and obesity in a population-based sample: The AusDiab study. *Int. J. Obes.* 31: 797–804.

Elbelt, U., T. Schuetz, I. Hoffmann et al. 2010. Differences of energy expenditure and physical activity patterns in subjects with various degrees of obesity. *Clin. Nutr.* 29: 766–772.

Flegal, K. M., M. D. Carroll, C. L. Ogden et al. 2010. Prevalence and trends in obesity among U.S. adults, 1999–2008. *JAMA* 303: 235–241.

Hill, J. O., H. R. Wyatt, G. W. Reed et al. 2003. Obesity and the environment: Where do we go from here? *Science* 299: 853–855.

Hu, F. B., T. Y. Li, G. A. Colditz et al. 2003. Television watching and other sedentary behaviors in relation to risk of obesity and type 2 diabetes mellitus in women. *JAMA* 289: 1785–1791.

Jakes, R. W., N. E. Day, K. T. Khaw et al. 2003. Television viewing and low participation in vigorous recreation are independently associated with obesity and markers of cardiovascular disease risk: EPIC-Norfolk population-based study. *Eur. J. Clin. Nutr.* 57: 1089–1096.

Janiszewski, P. M., and R. Ross. 2009. The utility of physical activity in the management of global cardiometabolic risk. *Obesity* 17: S3–S14.

Jeffery, R. W., M. T. McGuire, and S. A. French. 2002. Prevalence and correlates of large weight gains and losses. *Int. J. Obes. Relat. Metab. Disord.* 26(7): 969–972.

Kahn, H. S., and Y. J. Cheng. 2008. Longitudinal changes in BMI and in an index estimating excess lipids among white and black adults in the United States. *Int. J. Obes.* 32: 136–143.

Kant, A. K., B. I. Graubard, and S. K. Kumanyika. 2007. Trends in black–white differentials in dietary intakes of U.S. adults, 1971–2002. *Am. J. Health Promot.* 32: 264–272.

Lamonte, M. J., and B. E. Ainsworth. 2001. Quantifying energy expenditure and physical activity in the context of dose response. *Med. Sci. Sports Exerc.* 33: S370–S378; discussion S419–S420.

Lee, C. D., S. N. Blair, and A. S. Jackson. 1999. Cardiorespiratory fitness, body composition, and all-cause and cardiovascular disease mortality in men. *Am. J. Clin. Nutr.* 69: 373–380.

Lemmens, V. E., A. Oenema, K. I. Klepp et al. 2008. A systematic review of the evidence regarding efficacy of obesity prevention interventions among adults. *Obes. Rev.* 9: 446–455.

Levine, J. A. 2007. Nonexercise activity thermogenesis—liberating the life-force. *J. Intern. Med.* 262: 273–287.

Matthews, C. E., K. Y. Chen, P. S. Freedson et al. 2008. Amount of time spent in sedentary behaviors in the United States, 2003–2004. *Am. J. Epidemiol.* 167: 875–881.

McCrory, M. A., V. M. Suen, and S. B. Roberts. 2002. Biobehavioral influences on energy intake and adult weight gain. *J. Nutr.* 132: 3830S–3834S.

McTiernan, A., B. Sorensen, M. L. Irwin et al. 2007. Exercise effect on weight and body fat in men and women. *Obesity* 15: 1496–1512.

Miyatake, N., H. Nishikawa, A. Morishita et al. 2002. Daily walking reduces visceral adipose tissue areas and improves insulin resistance in Japanese obese subjects. *Diabetes Res. Clin. Proc.* 58: 101–107.

Mokdad, A. H., B. A. Bowman, E. S. Ford et al. 2001. The continuing epidemics of obesity and diabetes in the United States. *JAMA* 286: 1195–1200.

Mokdad, A. H., M. K. Serdula, W. H. Dietz et al. 1999. The spread of the obesity epidemic in the United States, 1991–1998. *JAMA* 282: 1519–1522.

Murphy, M. H., A. M. Nevill, E. M. Murtagh et al. 2007. The effect of walking on fitness, fatness and resting blood pressure: A meta-analysis of randomised, controlled trials. *Prev. Med.* 44: 377–385.

National Institutes of Health. 1998. *Clinical Guidelines on the Identification, Evaluation, and Treatment of Overweight and Obesity in Adults: The Evidence Report.* Rockville, MD: National Institutes of Health.

Pate, R. R., J. R. O'Neill, and F. Lobelo. 2008. The evolving definition of "sedentary." *Exerc. Sport Sci. Rev.* 36: 173–178.

Physical Activity Guidelines Advisory Committee. 2008. *Physical Activity Guidelines Advisory Committee Report, 2008.* Washington, D.C.: U.S. Department of Health and Human Services.

Raynor, D. A., S. Phelan, J. O. Hill et al. 2006. Television viewing and long-term weight maintenance: Results from the National Weight Control Registry. *Obesity* 14: 1816–1824.

Richardson, C. R., T. L. Newton, J. J. Abraham et al. 2008. A meta-analysis of pedometer-based walking interventions and weight loss. *Ann. Fam. Med.* 6: 69–77.

Slentz, C. A., B. D. Duscha, J. L. Johnson et al. 2004. Effects of the amount of exercise on body weight, body composition, and measures of central obesity: STRRIDE—a randomized controlled study. *Arch. Intern. Med.* 164: 31–39.

Tudor-Locke, C., and D. R. Bassett Jr. 2004. How many steps/day are enough? Preliminary pedometer indices for public health. *Sports Med.* 34: 1–8.

Tudor-Locke, C., D. R. Bassett Jr., W. J. Rutherford et al. 2008. BMI-referenced cut points for pedometer-determined steps per day in adults. *J. Phys. Act. Health* 5: S126–S139.

Tudor-Locke, C., M. Bittman, D. Merom et al. 2005. Patterns of walking for transport and exercise: A novel application of time use data. *Int. J. Behav. Nutr. Phys. Act.* 2: 5.

Tudor-Locke, C., and S. A. Ham. 2008. Walking behaviors reported in the American Time Use Survey 2003–2005. *J. Phys. Act. Health* 5: 633–647.

Tudor-Locke, C., and A. M. Myers. 2001. Challenges and opportunities for measuring physical activity in sedentary adults. *Sports Med.* 31: 91–100.

Tudor-Locke, C., W. D. Johnson, and P. T. Katzmarzyk. 2010. Frequently reported activities by intensity for U.S. adults: The American Time Use Survey. *Am. J. Prev. Med.* 39: e13–e20.

U.S. Department of Health and Human Services. 2001. *The Surgeon General's Call to Action to Prevent and Decrease Overweight and Obesity.* Rockville, MD: U.S. Department of Health and Human Services, Public Health Service, Office of the Surgeon General.

Wang, Y., M. A. Beydoun, L. Liang et al. 2008. Will all Americans become overweight or obese? Estimating the progression and cost of the U.S. obesity epidemic. *Obesity* 16: 2323–2330.

Wang, Y. C., G. A. Colditz, and K. M. Kuntz, 2007. Forecasting the obesity epidemic in the aging U.S. population. *Obesity* 15: 2855–2865.

Weiss, E. C., D. A. Galuska, L. Kettel Khan et al. 2007. Weight regain in U.S. adults who experienced substantial weight loss, 1999–2002. *Am. J. Prev. Med.* 33: 34–40.

Wing, R. R., J. Jakicic, R. Neiberg et al. 2007. Fitness, fatness, and cardiovascular risk factors in type 2 diabetes: Look ahead study. *Med. Sci. Sports Exerc.* 39: 2107–2116.

11 Physical Activity Measurement

Stephen D. Herrmann

CONTENTS

INTRODUCTION

This chapter provides an overview of methods used to measure physical activity in public health surveillance and to assess recommended levels of physical activity for health. As a health-enhancing behavior, researchers and public health professionals are interested in knowing how to measure physical activity to identify changes in physical activity following intervention studies and community programs and how to determine the prevalence of physical activity and inactivity for use in surveillance systems. Historically, physical activity was most commonly measured by subjective self-reports of structured exercise. The types of activities measured reflected knowledge about the dose and volume of vigorous intensity exercise that led to improvements in cardiorespiratory fitness. Following dissemination about the benefits of moderate-intensity exercise on reducing risks for chronic diseases and premature mortality, surveillance of physical activity expanded to include self-reports of moderate- and vigorous-intensity physical activity (Macera et al. 2005; Pate et al. 1995). Advances in the use of accelerometers (devices that measure accelerations, or movement) to record movement by intensity and duration has expanded the measurement of physical activity to include objective methods, in addition to subjective self-report questionnaires, to measure physical activity in surveillance settings. This chapter provides an overview of subjective and objective methods used to measure physical activity in public health surveillance and to assess recommended levels of physical activity for health.

SUBJECTIVE MEASURES

Self-reported physical activity instruments include activity logbooks, diaries, recall questionnaires, and voice recorders. These self-report options use a person's ability to recall their activities from a specified period (e.g., 24 h, 7 days, 1 year) or record their activities throughout the day (e.g., every 30 min). Self-report instruments are relatively inexpensive, generally easy to administer and complete, and oftentimes provide additional information about the context of the physical activity (i.e., information about when, why, and where activity occurs). Specific subjective instruments generally fall under a few broad types, including recall questionnaires, global questionnaires, quantitative history questionnaires, and logbooks.

RECALL QUESTIONNAIRES

Recall questionnaires are the most common form of physical activity assessment used in epidemiologic studies and in surveillance settings (Lamonte and Ainsworth 2001). In general, recall questionnaires provide information about physical activity over the past 24 h, week, or month, or about "usual" physical activity during a period. In about 10–20 items, recall questionnaires supply data about the type, frequency, duration, and intensity of activity (Craig et al. 2003). Such information has been used to assess physical activity in U.S. surveillance settings to include the Behavioral Risk Factors Surveillance System, the National Health Interview Survey, and the National Health and Nutrition Examination Survey (NHANES) to identify individuals who are meeting public health physical activity guidelines. Recall surveys are also frequently used in epidemiological studies to assess physical activity behaviors and health or disease outcomes (Paffenbarger, Kampert, and Lee 1997), to identify persons targeted for interventions to increase physical activity, or to assess success in improving or changing physical activity behaviors (Blair et al. 1985).

A recently developed and commonly used recall questionnaire is the International Physical Activity Questionnaire (IPAQ) (Craig et al. 2003). The IPAQ was developed to evaluate physical activity and sedentary behaviors in global surveillance settings by using a variety of physical activity domains with a short format (time in sedentary, moderate, and vigorous intensity activity and time spent walking) and a long format (time in leisure, work, household, yard, and sedentary activity, as well as self-powered transport) that could be used by telephone interview or self-administered

(Bauman et al. 2009; Craig et al. 2003). The IPAQ has been translated into approximately 20 languages and has been used in many countries worldwide (Bauman et al. 2009; Craig et al. 2003). Reliability studies have shown wide-ranging values for the test–retest reliability of the IPAQ (0.34 to 0.93) (Craig et al. 2003; Hagströmer, Oja, and Sjöström 2006). Multiple validation studies have been published on the IPAQ yielding generally positive yet relatively modest correlations with accelerometers ($r = 0.07$–0.71) (Fogelholm et al. 2006; Rzewnicki, Vanden Auweele, and De Bourdeaudhuij 2003). Resources for the IPAQ, including the questionnaire presented in several languages, can be obtained from www.ipaq.ki.se.

Some researchers have questioned the accuracy of the IPAQ as a recall questionnaire and have demonstrated substantial overreporting of physical activity levels by respondents. In 2003, Rzewnicki, Vanden Auweele, and De Bourdeaudhuij (2003) obtained physical activity information with the IPAQ and then followed up with probing participant interviews to better understand how participants responded to the questions. From these interviews, Rzewnicki, Vanden Auweele, and De Bourdeaudhuij (2003) found that nearly half of the participants reported some physical activity (walking, moderate- or vigorous intensity) on the IPAQ when they should have reported no physical activity. Therefore, approximately 50% of individuals were classified as meeting physical activity guidelines when in fact, they did not meet those guidelines because they overreported their activity. Furthermore, about 5% of respondents provided physical activity values so high that they were deemed not credible or impossible.

This overreporting of physical activity on physical activity recall questionnaires is not limited to the IPAQ. Self-reported instruments in general are often thought to suffer from inaccurate participant recall with associated errors ranging from 35% to 50% of recalled activities (Lagerros and Lagiou 2007). Overreporting of physical activity is an issue to consider when using recall questionnaires. However, other types of physical activity self-report measures have their own limitations, such as activity records and activity logs (to be described later in this chapter), which are oftentimes thought to influence the physical activity patterns being measured (Lamonte and Ainsworth 2001; Matthews et al. 2001).

Global Questionnaires

Global questionnaires are characterized by being rather short: having one to four items (Lamonte and Ainsworth 2001). The primary purpose of global questionnaires is to provide only broad classifications (e.g., active or inactive, meeting physical activity recommendations or not). Examples of global questionnaires include the Physical Activity Vital Sign (Greenwood, Joy, and Stanford 2010), the Exercise Vital Sign (Sallis 2011), the Short Telephone Activity Recall (Matthews et al. 2005), and the Stanford Brief Activity Survey (SBAS) (Taylor-Piliae et al. 2006). Although generally worded and presented differently, the one- to four-item measures aim to identify if individuals meet the physical activity recommendations for moderate- and/or vigorous-intensity physical activity (Pate et al. 1995; Haskell et al. 2007; U.S. Department of Health and Human Services 2008), rank individuals, or generally classify their behavior. The use of the Exercise Vital Sign is proposed for use in the American College of Sports Medicine's Exercise is Medicine™ campaign to increase physical activity counseling by primary care providers (Sallis 2011). The SBAS is a two-item self-administered physical activity questionnaire used to classify individuals' activity levels at work and during leisure time while reducing the burden on both the participant and administrative staff. Although global forms of subjective physical activity assessment lessen the participant burden, they also provide only limited information about a person's physical activity. What remains unknown with these global questionnaires are specific details regarding patterns of physical activity, specific time in different activity intensity levels, and the context in which the activity occurs.

Quantitative History

Quantitative history questionnaires use a more comprehensive format to acquire detailed information. These questionnaires typically evaluate physical activity using 15 to 60 items to assess frequency, intensity, and duration of activity during the past month, year, or lifetime (Taylor et al. 1978). The Minnesota Leisure Time Physical Activity Questionnaire (MNLTPAQ) was one of the first questionnaires to provide an extensive list of activities (63 sports, recreational, yard, and household activities) (Lagerros and Lagiou 2007; Taylor et al. 1978). Most of the activities are classified as moderate-intensity, ranging from 3.0 to 5.9 METs (metabolic equivalent). The MNLTPAQ was used in the Multiple Risk Factor Intervention Trial (MRFIT) to determine the relation between the dose of physical activity and the risk for all-cause mortality and cause-specific mortality (Leon et al. 1987). The 12,866 men enrolled in MRFIT were placed into three physical activity levels based on the average daily time spent in various physical activities in the past year as reported on the MNLTPAQ: low = 16 min; middle = 48 min; high = 134 min. After 7 years of follow-up, relative risks for all-cause mortality and coronary heart disease mortality were significantly higher for men with the low physical activity durations compared to the middle- and high physical activity durations, which were not different (see Figure 11.1) (Leon et al. 1987). This study shows the value of using subjective, quantitative history measures in epidemiological studies to identify the role of physical activity on morbidity and mortality outcomes.

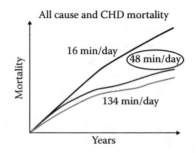

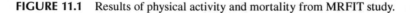

FIGURE 11.1   Results of physical activity and mortality from MRFIT study.

Although the purpose of quantitative history questionnaire format has its strength in obtaining the type and frequency of activities to calculate an estimate of energy expenditure and characterize chronic physical activity levels, the time and cost of training interviewers, contacting participants, and coding the data are significant drawbacks of this form of in-depth interviewer-assisted recall (Bouchard et al. 1983). Thus, quantitative history questionnaires are seldom used to measure physical activity in surveillance settings.

RECORDS AND LOGBOOKS

Physical activity logbooks, records, and/or diaries are used to obtain details on the type and duration of all the activities performed in a short period. Using records or diaries, individuals are instructed to keep a record of all the activities as they occur (Lamonte and Ainsworth 2001; Ainsworth et al. 2011) or at a specified time interval (e.g., 15 min) (Bouchard et al. 1983). This generated list of activities can be coded according to energy expenditure or MET value to identify physical activity patterns and understand behavior (Ainsworth et al. 2011). This format is burdensome to the participant and requires considerable effort by the researcher to code entries. Despite these limitations, physical activity records are often considered a criterion measure for subjective physical activity assessment.

A summary score can be created by summing the minutes performed at each of the 9 categories and associated MET intensity levels. This reduces some participant and researcher burden but may not be inclusive of all physical activities performed during the day, thus missing activities that are actually performed (Lagerros and Lagiou 2007; Lamonte and Ainsworth 2001). Bouchard et al. (1983) developed a checklist to identify nine physical activity behaviors performed during a 24-h period. The activities range from sleeping (#1) to vigorous exercise or work (#9) that differ by MET intensity. Every 15 min, an individual identifies the primary type of activity performed during that interval and records a number to reflect that activity in a space provided in the checklist. A summary score can be created by summing the minutes performed at each of the 9-MET intensity activities. Although an effective way to record physical activity behaviors with more detail and perceived accuracy than obtained with self-report recall questionnaires, logbooks and records can potentially alter participants' physical activity behaviors. Since the participants are more aware of their physical activity because they are recording the types of activity performed, this increased awareness may cause them to change their physical activity behavior.

OBJECTIVE MEASURES

Objective measures of physical activity include pedometers, accelerometers, heart rate monitors, indirect calorimetry, and doubly labeled water. These instruments and methods objectively quantify activity or physiological responses to physical activity. When used appropriately, objective measures are helpful in quantifying physical activity; however, there are some limitations in their abilities to record all aspects of physical activity, such as context or type and location of movement. The cost of these objective instruments can vary, ranging from only a couple of dollars, to thousands of dollars. Some instruments require expert knowledge and special software to use and evaluate the data. Additionally, these devices can increase the burden on an individual by requiring them to wear a monitor attached to their body or clothing or visit a laboratory where the measurements can be initiated.

ACTIVITY MONITORS

Pedometers and accelerometers have become an increasingly popular objective method for physical activity assessment. A recent search in PubMed returned 1696 articles for "accelerometer" and 603 articles for "pedometer" published from January 2001 to January 2011. The search during 1990 through 2000 returned only 75 articles for "pedometer" and 378 articles for "accelerometer."

PEDOMETERS

Pedometers have become a widely used tool for assessing walking (Bassett et al. 2010; Beets et al. 2010; Craig et al. 2010). These devices often range in price from only a few dollars up to $200 depending on the internal mechanism and device options (i.e., memory, software) (Schneider, Crouter, and Bassett 2004). The primary outcome measure is a step count that allows for some pedometers to estimate distance walked (from stride length [distance = steps × stride length]), energy expended in movement, and activity intensity (from step rate in steps min^{-1}). Pedometers are generally accurate in counting steps within 3% of actual steps taken (Schneider et al. 2003) and become less accurate for estimating distance, and even less accurate for estimating energy expenditure (Crouter et al. 2003). However, significant variation can be found because of the internal mechanism and sensitivity causing under- or overestimation by 25–45% (Schneider, Crouter, and Bassett 2004; Schneider et al. 2003). To minimize this error, it is important for researchers and clinicians to be aware of the reliability and validity evidence for the devices they use.

Pedometers function from a few different internal mechanisms: horizontal spring-lever, magnetic reed proximity switch, or a piezoelectric mechanism. The horizontal spring-lever mechanism responds to vertical movements at the hip by swinging the lever up and down to close an electrical circuit (Schneider et al. 2003). When the lever makes contact, it counts the steps and oftentimes produces an audible "click," which can be an easy way to distinguish this type of pedometer mechanism.

The magnetic reed proximity switch is composed of a magnet connected to a spring suspended horizontal lever arm that responds to vertical hip movement. Steps are counted when a magnetic field is created that activates a proximity switch inside of a glass cylinder (Schneider et al. 2003). These two mechanisms make use of coiled or hairspring mechanisms that have the potential to wear out over time, thereby affecting sensitivity.

The third common mechanism used in pedometers is a piezoelectric mechanism. The piezoelectric mechanism uses a strain gauge to measure inertia that interprets step count and is better than the previously described mechanisms at estimating activity intensity and energy expenditure. This type of device also improves

TABLE 11.1
Activity Classification Based on Steps per Day

Classification	Steps/Day
Sedentary	<5000
Low active	5000–7499
Somewhat active	7500–9999
Active	10,000–12,499
Highly active	>12,500

Source: Tudor-Locke, C., Bassett, D. R., *Sports Med.*, 34, 1–8, 2004. With permission.

measurement accuracy when walking at slower speeds that might fail to register steps with a spring-levered mechanism (Crouter et al. 2003).

A common public health message using pedometers is to encourage adults to achieve 10,000 steps/day (Hatano 1993). Walking for 10,000 step/day expends about 300 kcal of added energy expenditure, which reflects the dose of physical activity identified as optimal for reducing the risk of having a first heart attack (Paffenbarger, Kampert, and Lee 1997), and is generally associated with a healthy level of physical activity (Chan, Ryan, and Tudor-Locke 2004). Step count goals have also been compared to physical activity recommendations that encourage 30 min/day of moderate intensity activity. This recommendation can be achieved by accumulating 3000–4000 steps that are of moderate intensity (≥100 steps/min) (Tudor-Locke et al. 2005), accumulated in at least 10-min bouts, and are above a sedentary threshold level of physical activity (e.g., 5000 total steps/day) (Hatano 1993). In 2004, a "zone-based hierarchy" was identified for pedometer step count indices (Tudor-Locke and Bassett 2004). Table 11.1 displays the preliminary classifications for daily walking activity in healthy adults.

Using the step count function on accelerometers (described below) from the 2005–2006 NHANES, Tudor-Locke, Johnson, and Katzmarzyk (2009) identified the average steps per day in U.S. adults. Women, on average, took 5756 steps/day, whereas men took 7431 steps/day or a combined average of 6540 steps/day. This is far below the recommended 10,000 steps/day.

ACCELEROMETERS

Accelerometers are used to assess the body's motion (i.e., proper or physical accelerations) as a result of movement and physical activity. The majority of accelerometers fall into two categories (uniaxial and triaxial) based on their ability to assess activity in single or multiple movement planes. Uniaxial accelerometers measure accelerations in a single (i.e., vertical) axis. Triaxial accelerometers measure body accelerations in three planes of movement (i.e., vertical, horizontal, and lateral) planes. The accelerations are interpreted as intensity of movement.

Accelerometers are comparable in size to a pedometer and are a very useful tool when conducting free-living and field physical activity research. One advantage of accelerometers is that they are constantly sampling movement and lack of movement providing detailed (e.g., second-by-second or minute-by-minute) output on activity intensity. From this constant output, accelerometers offer information on the frequency and duration of movement by intensity levels. Several researchers have used accelerometer outputs in activity counts to develop thresholds to identify various activity intensities. These thresholds are typically called a "cut-point." For example, using the cut-points developed by Freedson, Melanson, and Sirard (1998), light intensity activity occurs below 1952 activity counts/min, moderate intensity activity occurs between 1952 and 5724, and vigorous intensity is identified above 5725 counts/min (Freedson, Melanson, and Sirard 1998). A cut-point of less than 100 denotes sedentary or inactive behaviors. Figure 11.2 provides an example of movements of varying intensities as recorded by an ActiGraph accelerometer.

Most accelerometers are designed to accurately measure ambulatory activity; thus, when worn on the waist, accelerometers may underestimate activities such as weight lifting, bicycling, isometric exercise, and other activities that produce less body movement but expend energy. The high cost of some accelerometers can limit their use in large-scale surveillance studies. The NHANES began using accelerometers in 2003 as part of its ongoing surveillance study to assess the health and nutritional status of adults and children in the United States. In 2008, Troiano et al. (2008) presented results from NHANES 2003–2004 using accelerometers in a sample of children and adults representing the U.S. population. These results provided the first objective measure of physical activity in the United States. Some of the results confirmed what was already known, that physical activity generally decreases with age and males are slightly more active than females. However, in rather strong contrast to physical activity survey data that generally show about 26% to 45% of the U.S. population meeting physical activity guidelines (Macera et al. 2005), Troiano found that less than 5% of adults meet these guidelines when physical activity is measured objectively with accelerometers (Troiano et al. 2008).

Accelerometers have also been used to identify sedentary behaviors or inactivity identified using cut-point threshold of about 100 counts/min or less. From the NHANES study, Matthews et al. (2008) identified that adults spent about 55% of their day (about 7.7 h) in sedentary behaviors. Recently, researchers have used accelerometers to investigate the associations of sedentary time and sedentary behaviors

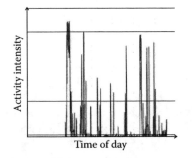

FIGURE 11.2 Sample accelerometer data showing the volume, intensity, and frequency of activity throughout a single day.

with other health outcomes. Associations have been observed for sedentary time and waist circumference along with other metabolic risk factors independent of moderate- to vigorous-intensity activity (Healy et al. 2008). This information from objective physical activity measures highlights the importance of both increasing time in physical activity and reducing sedentary time to optimize health.

Direct Observation

Assessing physical activity using direct observation involves a trained observer who records or codes the activity they witness. Because of the relatively high cost and potential intrusiveness of direct observation, it is impractical in large studies. However, this has often been a preferred method to assess physical activity in children (McKenzie, Sallis, and Nader 1992) and to observe the use of public spaces such as parks or sidewalks (McKenzie et al. 2006). Common observation systems used to classify physical activity behaviors include the System for Observing Play and Leisure in Youth and the System for Observing Play and Recreation in Communities. These measurement systems can be downloaded from www.activelivingresearch.org.

Direct/Indirect Calorimetry

Calorimetry is the measurement of the amount of heat produced by a subject. The heat produced is related to energy expenditure. This energy can be measured by direct or indirect calorimetry. Direct calorimetry is the directly measured heat produced by a person enclosed in a whole room calorimeter, which is typically a small room that can measure heat production. Although very accurate, whole room calorimetry does not always accurately reflect free-living conditions since it requires an individual to stay in a small (e.g., 10 ft × 10 ft) room. Indirect calorimetry measures energy expenditure by assessing the amount of oxygen consumed rather than heat production. Measuring energy expenditure is different than measuring physical activity. Energy expenditure can be assessed for a person's total daily energy expenditure by measuring resting metabolic rate, thermal effect of food, and physical activity energy expenditure. On the other hand, physical activity is a measure of physical movement or behavior and measured as frequency, duration, and intensity.

Doubly Labeled Water

The method of doubly labeled water is generally thought of as the "gold standard" for assessing energy expenditure (Taylor-Piliae et al. 2006). This method was first discovered and developed in mice in the 1940s and 1950s by Lifson et al. (Lifson et al. 1949; Lifson, Gordon, and McClintock 1955) but was not used in humans until the early 1980s (Schoeller and van Santen 1982). Doubly labeled water assesses total daily energy expenditure using two isotopes, ^2H (deuterium) and ^{18}O. The basic method is that a person is given an oral dose of these stable isotopes, a urinary sample is taken to establish the new levels of ^2H and ^{18}O, and then they are allowed to go about their normal activities for 1–2 weeks. After that time, the person returns and provides a urinary sample to reassess the ^2H and ^{18}O levels. The difference between ^2H and ^{18}O at this time indicates the amount of CO_2 production during the period used to determine total daily energy expenditure. Although this method is very accurate in assessing energy expenditure during free living activity, it can be rather expensive and does not differentiate between types of activity or the context in which that activity occurs.

Activity Space

An emerging area of interest in physical activity assessment is activity space, or where and when activity occurs. The premise of activity space has its origins in the 1960s and 1970s. During this time, researchers began to develop spatial concepts that have helped formulate our thinking today. In 1965, Haggett pioneered the idea of assessing locational geography and movement using nodes (locations), networks (travel paths), and areas, which is the foundation of much current research (Anderson 1971; Haggett 1965). Researchers in the 1970s and 1980s refined these ideas and focused on individual activity patterns and the value of space–time budgets (Palm 1981), the influence of environment (Lenntorp 1976), and the concept of Space–Time Paths and Prisms (Golledge and Stimson 1997) that map or predict potential travel. For example, this can be used to understand how a person got to a location, and if a person was in that location for 30 min, what were the possible locations and likelihood of them going to different places during that allotted time?

Physical Activity Space

Physical activity space is derived from "activity space" proposed by Golledge and Stimson (Golledge and Stimson 1997) and described as the area where a person spends time. Golledge also used this term to describe "spatial behavior," another term often used interchangeably with activity space today. Zhu is a more recent proponent of activity space and further refined the idea of activity space by calling it "Physical Activity Space" and defining it as "the area or space where an individual spends time *and engages in physical activity*" (Zhu 2003). This definition of physical activity space includes three components: *time*, *space*, and *activity*. Nearly all current physical activity measures only measure activity time; therefore, Zhu (2003) called for new measures of physical activity space that assess the interaction between an individual and the environment. At about the same time, Schönfelder and Axhausen (2002) were researching travel behavior and thought that spatial data analysis could help measure the concept of activity space and help identify how and why the environment influences behaviors. Recently, the built environment has been the focal point for the majority of health research using geospatial technology and its role in promoting physical activity. In 2008, Saarloos et al. proposed a bottom-up approach using activity-based modeling to understand how individuals interact in space and time with their environment and each other (Saarloos, Kim, and Timmermans 2009). This approach may be very helpful in shifting the paradigm from a built environment approach to better understand individual spatial behavior.

Subjective methods, such as time–budget diaries (Anderson 1971), have been used to assess activity space because direct measures have not been readily available. Of the three components of physical activity space (i.e., activity, space, and time), activity and time can be measured by activity logbooks or diaries via recording the time for every activity performed. An assessment of space could be appraised using a travel log. However, these types of methodologies are often limited by recall, classification difficulties, and participant burden.

Objective methods, such as pedometers and accelerometers, can be used in part to assess physical activity space. Recent advances in geospatial technology can assist in assessing space and time objectively using Global Positioning System (GPS) receivers that automatically record time at a location and detailed travel data. Geographic Information Systems (GIS) can then be used to apply spatial statistics to analyze the data gathered from motion sensors and GPS. In theory, these technologies should be able to quantify physical activity space, yet few people have proposed quantitative methodologies to do so. When GPS is combined with accelerometers, it is possible to identify the frequency, duration, and intensity of an individual's movement patterns in time and space.

Combining Technology to Assess Physical Activity

Efforts are underway to combine GPS and accelerometer technology to improve the assessment of physical activity space (Patrick et al. 2008; Rodríguez, Brown, and Troped 2005). One of the earliest concept devices of the integrated accelerometer and GPS receiver was designed in 1996 (Makikawa and Murakami 1997). More recently, Rodriguez et al. (2005) investigated the capabilities of combining a GPS receiver and accelerometer to assess physical activity behavior but provided limited conclusions. The study reported that the device was able to measure activity and could measure location (Rodríguez et al. 2005). Several researchers funded through the National Institute of Health Genes and Environment initiative are developing a system that uses multiple accelerometers and Bluetooth technology to send data to a smart phone (i.e., GPS-capable) to interpret activity type (Patrick et al. 2008). The use of GPS capabilities has been limited in this system because of issues relating to battery life and running multiple programs on the cellular phone platform. However, this method offers a vast amount of potential for assessing physical activity behaviors and interaction with the environment and could enrich our understanding of physical activity behavior.

The Movement and Activity in Physical Space (MAPS) score is a newly developed method to quantify and provide and index score for physical activity space by combining data from separate GPS and accelerometer devices (Herrmann et al. 2011). This method incorporates the spatial assessment of the GPS by measuring locations where activities occur and matching data by time with an accelerometer that measures characteristics of the activity (i.e., intensity, duration) (see Figure 11.3a and b). Initial work using MAPS scores has demonstrated evidence of reliability and the ability to assess known-group differences in individuals with a reduced functional capacity and evidence of responsiveness to monitor their recovery/improvements in function over time (Herrmann et al. 2011). Other researchers have adopted using MAPS scores to investigate different populations including individuals with multiple sclerosis (Snook et al. 2010).

(a)   (b)

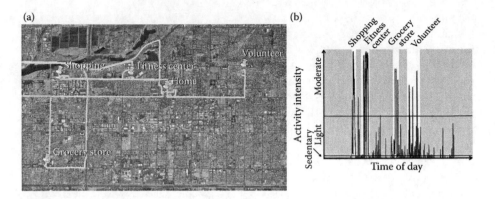

FIGURE 11.3 Combining GPS and accelerometry. (a) GPS data alone indicating travel pathways (white lines) and locations (white push pin icons. (b) Accelerometer and GPS data combined to identify volume, intensity, and frequency of activity and where activity occurs. Gray areas indicate time spent at home.

Limitations and Challenges in Physical Activity Space

Although technology is rapidly advancing and multiple researchers are working on incorporating accelerometers with GPS and smart phone technology to enhance physical activity research, limitations and challenges exist. One existing challenge is that physical activity researchers lack training in geospatial technology. Therefore, assessing spatial behavior may be best served through interdisciplinary approaches that include individuals from travel, geography, engineering, and physical activity fields. Another limitation of objectively measured activity space is that trip motives and/or purpose cannot always be easily assumed from GPS technology alone (Wolf, Guensler, and Bachman 2001). This provides an opportunity for researchers to include real-time querying of users (possibly with smart phones) to learn about activity (or trip) motives and/or purpose. In addition, Zhu (2003) identified that new spatial statistics need to be developed to better assess physical activity space. Last, practical problems also exist that include the relatively high cost of equipment and costly postprocessing of GPS data to assess purpose and location.

SUMMARY

At present, a variety of methods exist for physical activity assessment. These include subjective measures of questionnaires, records, and logs and objective measures of pedometers, accelerometers, heart rate monitors, GPS, and combinations of accelerometry and GPS. Indirect calorimetry and doubly labeled water are often used to measure the energy expenditure of physical activity. Although the validity and reliability evidence exists for many of these measurement methods, it is essential that these instruments and methodologies be continually improved upon to advance our understanding of physical activity assessment and behaviors. Doing so may provide more accurate assessments and help improve physical activity levels by developing and implementing more specific and targeted interventions.

STUDY QUESTIONS

1. Identify the two categories for physical activity assessment and, within each category, evaluate the strengths and limitations of each measurement method for use in physical activity surveillance activities.
2. Develop a strategy to measure physical activity for the following scenario. Adults are enrolled in a community level physical activity program for 8 weeks. The aim of the program is to achieve the National Physical Activity Guidelines for moderate- and/or vigorous-intensity aerobic physical activity for 150 min/week and at least 2 days of strength training during the 8-week program. Your goal is to assess if participants are meeting the program aim.
3. Pedometers are a popular way for individuals to track their physical activity achievements. Describe step goals for optimal physical activity and construct ways that individuals can track their physical activity improvements using pedometers.
4. Demonstrate how a public health practitioner can measure an individual's physical activity in a community setting using a combination of accelerometers, pedometers, and global position systems.
5. Discuss the options to measure energy expenditure and list the pros and cons of each method.

REFERENCES

Ainsworth, B. E., W. L. Haskell, S. D. Herrmann et al. 2011. 2011 Compendium of physical activities: A second update of codes and MET Values. *Med. Sci. Sports Exerc.* 43(8): 1575–1581.

Anderson, J. 1971. Space–time budgets and activity studies in urban geography and planning. *Environ, Plann.* 3: 353–368.

Bassett, D. R., H. R. Wyatt, H. Thompson et al. 2010. Pedometer-measured physical activity and health behaviors in U.S. adults. *Med. Sci. Sports Exerc.* 42: 1819–1825.

Bauman, A., F. Bull, T. Chey et al. 2009. The International Prevalence Study on Physical Activity: results from 20 countries. *Int. J. Behav. Nutr. Phys. Act.* 6: 21.

Beets, M. W., D. Bornstein, A. Beighle et al. 2010. Pedometer-measured physical activity patterns of youth: A 13-country review. *Am. J. Prev. Med.* 38: 208–216.

Blair, S. N., W. L. Haskell, P. Ho et al. 1985. Assessment of habitual physical activity by a seven-day recall in a community survey and controlled experiments. *Am. J. Epidemiol.* 122: 794–804.

Bouchard, C., A. Tremblay, C. Leblanc et al. 1983. A method to assess energy expenditure in children and adults. *Am. J. Clin. Nutr.* 37: 461–467.

Chan, C. B., D. A. J. Ryan, and C. Tudor-Locke. 2004. Health benefits of a pedometer-based physical activity intervention in sedentary workers. *Prev. Med.* 39: 1215–1222.

Craig, C. L., C. Cameron, J. M. Griffiths et al. 2010. Descriptive epidemiology of youth pedometer-determined physical activity: CANPLAY. *Med. Sci. Sports Exerc.* 42: 1639–1643.

Craig, C. L., A. L. Marshall, M. Sjöström et al. 2003. International Physical Activity Questionnaire: 12-country reliability and validity. *Med. Sci. Sports Exerc.* 35: 1381–1395.

Crouter, S. E., P. L. Schneider, M. Karabulut et al. 2003. Validity of 10 electronic pedometers for measuring steps, distance, and energy cost. *Med. Sci. Sports Exerc.* 35: 1455–1460.

Fogelholm, M., J. Malmberg, J. Suni et al. 2006. International Physical Activity Questionnaire: Validity against fitness. *Med. Sci. Sports Exerc.* 38: 753–760.

Freedson, P. S., E. Melanson, and J. Sirard. 1998. Calibration of the Computer Science and Applications, Inc. accelerometer. *Med. Sci. Sports Exerc.* 30: 777–781.

Golledge, R. G., and R. J. Stimson. 1997. *Spatial behavior: A geographic perspective.* New York: Guilford Press.

Greenwood, J. L., E. A. Joy, and J. B. Stanford. 2010. The Physical Activity Vital Sign: A primary care tool to guide counseling for obesity. *J. Phys. Act. Health* 7: 571–576.

Haggett, P. 1965. *Locational Analysis in Human Geography.* London: Edward Arnold.

Hagströmer, M., P. Oja, and M. Sjöström. 2006. The International Physical Activity Questionnaire (IPAQ): A study of concurrent and construct validity. *Public Health Nutr.* 9: 755–762.

Haskell, W. L., I. M. Lee, R. R. Pate et al. 2007. Physical activity and public health: updated recommendation for adults from the American College of Sports Medicine and the American Heart Association. *Circulation* 116: 1081–1093.

Hatano, Y. 1993. Use of the pedometer for promoting daily walking exercise. *Int. Counc. Health, Phys. Educ. Recreation* 29: 4–8.

Healy, G. N., K. Wijndaele, D. W. Dunstan et al. 2008. Objectively measured sedentary time, physical activity, and metabolic risk. *Diabetes Care* 31: 369–371.

Herrmann, S. D., E. M. Snook, M. Kang et al. 2011. Development and Validation of a Movement and Activity in Physical Space (MAPS) Score as a functional outcome measure. *Arch. Phys. Med. Rehabil* 92(10): 1652–1658.

Lagerros, Y. T., and P. Lagiou. 2007. Assessment of physical activity and energy expenditure in epidemiological research of chronic diseases. *Eur. J. Epidemiol.* 22: 353–362.

Lamonte, M. J., and B. E. Ainsworth. 2001. Quantifying energy expenditure and physical activity in the context of dose response. *Med. Sci. Sports Exerc.* 33: S370.

Lenntorp, B. 1976. *Paths in Space–Time Environments a Time–Geographic Study of Movement Possibilities of Individuals.* Lund Studies in Geography B: Human Geography ed. Lund: Gleerup.

Leon, A. S., J. Connett, D. R. Jacobs et al. 1987. Leisure-time physical activity levels and risk of coronary heart disease and death. *JAMA* 258: 2388–2395.

Lifson, N., G. B. Gordon, and R. McClintock. 1955. Measurement of total carbon dioxide production by means of D2O18. *J. Appl. Physiol.* 7: 704–710.

Lifson, N., G. B. Gordon, M. B. Visscher et al. 1949. The fate of utilized molecular oxygen and the source of the oxygen of respiratory carbon dioxide, studied with the aid of heavy oxygen. *J. Biol. Chem.* 180: 803–811.

Macera, C. A., S. A. Ham, M. M. Yore et al. 2005. Prevalence of physical activity in the United States: Behavioral Risk Factors Surveillance System, 2001. *Prev. Chronic Dis.* 2: A17.

Makikawa, M., and D. Murakami. 1997. Ambulatory behavior map, physical activity and biosignal monitoring system. *Methods Inf. Med.* 36: 360–363.

Matthews, C. E., B. E. Ainsworth, C. Hanby et al. 2005. Development and testing of a short physical activity recall questionnaire. *Med. Sci. Sports Exerc.* 37: 986–994.

Matthews, C. E., K. Y. Chen, P. S. Freedson et al. 2008. Amount of time spent in sedentary behaviors in the United States, 2003–2004. *Am. J. Epidemiol.* 167: 875–881.

Matthews, C. E., J. R. Hebert, P. S. Freedson et al. 2001. Sources of variance in daily physical activity levels in the seasonal variation of blood cholesterol study. *Am. J. Epidemiol.* 153: 987–995.

McKenzie, T. L., D. A. Cohen, A. Sehgal et al. 2006. System for Observing Play and Recreation in Communities (SOPARC): Reliability and feasibility measures. *J. Phys. Act. Health* 3: S208–S222.

McKenzie, T. L., J. F. Sallis, and P. R. Nader. 1992. SOFIT: System for Observing Fitness Instruction Time. *J. Teaching Phys. Educ.* 11: 195–205.

Paffenbarger, R. S., J. B. Kampert, and I. M. Lee. 1997. Physical activity and health of college men: longitudinal observations. *Int. J. Sports Med.* 18(Suppl 3): S200–S203.

Palm, R. 1981. Women in nonmetropolitan areas: A time-budget survey. *Environ. Plann. A* 13: 373–378.

Pate, R. R., M. Pratt, S. N. Blair et al. 1995. Physical activity and public health. A recommendation from the Centers for Disease Control and Prevention and the American College of Sports Medicine. *JAMA* 273: 402–407.

Patrick, K., W. G. Griswold, F. Raab et al. 2008. Health and the mobile phone. *Am. J. Prev. Med.* 35: 177–181.

Rodríguez, D. A., A. L. Brown, and P. J. Troped. 2005. Portable global positioning units to complement accelerometry-based physical activity monitors. *Med. Sci. Sports Exerc.* 37: S572–S581.

Rzewnicki, R., Y. Vanden Auweele, and I. De Bourdeaudhuij. 2003. Addressing overreporting on the International Physical Activity Questionnaire (IPAQ) telephone survey with a population sample. *Public Health Nutr.* 6: 299–305.

Saarloos, D., J. Kim, and H. Timmermans. 2009. The built environment and health: Introducing individual space–time behavior. *Int J Environ Res Public Health* 6(6): 1724–1743.

Sallis, R. 2011. Developing healthcare systems to support exercise: Exercise as the fifth vital sign. *Br. J. Sports Med.* 45: 473–474.

Schneider, P. L., S. E. Crouter, and D. R. Bassett. 2004. Pedometer measures of free-living physical activity: Comparison of 13 models. *Med. Sci. Sports Exerc.* 36: 331–335.

Schneider, P. L., S. E. Crouter, O. Lukajic et al. 2003. Accuracy and reliability of 10 pedometers for measuring steps over a 400-m walk. *Med. Sci. Sports Exerc.* 35: 1779–1784.

Schoeller, D. A., and E. van Santen. 1982. Measurement of energy expenditure in humans by doubly labeled water method. *J. Appl. Physiol.* 53: 955–959.

Schönfelder, S., and K. W. Axhausen. 2002. Measuring the size and structure of human activity spaces: The longitudinal perspective. *Arbeitsbericht Verkehrs-und Raumplanung* 135.

Snook, E. M., C. B. Scott, B. G. Ragan et al. 2010. Combining GPS and accelerometer data as a new functional outcome measure for multiple sclerosis: A case comparison study of the movement and activity in physical space (MAPS) score. 2010 Health Summit Conference, Washington, DC.

Taylor, H. L., D. R. Jacobs, B. Schucker et al. 1978. A questionnaire for the assessment of leisure time physical activities. *J. Chronic Dis.* 31: 741–755.

Taylor-Piliae, R. E., L. C. Norton, W. L. Haskell et al. 2006. Validation of a new brief physical activity survey among men and women aged 60–69 years. *Am. J. Epidemiol.* 164: 598–606.

Troiano, R. P., D. Berrigan, K. W. Dodd et al. 2008. Physical activity in the United States measured by accelerometer. *Med. Sci. Sports Exerc.* 40: 181–188.

Tudor-Locke, C., and D. R. Bassett. 2004. How many steps/day are enough? Preliminary pedometer indices for public health. *Sports Med.* 34: 1–8.

Tudor-Locke, C., W. D. Johnson, and P. T. Katzmarzyk. 2009. Accelerometer-determined steps per day in U.S. adults. *Med. Sci. Sports Exerc.* 41: 1384–1391.

Tudor-Locke, C., S. B. Sisson, T. Collova et al. 2005. Pedometer-determined step count guidelines for classifying walking intensity in a young ostensibly healthy population. *Can. J. Appl. Physiol.* 30: 666–676.

U.S. Department of Health and Human Services. 2008. Physical Activity Guidelines Advisory Committee Report. U.S. Department of Health and Human Services (USDHHS).

Wolf, J., R. Guensler, and W. Bachman. 2001. Elimination of the travel diary: Experiment to derive trip purpose from global positioning system travel data. *Transp. Res. Rec.: J. Transp. Res. Board* 1768: 125–134.

Zhu, W. 2003. Assessing physical activity space: Issues and challenges. *Proceedings II of 2003 Daegu Universiade Conference: Facing the Challenge*, pp. 601–608. Daegu Universiade Conference Organizing Committee, Daegu, Korea.

12 National Guidelines for Physical Activity

Richard P. Troiano and David M. Buchner

CONTENTS

INTRODUCTION

The U.S. Department of Health and Human Services (HHS) announced and released the *2008 Physical Activity Guidelines for Americans* (U.S. Department of Health and Human Services 2008) in October of that year, the first time that the Federal government had published comprehensive physical activity guidelines. The Guidelines development process began with a systematic review of epidemiologic literature and the resulting document extended earlier government recommendations and professional organization position statements. Since their release, the *Physical Activity Guidelines* have been widely disseminated and used in many ways. Other countries, including Canada, the United Kingdom, Ireland, Austria, and Finland, have used the *Physical Activity Guidelines Advisory Committee Report, 2008* and the *2008 Physical Activity Guidelines for Americans* to develop their national guidelines or recommendations. The documents produced by other nations present the same or very similar recommendations. The World Health Organization (2010) has also adapted the 2008 Guidelines for use in its member countries.

This chapter describes the background and context for the development of the *Physical Activity Guidelines*. It summarizes the process that led to the release of the Guidelines, as well as efforts to support the dissemination and application of the Guidelines. Because the Guidelines document is readily available, only the key guidelines are presented here. Issues that arose during the development of the Guidelines and contrasts with earlier recommendations are described. Finally, a perspective on the appropriate role of physical activity guidelines in improving public health is presented.

BACKGROUND

Development of physical activity recommendations to promote health has a long history in the United States (Physical Activity Guidelines Advisory Committee 2008). The need for guidance on recommended types, intensities, and amounts of physical activity was recognized as early as the 1960s and 1970s. Initially, recommendations had a primarily clinical and therapeutic focus on exercise prescription. Considerable attention was given to reducing the risk of exercise among those with existing coronary heart disease or who were considered at risk for it. Because of the clinical orientation and primary focus on those with impaired health status, the exercise prescriptions were generally based on relative intensity (e.g., percent of maximal heart rate). Recommendations were published in position stands and statements by professional organizations, such as the American College of Sports Medicine and the American Heart Association.

In the mid-1980s, the paradigm began to shift from a clinical to a public health basis for promoting physical activity. Accumulating epidemiologic data showed significant chronic disease risk reduction from moderate-intensity physical activities that were often carried out during activities of daily living, rather than in exercise training sessions, and in short episodes, such as climbing the stairs. The evolving chronic disease risk model contrasted with the prevailing exercise prescription/training model that emphasized extended bouts of higher intensity physical activity to increase aerobic capacity. The paradigm shift was exemplified by the American Heart Association's recognition of inactivity as a major coronary heart disease risk factor (Fletcher et al. 1992).

This new public health perspective culminated in the publication of several major reports in quick succession from U.S. and international agencies. An important year was 1995, which saw the publication of *Physical Activity and Public Health: A Recommendation from the Centers for Disease Control and Prevention and the American College of Sports Medicine* (Pate et al. 1995) and *Exercise for Health* (WHO/FIMS Committee on Physical Activity for Health 1995). These reports were followed by *Physical Activity and Cardiovascular Health* from the National Institutes of Health Consensus Development Panel on Physical Activity and Cardiovascular Health (1996), and *Physical Activity and Health: A Report of the Surgeon General* (U.S. Department of Health and Human Services 1996). All of the publications recommended that individuals accumulate at least 30 min/day of moderate-intensity physical activity on most, and preferably all, days of the week. Brisk walking became the typical example for recommending moderate-intensity physical activity.

The basic health promotion message of accumulating at least 30 min of moderate or greater intensity physical activity on most days of the week changed little for more than a decade. With increasing focus on the rising prevalence of obesity in the United States, the physical activity chapter in the *Dietary Guidelines for Americans, 2005* (U.S. Department of Health and Human Services and U.S. Department of Agriculture 2005) added recommendations of greater durations of physical activity to contribute to weight loss or maintenance of weight loss. Additionally, some of the original authors of the *Physical Activity and Public Health: A Recommendation from the Centers for Disease Control and Prevention and the American College of Sports Medicine* (Pate et al. 1995) developed two documents to update their original publication and clarify issues that had been misinterpreted in the media as well as scientific literature (Haskell et al. 2007; Nelson et al. 2007). The updated recommendations for adults (ages 18 to 64 years) (Haskell et al. 2007) explicitly stated that for health promotion and maintenance, adults needed a minimum of 30 min of moderate-intensity aerobic physical activity on 5 days per week, or 20 min of vigorous-intensity aerobic physical activity on 3 days per week, or a combination of moderate- and vigorous-intensity aerobic physical activity. These activities needed to occur in bouts of at least 10 min duration and be above and beyond the routine light activities of daily life. Additionally, muscle-strengthening activities that exercised all major muscle groups were recommended on at least 2 days per week. The benefits of amounts of activity beyond the minimum recommendations as well as bone-strengthening activities were noted.

The recommendations for older adults (ages older than 65 years or 50 to 64 years with clinically significant chronic conditions or physical activity limitations) (Nelson et al. 2007) were similar to the updated recommendations for adults, but had severable notable differences. In contrast to recommendations for adults that were based on absolute intensity expressed in terms of metabolic equivalents (METs), Nelson et al. (2007) noted that older adults should base their target intensity on relative intensity, which considers the aerobic fitness capacity of the individual. Furthermore, in addition to muscle-strengthening activities, older adults were recommended to engage in activities to maintain or increase their flexibility on at least 2 days per week and activities to improve balance if they were at risk of falls. Additional attention was given to integrating preventive and therapeutic physical activity for adults with chronic conditions. A clear statement was made that in all cases, older adults should attempt to reduce sedentary behavior.

DEVELOPMENT OF 2008 PHYSICAL ACTIVITY GUIDELINES

In May 2006, HHS Secretary Michael Leavitt announced his top priorities, one of which was disease prevention. The Secretary's Prevention Priority built on the George W. Bush Administration's HealthierUS initiative (The White House 2002). HealthierUS had four "pillars":

1. Be physically active every day.
2. Eat a nutritious diet.
3. Get preventive screenings.
4. Make healthy choices.

One of the government activities associated with the Prevention Priority was the development of Physical Activity Guidelines for Americans. The process that led up to the release of the *2008 Physical Activity Guidelines for Americans* is described in the *Physical Activity Guidelines Advisory Committee Report, 2008* (Physical Activity Guidelines Advisory Committee 2008). Briefly, the major steps in the process were

- Institute of Medicine Workshop and Report: Adequacy of Evidence for Physical Activity Guidelines Development (October 2006)
- Secretary Leavitt announces plans to develop Physical Activity Guidelines for Americans, to be released in 2008 (October 27, 2006)
- Recruitment and selection of Physical Activity Guidelines Advisory Committee (January–February 2007)
- Development and creation of *Physical Activity Guidelines for Americans* Scientific Database (January 2007–March 2008)
- Advisory Committee public meetings (June 26–27, 2007; December 6–7, 2007; and February 28–29, 2008)
- Preparation of *Physical Activity Guidelines Advisory Committee Report, 2008* (released June 2008)
- Development of the *2008 Physical Activity Guidelines for Americans* (June–September 2008)
- Development of communication and support materials, including *2008 Physical Activity Guidelines for Americans Toolkit* (June–September 2008)
- Official announcement and release of Physical Activity Guidelines (October 8, 2008)

OVERVIEW OF *2008 PHYSICAL ACTIVITY GUIDELINES FOR AMERICANS*

The key guidelines from the *2008 Physical Activity Guidelines for Americans* are shown for children, ages 6 to 17 years (Table 12.1), and for adults, ages 18 to 64

TABLE 12.1

Key Guidelines for Children

- Children and adolescents should do 60 min (1 h) or more of physical activity daily.
  - **Aerobic**: Most of the 60 min or more a day should be either moderate- or vigorous-intensity aerobic physical activity, and should include vigorous-intensity physical activity at least 3 days a week.
  - **Muscle-strengthening**: As part of their 60 min or more of daily physical activity, children and adolescents should include muscle-strengthening physical activity on at least 3 days of the week.
  - **Bone-strengthening**: As part of their 60 min or more of daily physical activity, children and adolescents should include bone-strengthening physical activity on at least 3 days of the week.
- It is important to encourage young people to participate in physical activities that are appropriate for their age, that are enjoyable, and that offer variety.

TABLE 12.2

Key Guidelines for Adults

- All adults should avoid inactivity. Some physical activity is better than none, and adults who participate in any amount of physical activity gain some health benefits.
- For substantial health benefits, adults should do at least 150 min (2 h and 30 min) a week of moderate-intensity, or 75 min (1 h and 15 min) a week of vigorous-intensity aerobic physical activity, or an equivalent combination of moderate- and vigorous-intensity aerobic activity. Aerobic activity should be performed in episodes of at least 10 min, and preferably, it should be spread throughout the week.
- For additional and more extensive health benefits, adults should increase their aerobic physical activity to 300 min (5 h) a week of moderate-intensity, or 150 min/week of vigorous-intensity aerobic physical activity, or an equivalent combination of moderate- and vigorous-intensity activity. Additional health benefits are gained by engaging in physical activity beyond this amount.
- Adults should also do muscle-strengthening activities that are moderate or high intensity and involve all major muscle groups on 2 or more days a week, as these activities provide additional health benefits.

years (Table 12.2). The older adult key guidelines include those for adults, as well as additional guidelines that apply to those who are 65 years and older (Table 12.3). These guidelines are generally consistent with previous recommendations. Notably, a person who does at least 30 min of moderate-intensity activity on five or more days per week meets guidelines. However, the 2008 Guidelines are comprehensive, and they have important, if not surprising, differences from previous recommendations.

DOSE–RESPONSE RELATIONSHIPS

The 2008 Guidelines reflect the full dose–response relationship between amount of physical activity and health benefits. A minimum level of physical activity required

TABLE 12.3

Key Guidelines Specific to Older Adults

- When older adults cannot do 150 min of moderate-intensity aerobic activity a week because of chronic conditions, they should be as physically active as their abilities and conditions allow.
- Older adults should do exercises that maintain or improve balance if they are at risk of falling.
- Older adults should determine their level of effort for physical activity relative to their level of fitness.

to meet guidelines is specified. The guidelines also explicitly recommend that people avoid inactivity because even insufficient amounts of activity are better than none, and further note that people who do amounts of activity beyond the minimum recommended level attain additional health benefits.

Combining Moderate- and Vigorous-Intensity Activity

The 2008 Guidelines specify how people can meet the guidelines by combining moderate-intensity and vigorous-intensity activity. The rule of thumb is 2 min of moderate-intensity activity is equivalent to 1 min of vigorous-intensity activity.

Frequency of Aerobic Activity

The Guidelines allow adults more flexibility in frequency of aerobic physical activity than earlier recommendations. This change was based on the observation by the Federal Advisory Committee that the chronic disease epidemiology literature does not present information to separate frequency of activity from volume. That is, there is no clear evidence that 50 min of moderate-intensity activity on 3 days per week has different health benefits from 30 min of activity on 5 days per week. The 2008 Guidelines do specify that, preferably, adults should be active on at least 3 days per week. The benefits of 3 to 7 days per week of activity are more extensively documented than those of 1 to 2 days per week, and there are concerns about injury risk from high amounts of activity concentrated on 1 to 2 days per week.

Absolute versus Relative Intensity

Children and adults can monitor the intensity of aerobic activity using either the absolute or relative intensity of the activity. The absolute intensity of physical activity refers to the rate of energy expenditure in METs when performing the activity. A MET is the rate of energy expenditure when awake and resting. Moderate-intensity activities are in the range of 3.0–5.9 METs, and vigorous intensity activities are in the range of 6.0 METs and higher.

The relative intensity of physical activity is related to a person's level of fitness. Relative intensity can be estimated using a 0 to 10 scale, where sitting is 0 and the highest level of effort possible is 10. With this scale, moderate-intensity activity is a 5 or 6, and vigorous-intensity activity is a 7 or 8.

MUSCLE-STRENGTHENING ACTIVITIES

The 2008 Guidelines recommend muscle strengthening activities on at least 3 days per week for children and at least 2 days per week for adults and older adults. Muscle-strengthening activities have additional health benefits beyond those of aerobic activity. Accordingly, the Guidelines clarify that, for adults, time spent on muscle-strengthening activity does not count toward meeting aerobic activity guidelines. The Guidelines do not specify that the 2 or more days each week should be nonconsecutive, because of lack of evidence that nonconsecutive days have greater health benefits or less injury risk than consecutive days.

BALANCE TRAINING

The 2008 Guidelines recommend balance training to reduce falls in older adults who are at increased risk of falls. Strong evidence from randomized trials shows that regular physical activity reduces fall risk. Most evidence supports an exercise program with at least 3 days per week of balance training and moderate-intensity muscle-strengthening activities for 30 min per session, with additional encouragement to participate in moderate-intensity walking 2 or more times per week for 30 min per session. Current evidence is insufficient to recommend balance training for all older adults because most research is conducted only among those at high risk of falls, which is generally indicated by having already experienced a fall.

FLEXIBILITY ACTIVITIES

Flexibility activities are acceptable, but not specifically recommended in the 2008 Guidelines. Flexibility activities do not have documented health benefits, and evidence is even lacking that stretching reduces risk of injury. However, stretching is a common component of physical activity programs with demonstrated benefits. Similarly, warm-up and cool-down activities are acceptable, but do not have documented distinct health benefits unless they involve moderate- to vigorous-intensity aerobic activity or muscle-strengthening activity.

MEDICAL CONSULTATION

The 2008 Guidelines make a clear statement that healthy children and adults do not need physician approval or a medical consultation before engaging in physical activity. Evidence is insufficient that a medical consultation reduces risk of adverse events such as heart attacks or musculoskeletal injury. Of course, people should gradually increase physical activity over time, and acclimate to regular moderate-intensity activity before attempting vigorous-intensity activity. People should consult with a healthcare provider if new symptoms develop during activity, if they have undiagnosed symptoms (e.g., chest pain), or have chronic medical conditions that may affect their choice of types and amounts of physical activity.

HEALTHY WEIGHT

The guidelines for the role of physical activity in attaining a healthy body weight from the *Dietary Guidelines for Americans, 2005* (U.S. Department of Health and Human Services and U.S. Department of Agriculture 2005) were not endorsed by the *2008 Physical Activity Guidelines*. There is no "one size fits all" guideline, such as at least 60 min/day of moderate-intensity activity for weight control. Rather, the 2008 Guidelines recommend that people first attain at least 150 min/week of moderate-intensity aerobic activity. If a person does not achieve a healthy body weight with this amount of aerobic physical activity, he/she should increase physical activity and decrease caloric intake to the point that is individually effective in maintaining a healthy weight. Furthermore, the 2008 Guidelines note that light-intensity physical activity expends calories, and can play a role in maintaining a healthy weight. The 2008 Guidelines also note that physical activity has health benefits regardless of body weight and independent of weight loss.

PHYSICAL ACTIVITY FOR CHILDREN AND ADOLESCENTS

The 2008 Guidelines specify that children and adolescents should be active every day (not just 5 or more days per week) for at least 1 h. In addition to this general activity recommendation, the guidelines specify minimum amounts of vigorous aerobic activity, muscle-strengthening activity, and bone-strengthening activity within the overall guideline. In contrast to adults, muscle-strengthening activity is included in the recommended daily amount of physical activity. The Guidelines apply only to children aged 6 years and older because the evidence relating physical activity to health outcomes for younger children was insufficient. However, the guidelines recognize that physical activity is important for healthy growth and development and encourage young children to be physically active in age- and developmentally appropriate ways.

PHYSICAL ACTIVITY FOR WOMEN DURING PREGNANCY
AND THE POSTPARTUM PERIOD

The 2008 Guidelines also provide specific guidance for women during pregnancy and the postpartum period (Table 12.4). Physical activity provides benefits to general health and pregnancy-related conditions and has low risk during a healthy pregnancy and normal postpartum period.

PHYSICAL ACTIVITY FOR PEOPLE WITH CHRONIC CONDITIONS AND DISABILITIES

The 2008 Guidelines state that regular physical activity is appropriate for people with disabilities and chronic conditions (Table 12.5). People with disabilities or

TABLE 12.4

Key Guidelines for Women during Pregnancy and Postpartum Period

- Healthy women who are not already highly active or doing vigorous-intensity activity should get at least 150 min (2 h and 30 min) of moderate-intensity aerobic activity per week during pregnancy and the postpartum period. Preferably, this activity should be spread throughout the week.
- Pregnant women who habitually engage in vigorous-intensity aerobic activity or are highly active can continue physical activity during pregnancy and the postpartum period, provided that they remain healthy and discuss with their healthcare provider how and when activity should be adjusted over time.

TABLE 12.5

Key Guidelines for Adults with Disabilities or Chronic Conditions

- Adults with disabilities, who are able to, should get at least 150 min/week (2 h and 30 min) of moderate-intensity, or 75 min (1 h and 15 min) per week of vigorous-intensity aerobic activity, or an equivalent combination of moderate- and vigorous-intensity aerobic activity. Aerobic activity should be performed in episodes of at least 10 min, and preferably, it should be spread throughout the week.
- Adults with disabilities, who are able to, should also do muscle-strengthening activities of moderate or high intensity that involve all major muscle groups on 2 or more days per week as these activities provide additional health benefits.
- When adults with disabilities are not able to meet the above Guidelines, they should engage in regular physical activity according to their abilities and should avoid inactivity.
- Adults with disabilities should consult their healthcare providers about the amounts and types of physical activity that are appropriate for their abilities.
- Adults with chronic conditions obtain important health benefits from regular physical activity.
- When adults with chronic conditions do activity according to their abilities, physical activity is safe.
- Adults with chronic conditions should be under the care of healthcare providers. People with chronic conditions and symptoms should consult their healthcare providers about the types and amounts of activity appropriate for them.

chronic conditions should follow the guidelines appropriate for their age if they are able. If not, they should engage in regular physical activity according to their abilities, and avoid inactivity.

ADVERSE EVENTS AND SAFETY

The 2008 Guidelines give substantial attention to prevention of adverse events of physical activity. The key guidelines for safe physical activity are shown in Table 12.6.

TABLE 12.6

Key Guidelines for Safe Physical Activity

To do physical activity safely and reduce the risk of injuries and other adverse events, people should:

- Understand the risks and yet be confident that physical activity is safe for almost everyone.
- Choose to do types of physical activity that are appropriate for their current fitness level and health goals, because some activities are safer than others.
- Increase physical activity gradually over time whenever more activity is necessary to meet guidelines or health goals. Inactive people should "start low and go slow" by gradually increasing how often and how long activities are done.
- Protect themselves by using appropriate gear and sports equipment, looking for safe environments, following rules and policies, and making sensible choices about when, where, and how to be active.
- Be under the care of a healthcare provider if they have chronic conditions or symptoms. People with chronic conditions and symptoms should consult their healthcare provider about the types and amounts of activity appropriate for them.

CHALLENGES OF COMMUNICATING PHYSICAL ACTIVITY GUIDELINES

The Physical Activity Guidelines Advisory Committee and HHS were aware of the challenge of communicating health information about physical activity to the public. Importantly, experts in communication participated in the writing of the guidelines. Some of the key challenges and their solutions are detailed in the following subsections.

APPROPRIATELY TARGETING THE INTENDED AUDIENCE

Traditionally, health recommendation documents attempt to communicate with scientists, policy makers, and consumers in the same document. This multiple audience approach overlooks the specific needs of each group. In developing the *2008 Physical Activity Guidelines for Americans*, a conscious effort was made to consider specific audiences. The *Physical Activity Guidelines Advisory Committee Report, 2008* was primarily intended for scientists, whereas the *2008 Physical Activity Guidelines for Americans* targeted health professionals and policy makers. In keeping with the principles of "plain language," the 2008 Guidelines provided a glossary of terms, and minimized use of technical terms, such as MET and MET-minutes. The 2008 Guidelines project also produced a consumer-targeted document, *Be Active Your Way: A Guide for Adults*, which took a step-by-step approach to increasing physical activity, depending on current activity levels. This document included example scenarios: a question-and-answer format, checklists, and behavior monitoring forms.

CLARIFYING TARGET AMOUNTS OF ACTIVITY

People commonly misinterpret the minimum recommended amount of activity (i.e., 150 min/week) as the target. Therefore, the key guidelines emphasized that more physical activity has greater health benefits. The 2008 Guidelines provided a variety of examples of how to meet guidelines—all involved doing more than 150 min/week of aerobic activity. The guidelines advised that people should set individualized goals for the amounts and types of activity appropriate for them.

DEFINING LEVELS OF INTENSITY

It is difficult for the public to understand what is meant by the term "moderate-intensity" activity. Therefore, the 2008 Guidelines provided many examples of moderate-intensity and vigorous-intensity activity. It also provided a rule of thumb (described above) that, on a scale of 0 to 10, moderate intensity is a 5 or 6, and vigorous intensity is a 7 or 8.

SUPPORTING DISSEMINATION AND MAINTAINING PUBLIC AWARENESS

The *2008 Physical Activity Guidelines for Americans* incorporated novel efforts to support engagement of many organizations in dissemination of the guidelines. Two efforts of the Office of Disease Prevention and Health Promotion (2008) are particularly noteworthy. Before the guidelines were launched, an online supporter network was initiated and developed. Supporter organizations commit to taking action to help individuals and communities become physically active. Within months after the launch, more than 2000 supporting organizations had signed up. Upon becoming a supporter, organizations received a toolkit with communication materials to help disseminate the guidelines. Supporters are also involved in the second novel dissemination effort, the Be Active Your Way blog. This blog provides a forum for supporters to share best practices and plan collaborative efforts. It is also an information resource for the public and provides an Internet presence for the *Physical Activity Guidelines*. Information about the *Be Active Your Way* Supporter Network and blog are available at the Physical Activity Guidelines for Americans web site, http://www.health.gov/PAGuidelines.

MOVING FORWARD WITH GUIDELINES WHEN EVIDENCE IS INCOMPLETE

Public health recommendations are often supported with a rationale of "We don't know everything, but we know enough to act." Gaps certainly exist in the evidence about how physical activity affects health, and that created a challenge for writing guidelines. As a result of these gaps, the guidelines did not endorse:

- A specified frequency of physical activity of 5 or more days per week in adults
- Flexibility and stretching activity
- Warm-ups and cool-downs
- Aerobic bouts of activity shorter than 10 min in adults
- Reducing sitting time
- An "optimal" level of physical activity

- Medical consultation in healthy people (of any age) before starting an exercise program
- A target step count on pedometers (all steps do not count, only moderate- to vigorous-intensity steps)
- Balance training for all older adults
- A minimum number of minutes of vigorous-intensity activity for youth

However, insufficient evidence is NOT the same as evidence against, and the *Physical Activity Guidelines Advisory Committee Report, 2008* includes a chapter (Part H) that summarizes research needed to address questions the committee identified during their review of the science. For example, future studies may indeed demonstrate that warm-ups and cool-downs are important for healthy physical activity.

Perhaps the most critical gap is the incomplete understanding of the role of caloric expenditure from light-intensity activity, referred to as "baseline" activity in the 2008 Guidelines. The lack of evidence regarding light-intensity activity also relates to questions about the importance of nonexercise activity thermogenesis and of reducing sedentary time. More broadly, the issue is the importance of total caloric expenditure from any intensity level of physical activity versus the importance of caloric expenditure from only moderate- or vigorous-intensity activity. It is not widely appreciated that the 1996 Surgeon General's report, *Physical Activity and Health* (U.S. Department of Health and Human Services 1996), provided a total caloric expenditure physical activity recommendation, even as it endorsed the recommended levels in *Physical Activity and Public Health: A Recommendation from the Centers for Disease Control and Prevention and the American College of Sports Medicine* (Pate et al. 1995). According to the Surgeon General's report, a person could do sufficient amounts of activity by performing 30 min of brisk walking, 15 min of running, or 45 min of playing volleyball. It is noteworthy that in the first epidemiologic study to measure caloric expenditure using doubly labeled water, total activity energy expenditure was strongly related to lower risk of premature mortality in older adults (Manini et al. 2006). As evidence accumulates, it is possible that future versions of physical activity guidelines will specify amounts of moderate- or vigorous-intensity physical activity as well as minimal amounts of light-intensity activity (or, equivalently, specify maximal amounts of sitting time).

ROLE OF PHYSICAL ACTIVITY GUIDELINES IN IMPROVING HEALTH

Physical activity guidelines are necessary, but not sufficient, to increase levels of health-enhancing physical activity. Physical activity is a complex behavior with multiple determinants. Therefore, it is important to consider how factors such as organizations, communities, and national policies can impede or facilitate choosing a physically active lifestyle (see Chapter 18 of this text). The last chapter of the *2008 Physical Activity Guidelines for Americans* presents a socioecologic approach to help make regular physical activity the easy choice for all. A similarly multifactorial approach is also evident in such efforts as the U.S. National Physical Activity Plan (2010), the Toronto Charter for Physical Activity (Global Advocacy Council for

Physical Activity 2010), and other national plans (see National Plan website for links to plans of other countries http://www.physicalactivityplan.org/history/resources.php). These plans provide guidance on how to develop and implement actions to increase the level of physical activity in populations. The plans share several aspects, including a focus on increasing opportunities for physical activity; recommended engagement and partnerships of governments, nongovernment organizations, professional organizations, and other agencies within health, transportation, planning, and other sectors; recommended broad involvement of affected and targeted constituencies; and an evidence-based approach.

Historically, in the case of guidelines for both physical activity and diet, a major assumption has been that provision of science-based recommendations would lead individuals to healthier behavior. Data on population trends in physical activity and dietary intake do not support this assumption, which raises the question, "If providing guidance is insufficient, what is the role of physical activity guidelines in preventing inactivity?"

It is increasingly recognized that systematic change in policies and environmental factors at multiple levels is necessary if individuals are to make healthy physical activity and diet choices. For a variety of reasons, physical activity guidelines based on an extensive scientific review should be the foundation for efforts to make these policy and environmental changes to prevent inactivity. First of all, science-based physical activity guidelines are needed to justify the expenditure of public funds for promotion and programming. A scientifically sound and practical set of guidelines is critical for establishing the legitimacy of physical activity among other public health interventions. Second, the guidelines are needed to specify the benefits to be expected by various population groups and the dose of activity considered necessary to achieve these benefits. Third, physical activity guidelines can support a unified message and provide behavior targets that can be used as consistent metrics for short- and long-term evaluation. Finally, the documented health benefits of physical activity can be used to help support economic arguments in terms of healthcare cost savings as well as moral justification based on equity and human rights.

CONCLUSION

The publication of the *2008 Physical Activity Guidelines for Americans* represented an evolution from clinical recommendations of professional organizations for cardiac patients to public health recommendations to reduce chronic disease risk. The development of the guidelines incorporated many steps including a systematic literature review, deliberations among a scientific advisory group, and consideration of plain language and communication science in presenting the Guidelines. The Guidelines document is consistent with previous physical activity recommendations in many ways, but also includes important changes and novel aspects. The 2008 Guidelines and their supporting science form the basis of other national physical activity recommendations, leading to a consistent message across multiple initiatives in the United States and other countries. The Guidelines provide a strong foundation for policy and environmental actions that will facilitate increased physical activity and health benefits for all.

STUDY QUESTIONS

1. Compare and contrast the 2008 Physical Activity Guidelines for youth, adults, and older adults.
2. Design a 6-week, physical activity program for adults using the 2008 Physical Activity Guidelines.
3. List at least five important areas that have gaps in the evidence related to details about the health benefits of physical activity. Defend the use of these physical activity modalities in an exercise prescription despite the gaps.
4. Describe at least two situations when it would be appropriate to use (a) absolute intensity and (b) relative intensity to describe aerobic physical activity.
5. What are two common challenges in communicating physical activity guidelines to the public? Suggest at least three ways to overcome these challenges.

REFERENCES

Fletcher, G. F., S. N. Blair, J. Blumenthal et al. 1992. Statement on exercise. Benefits and recommendations for physical activity programs for all Americans. A statement for health professionals by the Committee on Exercise and Cardiac Rehabilitation of the Council on Clinical Cardiology, American Heart Association. *Circulation* 86: 340–344.

Global Advocacy Council for Physical Activity, International Society for Physical Activity and Health. 2010. The Toronto Charter for Physical Activity: A Global Call to Action. http://www.globalpa.org.uk/pdf/torontocharter-eng-20may2010.pdf (accessed January 31, 2011).

Haskell, W. L., I. M. Lee, R. R. Pate et al. 2007. Physical activity and public health: Updated recommendation for adults from the American College of Sports Medicine and the American Heart Association. *Med. Sci. Sports Exerc.* 39: 1423–1434.

Manini, T. M., J. E. Everhart, K. V. Patel et al. 2006. Daily activity energy expenditure and mortality among older adults. *JAMA* 296: 171–179.

Nelson, M. E., W. J. Rejeski, S. N. Blair et al. 2007. Physical activity and public health in older adults: Recommendation from the American College of Sports Medicine and the American Heart Association. *Med. Sci. Sports Exerc.* 39: 1435–1445.

NIH Consensus Development Panel on Physical Activity and Cardiovascular Health. 1996. Physical activity and cardiovascular health. *JAMA* 276: 241–246.

Office of Disease Prevention and Health Promotion. 2008. *Be Active Your Way: A Guide for Adults.* Washington, DC: U.S. Government Printing Office. ODPHP Publication No. U0037.

Pate, R. R., M. Pratt, S. N. Blair et al. 1995. Physical activity and public health: A recommendation from the Centers for Disease Control and Prevention and the American College of Sports Medicine. *JAMA* 273: 402–407.

Physical Activity Guidelines Advisory Committee. 2008. *Physical Activity Guidelines Advisory Committee Report, 2008.* Washington, DC: U.S. Department of Health and Human Services. Part D: Background.

The White House (President George W. Bush). 2002. Fact Sheet: President Bush Launches HealthierUS Initiative. http://georgewbush-whitehouse.archives.gov/news/releases/2002/06/20020620-6.html (accessed January 31, 2011).

U.S. Department of Health and Human Services. 2008. *2008 Physical Activity Guidelines for Americans.* Washington, DC: U.S. Department of Health and Human Services. http://www.health.gov/PAGuidelines (accessed February 18, 2011).

U.S. Department of Health and Human Services. 1996. *Physical Activity and Health: A Report of the Surgeon General*. Atlanta, GA: U.S. Department of Health and Human Services, Centers for Disease Control and Prevention.

U.S. Department of Health and Human Services and U.S. Department of Agriculture. 2005. *Dietary Guidelines for Americans, 2005*. 6th Edition, Washington, DC: U.S. Government Printing Office.

U.S. National Plan for Physical Activity. 2010. National Physical Activity Plan. http://www.physicalactivityplan.org/ (accessed January 31, 2011).

WHO/FIMS Committee on Physical Activity for Health. 1995. Exercise for health. *Bull. World Health Organ.* 73: 135–136.

World Health Organization. 2010 *Global Recommendations on Physical Activity for Health*. Geneva: WHO Press.

13 Surveillance of Physical Activity

Janet E. Fulton and Susan A. Carlson

CONTENTS

INTRODUCTION

Surveillance of physical activity is an important and vital function of physical activity epidemiology and, in turn, of public health. This chapter will introduce and define several key concepts of physical activity surveillance: (1) definition of epidemiology; (2) definition and characteristics of surveillance systems; (3) surveillance of the behavior of physical activity; (4) surveillance of environmental and policy supports for physical activity; and (5) uses of surveillance data. The chapter concludes with thoughts about the challenges and opportunities awaiting surveillance of physical activity in the United States.

EPIDEMIOLOGY

Epidemiology is the science of public health and has been defined as "the study of the distribution and determinants of health-related states and events in populations, and the application of this study to the control of health problems" (Last and International Epidemiological Association 1983). Translating and disseminating information about the proportion of the population that is sufficiently physically active, for example, is one key step to determine where it is best to intervene. Thus, not only is it important to understand the distribution and determinants of disease—it is also important to use that information to make improvements to the health of the population. These improvements can be made by controlling or delaying the development of risk factors and diseases and also by attempting to prevent risk factors and diseases from occurring in the first place. Translation and dissemination of information to stakeholders therefore is one of the hallmarks of epidemiology and therefore of effective public health practice.

SURVEILLANCE

Surveillance is a vital component of the science of epidemiology. Public health surveillance has been defined as the "Ongoing, systematic collection, analysis, and interpretation of outcome-specific data for use in the planning, implementation, and evaluation of public health practice" (Thacker and Berkelman 1988). Two components of this definition are particularly important to consider. First, surveillance is ongoing and systematic. Ongoing refers to the assessment of the outcomes of interest over time. In this way, surveillance differs from the one-time survey (Galuska and Fulton 2009).

Because data collection for surveillance is done multiple times, it must be systematic; the same information needs to be collected in the same manner over time. Even slight changes in survey questions or data collection methodologies can alter the interpretation of the findings both within a surveillance system and across systems.

For example, the National Health Interview Survey (NHIS) has collected physical activity information using the same questions and the same methodology from 1998 through the to present. NHIS data are essential for evaluating national indicators defined by U.S. the Department of Health and Human Services, such as the *Healthy People* objectives.

Second, data from public health surveillance systems need to be used. That is, the data need to be readily available to those who make decisions about public health issues such as the implementation of physical activity programs. Furthermore, the information collected must be of sufficient specificity and quality to address the information needs of the decision maker and must be able to be communicated in a timely manner (Galuska and Fulton 2009). For example, the Behavioral Risk Factor Surveillance System (BRFSS) collects physical activity information from all 50 states in odd-numbered years to determine the national and state-specific prevalence of U.S. adults meeting the *2008 Physical Activity Guidelines for Americans* (Loustalot et al. 2009; U.S. Department of Health and Human Services 2008; Centers for Disease Control and Prevention 2010a). This information is available within about 6 months of data collection and is used to inform state physical activity coordinators of the status of adult physical activity levels in their state.

Finally, because surveillance systems have specific characteristics that serve a specific purpose (to provide ongoing and systematic information to enhance the public health), it is important to remember that not all surveys constitute surveillance. For example, in 2003–2006 and again beginning in 2011, the National Health and Nutrition Examination Survey (NHANES) has assessed physical activity using accelerometers that provide a snapshot of physical activity. If accelerometers are incorporated on an ongoing, systematic fashion, then this method would constitute a physical activity surveillance system.

For chronic disease prevention and health promotion, once a behavior has been established as beneficial for health, such as physical activity (Physical Activity Guidelines Advisory Committee 2008), then it is reasonable to include this in a public health surveillance system. Figure 13.1 shows a conceptual rendering of "The life cycle of

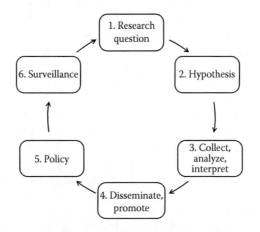

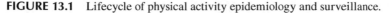

FIGURE 13.1 Lifecycle of physical activity epidemiology and surveillance.

physical activity epidemiology and surveillance." The physical activity lifecycle begins with a research question and corresponding hypothesis. The question can be addressed by choosing from a variety of study designs (e.g., cross-sectional, prospective, experimental), data collection methodologies, and analytic techniques. Once the research question is answered and the hypothesis supported or refuted in multiple studies, an evidence base begins to emerge in response to the research question. From this body of knowledge, the evidence is then translated and disseminated to a variety of audiences (e.g., policy makers, educators, healthcare professionals, caregivers, and the general public), where the choice of the audience largely depends on the intent of the message to be communicated. Policy makers, for example, may be most influenced by data showing cost savings when physical activity programs are implemented. Conversely, parents and care givers may be most interested in health or academic achievement benefits for children and adolescents. Advancing the research findings into policies to support physical activity may occur once the findings are translated and disseminated, although policy development is not always carried out in a systematic, linear fashion.

Surveillance of physical activity is conducted for different reasons and often with limited resources. Because of this, it is important to have a good rationale to collect physical activity information in surveillance systems. One rationale is that there is evidence that changing a behavior or policy will have an impact on public health. Another rationale is that policy makers want the data to make decisions (e.g., data on the cost-effectiveness of introducing physical activity programs). It is important therefore to recognize from Figure 13.1 that surveillance may be most useful if it occurs toward the end of the physical activity lifecycle (step 6) so that precious resources are reserved to systematically monitor physical activity over time that have a direct link to the public health and to key stakeholders.

KEY CHARACTERISTICS OF PHYSICAL ACTIVITY SURVEILLANCE SYSTEMS

Physical activity surveillance systems are typified by seven key characteristics (i.e., simplicity, flexibility, acceptability, sensitivity, representativeness, timeliness, and cost) as shown in Table 13.1 (Centers for Disease Control and Prevention 1988). Taken together, these characteristics provide the framework from which a public health surveillance system is developed, carried out, and evaluated. It is unlikely that a surveillance system will rank highly on all elements, but the goal is to maximize the capacity of the system to capture the outcome of interest (in this case, physical activity behaviors or environmental/policy supports) in the best way possible to provide the most relevant information for the end user. Efforts to improve certain attributes, such as the ability of a system to accurately detect physical activity (sensitivity), may detract from other attributes, such as the simplicity of collecting physical activity information from a population or timeliness in transferring physical activity data into a usable form for researchers and practitioners alike. Thus, the success of an individual physical activity surveillance system depends on having the proper balance of the characteristics the user considers most essential (Centers for Disease Control and Prevention 1988).

TABLE 13.1

Key Criteria to Consider When Developing or Evaluating Public Health Surveillance Systems

Criteria	Definition	Key Question(s) to Address	Physical Activity Example
Simplicity	Refers to both its structure and ease of operation. Surveillance systems should be as simple as possible while still meeting their objectives.	Are procedures, training, data collection, computer requirements, etc., simple to use?	Training telephone interviewers or household data collectors does not take excessive time. Physical activity questions are not overly burdensome for the interviewer or the participant.
Flexibility	Can adapt to changing information needs or operating conditions with little additional cost in time, personnel, or allocated funds. Can accommodate, for example, changes in definitions and variations in reporting sources.	Does the system have the ability to adapt to changing needs?	Able to adapt to changes in *Guideline* definitions. For example, two definitions of "sufficiently active" (e.g., *Healthy People* 2010 and the *2008 Physical Activity Guidelines*) can be assessed in the surveillance system.
Acceptability	Reflects the willingness of individuals and organizations to participate in the surveillance system.	Will drop out be a factor? Does the system, because of its characteristics, discourage participation?	Participants are willing to complete a physical activity questionnaire or wear a monitor for the prespecified period.
Sensitivity	The system should be able to accurately classify participants according to the health outcome of interest (e.g., prevalence of meeting the Guidelines) and should also be able to detect change in the prevalence of the health outcome.	Does the instrument measure what you want it to measure?	Physical activity surveillance questions have known validity (Yore et al. 2007)

(continued)

TABLE 13.1 (Continued)
Key Criteria to Consider When Developing or Evaluating Public Health Surveillance Systems

Criteria	Definition	Key Question(s) to Address	Physical Activity Example
Representativeness	Assessed by comparing the characteristics of reported health outcomes to all such actual outcomes.	Are those who participate (or who are included for environmental systems) different from those who are not?	The proportion of adults meeting Guidelines who complete the physical activity interview should be similar to adults who do not complete the interview or who are unable to be contacted.
Timeliness	Reflects the speed or delay between steps in a surveillance system. Timeliness is evaluated in terms of availability of information—either for immediate efforts or for long-term program planning.	Is time from data collection to dissemination reasonable?	In the BRFSS, time from data collection to having data available for analysis is about 6 months.
Cost	Covers only the resources directly required to operate a surveillance system. These "direct costs" include the personnel and financial resources expended in collecting, processing, analyzing, and disseminating the data.	What are the total costs to obtain population-based estimates of physical activity and environmental and policy supports for physical activity?	It is difficult to estimate the specific cost for physical activity surveillance because physical activity is only one part of most population-based surveillance systems.

Source: Centers for Disease Control and Prevention, *MMWR Morb. Mortal. Wkly. Rep.*, 37, Suppl. 5, 1–18, 1988. With permission.

SURVEILLANCE OF PHYSICAL ACTIVITY BEHAVIOR

Surveillance systems most often assess the physical activity behaviors of individuals. For example, current U.S. systems measure the frequency and duration of moderate- and vigorous-intensity physical activity (Table 13.2). Table 13.2 presents characteristics of two U.S. surveillance systems for adults, the NHIS and the BRFSS (Carlson et

TABLE 13.2

Characteristics and Physical Activity Assessment of National Health Interview Survey (NHIS) and Behavioral Risk Factor Surveillance System (BRFSS)

Category	NHIS	BRFSS
Mode	In person	Telephone
Sampling frame	Addresses compiled from the 1990 U.S. census	Random digit dialing
Response rate	62.6% (2008)[a]	52.5 % (2009)[a]
Number of responders	21,781 (2008)	432,607 (2009)
Can produce state-based estimates?	No	Yes
Physical activity assessment		
Survey years current physical activity questions asked	1998–2009[b]	2001–2009 (odd years)
Recall period	Respondent selects recall period[a]	Usual week
Domain(s) of PA assessed	Leisure-time physical activity	Nonoccupational physical activity[c]
Assesses moderate-intensity PA	Yes, but includes light-intensity	Yes
Assesses vigorous-intensity PA	Yes	Yes
Which intensity level is asked about first?	Vigorous	Moderate
Definition for moderate-intensity of physical activity	Light sweating or a slight to moderate increase in breathing or heart rate	Small increases in breathing or heart rate
Definition for vigorous-intensity of physical activity	Heavy sweating or large increases in breathing or heart rate	Large increases in breathing or heart rate

Source: Carlson, S.A. et al., *J. Phys. Act. Health*, 6, Suppl. 1, S18–S27, 2009. With permission.

[a] Response rate reported for NHIS is the final unconditional sample adult response rate. Response rate reported for BRFSS is the Council of American Survey and Research Organization median state response rate. These two response rates are not directly comparable.

[b] NHIS physical activity questions allow respondents to select recall period. To define physical activity levels, average number of times/week (rounded to the nearest time) were calculated for those respondents who selected monthly or yearly periods.

[c] BRFSS has a separate question about monthly participation (yes/no) in any physical activities or exercises such as running, calisthenics, golf, gardening, or walking for exercise that was not included as part of this analysis.

al. 2009). In the table, comparable information on survey sampling and information on physical activity assessment is presented for these two surveillance systems. Data from these surveys are often used to categorize an individual's behavior as meeting (or not meeting) physical activity guidelines to estimate the prevalence of meeting physical activity guidelines in the population.

SURVEILLANCE OF CHILDREN AND ADOLESCENTS

In children and adolescents, regular physical activity promotes stronger bones, higher cardiovascular fitness, better blood pressure, and a healthy weight (Strong et al. 2005; Physical Activity Guidelines Advisory Committee 2008). Active youth may also be more likely to remain active as they mature into adulthood (Malina 1996). Guidelines for physical activity for children and adolescents include three components: aerobic, muscle-strengthening, and bone-strengthening. The U.S. surveillance system that currently assesses the percentage of high school students who meet the aerobic guideline for 60 min on 7 days/week is the Youth Risk Behavior Surveillance System (YRBSS). Muscle-strengthening and bone-strengthening are not currently assessed in U.S. surveillance systems, although a muscle strengthening question will be included on the 2011 YRBSS.

SURVEILLANCE OF ADULTS

For adults, participation in regular physical activity has many health benefits. Physically active adults, compared to their inactive counterparts, are less likely to develop many chronic conditions and diseases (including coronary heart disease, stroke, hypertension, osteoporosis, depression, colon and breast cancers) and death from all causes (Physical Activity Guidelines Advisory Committee 2008). The *2008 Physical Activity Guidelines for Americans* (Guidelines) suggest that the minimum amount of aerobic physical activity that provides sufficient health benefits is 150 min/week of moderate-intensity physical activity, 75 min/week of vigorous-intensity activity, or an equivalent combination of the two (U.S. Department of Health and Human Services 2008). For additional and more extensive health benefits, adults should increase their aerobic activity to 300 or more min a week of moderate-intensity activity, or 150 or more min a week of vigorous-intensity activity, or an equivalent combination of the two. In addition to the aerobic guidelines, the Guidelines also recommend that adults do muscle-strengthening activities that involve all major muscle groups on 2 or more days a week. Fully meeting the physical activity Guidelines includes meeting both the aerobic and muscle-strengthening components of the Guidelines.

EXAMPLES OF U.S. GOVERNMENT SURVEILLANCE SYSTEMS THAT MEASURE PHYSICAL ACTIVITY BEHAVIOR

There are many surveillance systems that measure physical activity behavior at the individual level. This section will focus on four systems that are the data sources to track the national physical activity objectives related to individual behavior from *Healthy People* 2020 (U.S. Department of Health and Human Services 2010a) and/or the state-equivalents of these objectives: (1) YRBSS; (2) NHIS; (3) BRFSS; (4) National Household Travel Survey (NHTS).

YOUTH RISK BEHAVIOR SURVEILLANCE SYSTEM

The YRBSS has been conducted every other year since its beginning in 1991. The YRBSS monitors priority health-risk behaviors and the prevalence of obesity and asthma among youth and young adults. The YRBSS includes a national school-based survey conducted by the Centers for Disease Control and Prevention (CDC) and state, territorial, tribal, and district surveys conducted by state, territorial, and local education and health agencies and tribal governments. The national, state, and local Youth Risk Behavior Surveys (YRBS) are administered to 9th through 12th grade students drawn from probability samples of schools and students. Each national school-based YRBS conducted by the CDC in odd years from 1999 to 2009 uses a similar three-stage cluster-sample design to obtain a nationally representative sample of private and public high school students in the United States. Primary sampling units (PSUs), consisting of large counties or groups of smaller adjacent counties, are selected from 16 strata formed according to the degree of urbanization and the relative percentages of black and Hispanic students in the PSU. The second stage of sampling is schools and the final stage of sampling consists of randomly selecting from each chosen school and grade level 1 or 2 intact classes of a required subject, such as English or social studies. The questionnaire is anonymous and self-administered usually during the spring. In 2009, the national YRBSS sample size was 16,410, and the overall response rate was 71% (Centers for Disease Control and Prevention 2009b).

The question that will be used to monitor the proposed *Healthy People* 2020 aerobic physical activity objective for adolescence has been asked since 2005 on the biannual YRBSS. In addition, high school students have been asked about days per week of physical education classes (1991–2009) and about whether they played on sports teams (1999–2009).

YRBSS PHYSICAL ACTIVITY QUESTIONS:

- During the past 7 days, on how many days were you physically active for a total of at least 60 minutes per day? (Add up all the time you spent in any kind of physical activity that increased your heart rate and made you breathe hard some of the time.)
- In an average week when you are in school, on how many days do you go to physical education (PE) classes?
- During the past 12 months, on how many sports teams did you play? (Include any teams run by your school or community groups.)

NATIONAL HEALTH INTERVIEW SURVEY

The NHIS has been conducted continuously since 1957. The NHIS collects information on a variety of health measures and is used to track progress on many national health objectives. NHIS is a face-to-face household survey of a random sample of civilian, noninstitutionalized persons living in the United States. It is conducted continuously throughout the year. The survey is a multistage design that starts by selecting PSUs from a list of geographically defined PSUs that cover the 50 states and the District of Columbia. The next level of sampling involves selecting households. Basic health and demographic information are collected for all household members; additional information, such as physical activity, is collected on one randomly selected adult (≥18 years of age). In 2008, the NHIS sample sizes for completed interviews of sampled adults was 21,781 and the final unconditional sample adult response rate was 62.6% (National Center for Health Statistics 2008).

The NHIS first asked questions about leisure-time physical activity in 1975 (National Center for Health Statistics 2010). From 1998 to 2009, the same series of leisure-time physical activity questions have been asked annually on the sample adult questionnaire of the NHIS. These questions have been almost identical since 1998 except that before 2004, the leisure-time qualifier was included only in the introduction to the physical activity section and beginning in 2004, the leisure-time qualifier was embedded in each question.

NHIS PHYSICAL ACTIVITY QUESTIONS:

The next questions are about physical activities (exercises, sports, physically active hobbies, etc.) that you may do in your LEISURE time.

- How often do you do VIGOROUS leisure-time physical activities for AT LEAST 10 MINUTES that cause HEAVY sweating or LARGE increases in breathing or heart rate?
  - About how long do you do these vigorous leisure-time physical activities each time?
- How often do you do LIGHT OR MODERATE leisure-time physical activities for AT LEAST 10 MINUTES that cause ONLY LIGHT sweating or a SLIGHT to MODERATE increase in breathing or heart rate?
  - About how long do you do these light or moderate leisure-time physical activities each time?

BEHAVIORAL RISK FACTOR SURVEILLANCE SYSTEM

The BRFSS began in 1984 and is a state-based system of health surveys that collects information on health risk behaviors, preventive health practices, and health-care access primarily related to chronic disease and injury. BRFSS is a state-based, random digit–dialed telephone survey of the civilian, noninstitutionalized U.S. adult population ≥18 years of age. It is conducted in all 50 states, the District of Columbia, Guam, Puerto Rico, and the U.S. Virgin Islands. Each state works with the CDC to develop a sampling protocol to select households, and one adult is selected from each household. In 2009, the BRFSS sample size was 432,607, and the median state response rate calculated using Council of American Survey and Research Organization guidelines was 52.5% (Centers for Disease Control and Prevention 2009a).

In 1984, 35 states included on their BRFSS core a question about monthly participation (yes/no) in any physical activities or exercises. By 1996, all states had incorporated this one question as part of the BRFSS core, and this question is often referred to as the BRFSS Physical Activity Tracking Question. From 2001 to 2009, the same seven physical activity questions (the one tracking question plus six additional questions shown below) have been asked on the BRFSS rotating core (i.e., every other year in odd-numbered years) to assess the amount of all nonoccupational physical activity. In 2011 and beyond, the six questions following the initial tracking question will be modified to include the questions used before 2001 (shown below). This series of questions will also assess all nonoccupational physical activity and is also able to estimate the proportion of U.S. adults meeting physical activity guidelines. One advantage of the 2011 questions is they will also measure the mode of physical activity as they assess the types of physical activity in which U.S. adults most frequently participate—such as walking. In 2011 and beyond, the BRFSS will also measure muscle strengthening as it is an important component of the Physical Activity Guidelines and also an objective of *Healthy People* 2010.

BRFSS PHYSICAL ACTIVITY QUESTIONS (2001–2009):

- During the past month, other than your regular job, did you participate in any physical activities or exercises such as running, calisthenics, golf, gardening, or walking for exercise? (Tracking question.)
- We are interested in two types of physical activity—vigorous and moderate. Vigorous activities cause large increases in breathing or heart rate while moderate activities cause small increases in breathing or heart rate.
  - Now, thinking about the moderate activities you do when you are not working in a usual week, do you do moderate activities for at least 10 minutes at a time, such as brisk walking, bicycling, vacuuming, gardening, or anything else that causes some increase in breathing or heart rate?
    - How many days per week do you do these moderate activities for at least 10 minutes?
    - On days when you do moderate activities for at least 10 minutes at a time, how much total time per day do you spend doing these activities?
  - Now, thinking about the vigorous activities you do when you are not working in a usual week, do you do vigorous activities for at least 10 minutes at a time, such as running, aerobics, heavy yard work, or anything else that causes large increases in breathing or heart rate?
    - How many days per week do you do these vigorous activities for at least 10 minutes at a time?
    - On days when you do vigorous activities for at least 10 minutes at a time, how much total time per day do you spend doing these activities?

BRFSS PHYSICAL ACTIVITY QUESTIONS (2011 AND BEYOND):

- During the past month, other than your regular job, did you participate in any physical activities or exercises such as running, calisthenics, golf, gardening, or walking for exercise? (Tracking question.)

- What type of physical activity or exercise did you spend the most time doing during the past month?
- How many times per week or per month did you take part in this activity during the past month?
- And when you took part in this activity, for how many minutes or hours did you usually keep at it?
- What other type of physical activity gave you the next most exercise during the past month?
- How many times per week or per month did you take part in this activity during the past month?
- And when you took part in this activity, for how many minutes or hours did you usually keep at it?

- During the past month, how many times per week or per month did you do physical activities or exercises to STRENGTHEN your muscles? Do NOT count aerobic activities like walking, running, or bicycling. Count activities using your own body weight like yoga, sit-ups or push-ups and those using weight machines, free weights, or elastic bands.

NATIONAL HOUSEHOLD TRAVEL SURVEY

The NHTS provides information to assist transportation planners and policy makers who need comprehensive data on travel and transportation patterns in the United States. The 2009 NHTS updates information gathered in the 2001 NHTS and in previous Nationwide Personal Transportation Surveys conducted in 1969, 1977, 1983, 1990, and 1995. The survey includes demographic characteristics of households, people, vehicles, and detailed information on daily and longer-distance travel for all purposes by all modes. NHTS survey data are collected from a sample adult in a U.S. household to provide national estimates of trips and miles by travel mode, trip purpose, and a host of household attributes. The 2009 NHTS included about 26,000 households (Federal Highway Administration 2009).

In NHTS, data are collected on daily trips taken in a 24-h period, and includes the following information: purpose of the trip (work, shopping, etc.), means of transportation used (car, bus, subway, walk, etc.), how long the trip took, and time of day when the trip took place. NHTS data can be used to examine trips that were made using active transportation (i.e., means of transportation was walking and/or bicycling) and can also be used to examine the mode of transportation used to get to school for children and adolescents. The NHTS is the data source for monitoring the *Healthy People* 2020 objectives related to increasing the proportion of trips made by walking and bicycling.

OTHER SURVEILLANCE SYSTEMS

Other U.S. government surveillance systems that may be of interest are the National Survey of Children's Health (NSCH) and the NHANES. The NSCH is a national survey that was conducted by telephone in English and Spanish during 2003–2004 and for a second time in 2007–2008. The survey provides a broad range of information about children's health and well-being collected in a manner that allows for comparisons between states and at the national level (National Center for Health Statistics 2007). NHANES is a program designed to assess the health and nutritional status of adults and children in the United States and is unique because it combines interviews and physical examinations. Both the NSCH and NHANES collect information about sedentary behavior (e.g., television viewing). Over the years, NHANES has used different physical activity questions (i.e., a different set of questions was used in 1999–2006, 2007–2008, and 2009–2010), therefore making it less useful for surveillance of physical activity over time. NHANES also introduced accelerometers to measure physical activity as part of the 2003–2006 study (Troiano et al. 2008) and also began including accelerometers again in 2011.

Comparing Estimates from Different Surveillance Systems

When examining estimates from a surveillance system, it is important to understand the design of the system and the method used to assess physical activity. Before comparing prevalence estimates from different surveillance systems, all aspects of data collection and data analysis must be examined. It is also important to understand the strengths and limitations inherent in each system to determine if comparisons are appropriate. To illustrate this point, a comparison of the BRFSS and the NHIS system's characteristics and physical activity assessment methods is provided in Table 13.2 (Carlson et al. 2009).

SURVEILLANCE OF ENVIRONMENTAL AND POLICY SUPPORTS FOR PHYSICAL ACTIVITY

In addition to strategies to improve physical activity behavior such as informational approaches (e.g., using point of decision prompts to encourage stair use) or behavioral and social approaches (e.g., improving school based physical education), strategies to improve the environment for physical activity or enact policies that promote physical activity have also been identified (Heath et al. 2006).

Environmental and policy-level strategies are used to improve the environment for physical activity (e.g., converting abandoned railroads to bicycle trails) or enact and implement policies that enhance an individual's ability to be physically active (e.g., authorizing a policy to support a 30-min physical activity break in the workplace). These indicators normally focus on environmental and policy supports related to recommendations found in *The Guide to Community Preventive Services* (Heath et al. 2006; Guide to Community Preventive Services 2010; Task Force on Community Preventive Services 2002; Kahn et al. 2002), *CDC's Guide to Strategies for Increasing Physical Activity in the Community* (Resources for State and Community Programs March 2010), *The Surgeon General's Vision for a Healthy and Fit Nation* (U.S. Department of Health and Human Services 2010b), and *The National Physical Activity Plan* (Pate 2009).

Environmental and policy-level indicators measure different aspects of physical activity supports available for a group of people, normally defined by a geographical area or within a certain setting (e.g., school, worksite, community). These types of strategies seek to make physical activity the easy choice!

Surveillance of indicators of the physical activity environment or of physical activity policies can be conducted in several ways: (1) by directly asking an individual about their perceptions (e.g., asking individuals about their neighborhood physical activity environment); (2) by asking key informants in the setting (e.g., interviewing a school principal about their school's physical activity policies); and (3) by using information already collected within the setting (e.g., as an indicator of high school sport participation, the number of students enrolled in school sports teams). Table 13.3 provides examples of environmental and policy indicators that have been used to provide state-level estimates.

QUESTIONNAIRES THAT MEASURE ENVIRONMENTAL AND POLICY SUPPORTS FOR PHYSICAL ACTIVITY

Questions about an individual's perceptions about policy and environmental supports can be added to surveillance systems that assess individual behavior. One example of this method of assessment from a state and national level is from the NSCH (National Center for Health Statistics 2007). This survey asks parents about whether certain environmental supports (e.g., park or playground area; recreation center, community center, or boys' or girls' club; sidewalks or walking paths) are available to children in their neighborhood. Other surveillance systems have not incorporated these types of questions but questionnaires have been developed to assess some environmental characteristics, including the Physical Activity Neighborhood Environment Survey and the Abbreviated Neighborhood Environment Walkability Scale (Cerin et al. 2006; Sallis et al. 2009, 2010). It is unclear, however, whether these two questionnaires are applicable for surveillance of the physical activity environment because they have not yet been used in the same population over time.

Currently, at state and national levels in the United States, surveillance that interviews officials in a specific setting about environmental and policy-level supports of physical activity is limited to the school setting, where there are two data sources (discussed in the following subsections).

SCHOOL HEALTH PROFILES (PROFILES)

The School Health Profiles (Profiles) is a system of surveys assessing school health policies and programs in states, large urban school districts, and territories. Since 1994, Profiles surveys have been conducted biennially by education and health agencies among middle and high school principals and lead health education teachers. Profiles uses random, systematic, equal-probability sampling strategies to produce representative samples of schools that serve students in grades 6 through 12 in each jurisdiction. In most jurisdictions, the sampling frame consists of all regular secondary public schools with one or more of grades 6 through 12. Profiles data are

TABLE 13.3
Examples of Policy and Environmental Indicators at State Level

Physical Activity Support	Policy/Environmental	Example of a State-Level Indicator and Data Source
Create or enhance access to places for physical activity	Environmental	Percentage of census blocks that have at least one fitness or recreation center located within the block or ½ mile from the block boundary *Source:* InfoUSA
	Environmental	Percentage of census blocks that have at least one park located within the block or 1/2 mile from the block boundary *Source:* Geographic Data Technology Database
	Policy	Percentage of middle and high schools that allow community-sponsored use of physical activity facilities by youth outside of normal school hours *Source:* School Health Profiles
Enhance physical education and activity in schools	Policy	State requires or recommends regular elementary school recess *Source:* School Health Policies and Programs Study
	Policy	State policy requiring elementary, middle, and high schools to teach physical education. *Source:* School Health Policies and Programs Study
	Policy	Percentage of middle and high schools within each state that support or promote walking or biking to and from school *Source:* School Health Policies and Programs Study
Support urban design, land use, and transportation policies	Policy	Existence of at least one state-level enacted street-scale urban design/land use policy *Source:* CDC Nutrition, Physical Activity and Obesity Legislative Database and National Conference of State Legislatures Healthy Community Design and Access to Healthy Food Legislation Database
	Policy	Existence of at least one state-level enacted transportation and travel policy *Source:* CDC Nutrition, Physical Activity and Obesity Legislative Database and National Conference of State Legislatures Healthy Community Design and Access to Healthy Food Legislation Database

collected from self-administered questionnaires from the principal and the lead health education teacher at each sampled school. In 2008, estimates were reported for 47 states, 18 cities, and 4 territories (Centers for Disease Control and Prevention 2008).

SCHOOL HEALTH POLICIES AND PROGRAMS STUDY

School Health Policies and Programs Study (SHPPS) is a state- and national-level survey periodically conducted to assess school health policies and programs at the state, district, school, and classroom levels. SHPSS has been conducted in 1994, 2000, and 2006. In 2006, telephone interviews or self-administered mail questionnaires were completed by state education agency personnel in all 50 states plus the District of Columbia and among a nationally representative sample of districts (n = 538). In-person interviews at the school and classroom levels were conducted with personnel in a nationally representative sample of elementary, middle, and high schools (n = 1103) and with a nationally representative sample of teachers of classes covering required health instruction in elementary schools and required health education courses in middle and high schools (n = 912) and teachers of required physical education classes and courses (n = 1194) (Centers for Disease Control and Prevention 2006).

Examples of indicators collected by each of the systems are provided in Table 13.3.

OBSERVATIONS OF A PHYSICAL ENVIRONMENT THAT MEASURE ENVIRONMENTAL AND POLICY SUPPORTS FOR PHYSICAL ACTIVITY

Researchers have developed several audit tools in recent years to measure the physical environment as it relates to physical activity (Brownson et al. 2009). Audit tools are used to collect primary data on physical features that are not commonly available via other data sources (e.g., street trees, sidewalk width) and are used for measuring physical features that are best assessed through direct observation (e.g., architectural character, landscape maintenance) (Brownson et al. 2009). Although audit tools can provide much information about an environment, from a surveillance perspective they are not feasible if the goal is to do surveillance on a large-scale because in-person observation is time-consuming and audits can be costly.

SECONDARY DATA SOURCES AND TOOLS USED TO MEASURE ENVIRONMENTAL AND POLICY SUPPORTS FOR PHYSICAL ACTIVITY

Surveillance of environmental and policy supports for physical activity has been conducted using a broad range of available data sources. Secondary data sources are often used to obtain this type of information. Examples of available secondary data sources include geographical data, commercial data, and the systematic collection of legislation or policy for a certain geographic area or setting (Table 13.3).

Policy or legislation can be systematically collected for certain geographic areas or settings, and there are different ways of obtaining data on physical activity policies. This can be done, for example, by directly contacting a certain setting or jurisdiction for their policy and/or legislation documents, conducting a web search for policy and/or legislation, or locating a data source that has already compiled the information. For example, there are two publicly available sources that system-atically collect state legislation related to the main subjects of nutrition, physical activity, and the combination of the two: CDC Nutrition, Physical Activity and Obesity Legislative Database (http://apps.nccd.cdc.gov/DNPALeg/) and National Conference of State Legislatures Healthy Community Design and Access to Healthy Food Legislation Database (http://www.ncsl.org/).

Data sources examining environmental data are often analyzed using geographic information systems (GIS), a platform for capturing, managing, manipulating, and visualizing geographic information (Schreier 2010). GIS provides a framework for gathering and organizing spatial data, and for analyzing spatial relationships.

GIS allows users to examine state, regional, and local trends for physical activity supports. Spatial data are often paired with census data to create an indicator that can be compared across geographical areas. For example, spatial data describing the location of national, state, or local parks can be linked with demographic data from the census (e.g., age, sex, or race/ethnicity) to further describe the demographic characteristics of persons living near parks. Sources of spatial data can vary from data that indicate the geographic location of physical activity supports such as state, national, and local parks (e.g., Geographic Data Technology Database) to commer-cial data that can provide information about the spatial location of commercial sup-ports such as fitness and recreation facilities (e.g., InfoUSA).

USES OF PHYSICAL ACTIVITY SURVEILLANCE DATA

Physical activity is a health behavior tracked at national and state levels and is begin-ning to be collected at local levels. Environmental and policy level surveillance efforts are just beginning to occur, but do not yet have a systematic method of col-lection in place. There are many ways, however, that surveillance systems measure and track changes in physical activity behavior that can be used for the following purposes.

SET HEALTH GOALS OR OBJECTIVES

One way to set a health goal or objective is to examine baseline estimates and use this information to base the target for a goal or objective. For example, the target may be a specific percent increase or decrease in baseline. This method was used for many of the physical activity objectives proposed for *Healthy People* 2020 (U.S. Department of Health and Human Services 2010a), where baseline data from the 2008 NHIS and the 2007 YRBSS data were used to inform the target for these national objectives (Table 13.4).

MONITOR TRENDS IN PHYSICAL ACTIVITY OVER TIME

This allows users to monitor progress in meeting national, state, and local goals and health objectives. Different systems assess physical activity in different ways; therefore, when monitoring physical activity over time, it is important that the data are from a single data source that has assessed physical activity in the same manner

TABLE 13.4
Healthy People **2020 Objectives**

Age Group	*Healthy People* 2020 Physical Activity Objective	Data Source	Baseline (%)	Target (%)
Adults	Increase the proportion of adults that meet current Federal physical activity guidelines for aerobic physical activity and for muscle strength training			
	(a) Aerobic, 150+ min/week of moderate-intensity equivalent activity	NHIS 2008	43.5	47.9
	(b) Aerobic, 300+ min/week moderate-intensity equivalent activity	NHIS 2008	28.4	31.3
	(c) Muscle strengthening, 2 days/week	NHIS 2008	21.9	24.1
	(d) Aerobic (150+ min/week of moderate-intensity equivalent activity) + muscle strengthening	NHIS 2008	18.2	20.1
Youth	Increase the proportion of adolescents that meet current physical activity guidelines for aerobic physical activity and for muscle-strengthening activity			
	(a) Aerobic, 60+ min/day, 7 days/week	YRBSS 2009	18.4	20.2
	(b) Muscle strengthening, 3+ days/week (developmental)	Data not available		
	(c) Aerobic + muscle strengthening (developmental)	Data not available		

throughout the period being monitored. Figure 13.2 provides an example of monitoring physical activity (using *Healthy People* 2010 criteria) using three surveillance systems (i.e., NHIS, NHANES, BRFSS) (Carlson et al. 2009). Data from the three surveillance systems yield slightly different conclusions about the trends over time in physical activity. When examining trends using the full period available from each system, in NHIS 1998 to 2007, there was a significant quadratic trend for being physically active. However, the prevalence of being physically active exhibited a small but significantly increasing linear trend only in BRFSS 2001 to 2007.

IDENTIFY POPULATIONS AT HIGH RISK

By analyzing data according to characteristics of the respondents' (e.g., age, sex, education, income, race/ethnicity) populations at highest risk and in need of intervention can be identified. This is often done by presenting data stratified by different demographic characteristics and comparing the subgroups (Table 13.5) (Carlson et al. 2010).

CREATE AWARENESS

Surveillance data are important for creating awareness about physical activity among varied audiences, including the general public, media, legislators, community

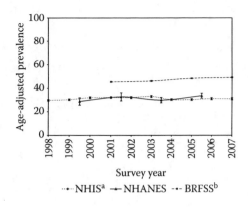

FIGURE 13.2 Age-adjusted prevalence of being physically active based on *Healthy People* 2010 criteria, National Health Interview Survey 1998–2007, National Health and Nutrition Examination Survey 1999–2006, and Behavioral Risk Factor Surveillance System 2001–2007. [a]Significant quadratic effect ($P < 0.05$). [b]Significant linear effect ($P < 0.05$). (From Carlson, S. A. et al., *J. Phys. Act. Health*, 6, Suppl. 1, S18–S27, 2009. With permission.)

leaders, parents, school administrators, and health professionals. Data can be presented in different forms that can be aimed at different audiences. For example, when CDC released the *State Indicator Report for Physical Activity*, an action guide for each state was included that provided surveillance estimates along with specific actions that persons (e.g., school officials, legislatures, urban planners, community leaders) within the state could take to improve physical activity in their state (Centers for Disease Control and Prevention 2010b). The *State Indicator Report for Physical Activity* is intended to be released periodically and will thus be an ongoing, state-specific source for information on physical activity behaviors as well as policy and environmental supports for physical activity.

DEVELOP AND EVALUATE PROGRAMS

Surveillance data can be used during the development and evaluation of programs. For example, the Racial and Ethnic Approaches to Community Health (REACH) 2010, launched in 1999, supports community coalitions in designing, implementing, and evaluating community-driven strategies to eliminate health disparities in six priority areas: cardiovascular diseases, diabetes, human immunodeficiency virus (HIV) infection and acquired immunodeficiency syndrome (AIDS), infant mortality, breast and cervical cancer screening and management, and child and adult immunization. A risk factor survey is conducted annually as part of REACH 2010, and baseline data provide important information for assessing, prioritizing, and planning intervention efforts, whereas the follow-up surveys will serve as an evaluation of the intervention programs within the demonstration communities (Liao et al. 2004).

TABLE 13.5
Estimated[a] Prevalence of Four Levels of Aerobic Activity among U.S. Adults as Defined in 2008 Guidelines, by Sex, Race/Ethnicity, and Education Level, NHIS 2008

	2008 Guidelines[b]							
	Active							
	Highly Active		Sufficiently Active		Insufficiently Active		Inactive	
Characteristic	%	95% CI	%	95% CI	%	95% CI	%	95% CI
Sex								
Male	33.0	(31.8, 34.3)	14.3	(13.4, 15.3)	18.4	(17.4, 19.4)	34.3	(32.7, 36.0)
Female	24.2	(23.2, 25.2)	15.5	(14.8, 16.3)	21.8	(20.8, 22.8)	38.5	(37.2, 39.8)
Race/ethnicity								
White, non-Hispanic	31.5	(30.3, 32.7)	16.0	(15.2, 16.8)	20.2	(19.4, 21.2)	32.3	(30.9, 33.7)
Black, non-Hispanic	21.3	(19.4, 23.4)	12.5	(11.2, 13.9)	18.7	(17.0, 20.5)	47.5	(45.1, 50.0)
Hispanic	21.0	(19.3, 22.9)	12.3	(10.9, 13.8)	19.1	(17.4, 20.8)	47.7	(45.1, 50.2)
Other, non-Hispanic[c]	27.0	(24.1, 30.1)	14.9	(12.8, 17.3)	23.1	(20.5, 26.1)	35.0	(31.6, 38.5)
Education level								
Less than HS graduate	16.5	(14.9, 18.3)	9.1	(7.9, 10.5)	17.0	(15.4, 18.8)	57.4	(55.1, 59.7)
High school graduate[d]	23.5	(22.1, 25.1)	11.9	(10.9, 13.0)	18.6	(17.2, 20.0)	46.0	(44.0, 48.0)
Some college	29.4	(27.9, 30.9)	16.0	(14.9, 17.1)	22.8	(21.6, 24.0)	31.9	(30.3, 33.5)
College graduate	38.2	(36.4, 40.0)	20.7	(19.2, 22.3)	21.0	(19.4, 22.7)	20.1	(18.6, 21.7)

Source: Carlson, S. A. et al., *Am. J. Prev. Med.*, 39, 4, 305–313, 2010. With permission.

[a] Estimates are age-adjusted to the 2000 U.S. projected population using five age groups (18–24, 25–34, 35–44, 45–64, and ≥65 years).

[b] Highly active was defined as more than 300 min of moderate-intensity aerobic activity, more than 150 min of vigorous-intensity aerobic activity, or an equivalent combination of moderate and vigorous-intensity physical activity per week. Sufficiently active was defined as 150–300 min of moderate-intensity aerobic activity, 75–150 min of vigorous-intensity aerobic activity, or an equivalent combination of moderate and vigorous-intensity aerobic activity per week. Insufficiently active was defined as some aerobic activity but not enough to meet the highly or sufficiently active definition. Inactive was defined as no moderate or vigorous-intensity aerobic activity for at least 10 min.

[c] "Other" race includes American Indian, Alaska Native, Asian, Native Hawaiian, and Other Pacific Islander.

[d] Includes individuals with a General Educational Development (GED) or equivalent.

SUPPORT HEALTH-RELATED POLICY OR LEGISLATION

Surveillance data can be provided to state and local government officials to support health-related public policy or legislation. For example, states use BRFSS data as part of their reports to their state legislatures so that the data can be used for planning state policy and legislation (http://www.cdc.gov/brfss/dataused.htm).

Examine Relations between Policy Changes and Changes in Behavior

An example of physical activity policy implementation to improve physical activity is illustrated in a study from the transportation sector. For transportation planners, implementing policies that improve access to active transportation is one way to reduce traffic congestion as well as increase physical activity. One study (Meyer and Beimborn 1998) examined the effect of implementing a transit pass program to encourage active transportation. The findings showed the proportion of university students who walked to school rather than driving increased when free transit was made available. Six months after the intervention began 57% more students chose walking with a sustained effect of 14% 1 year later (Meyer and Beimborn 1998).

CHALLENGES AND OPPORTUNITIES

There are many challenges and accompanying opportunities facing physical activity surveillance. These include the following: (1) gaining access to representative samples and maintaining acceptable response rates over time; (2) collecting data on behavioral, environmental and policy supports at the state, community, or local level; (3) collecting information on sedentary behaviors; and (4) capitalizing on advances in measurement technologies.

Gaining access to participants is becoming increasingly difficult, especially when a survey is administered by telephone as is done in the BRFSS (Blumberg and Luke 2009). New sampling and weighting procedures for the BRFSS therefore have been developed to provide a representative sample and will be implemented in 2010 (Centers for Disease Control and Prevention 2009a) (http://www.cdc.gov/brfss/dataused.htm). These new procedures will likely provide a more representative sample although they will preclude comparisons of the data collected in 2010 and beyond with data collected before 2010. This is an important trade-off to consider when surveillance system methodologies or survey questions are changed. When changes are made to surveillance systems, comparisons between "old" and "new" survey administrations must be done with caution and with an understanding of how the changes will affect established trends. Although some modifications are small and do not need to stop examination of surveillance trends (e.g., modifications to NHIS questions in 2004), others are large (e.g., changing nearly all BRFSS questions between 2000 and 2001) and do not allow valid comparisons of surveillance data before and after the changes.

Surveillance of environmental and policy supports for physical activity is an emerging area for public health. As described earlier, information about school programs and policies can be obtained from the SHPPS. Geographic characteristics thought to promote physical activity such as having access to parks or walking or bicycling paths can be obtained using GIS. Missing are data for settings other than schools and comprehensive data collection systems that provide information at national, state, and local levels on environmental and policy supports for physical activity.

The health effects of sedentary behavior apart from physical activity are increasingly becoming a distinct area of investigation (Hamilton, Hamilton, and Zderic

2007). Some measures or proxies of sedentary behavior (e.g., television viewing and computer use) are collected among youth in the YRBSS and the NSCH. Other measures of adult sedentary behavior (e.g., classification of occupational activity as either mostly sitting or standing, mostly walking, or mostly heavy labor or physically demanding work) have been previously collected in the BRFSS, and the NHIS has collected data about sedentary behavior every 5 years as part of the Cancer Supplement (National Center for Health Statistics 2008). Whether sedentary behavior *per se* is related to the development of chronic disease or its risk factors independent of physical activity is an important research question. Therefore, whether measures of sedentary behavior should be included in national surveillance systems for physical activity is an important issue to consider in the future.

Capitalizing on advances in measurement technologies (e.g., accelerometry) is an important area to carefully consider for physical activity surveillance. Historically, physical activity information has been collected in surveillance systems using self-report questionnaires primarily because of several feasibility issues: (1) requiring large nationally or state-representative samples, (2) having limited or no contact with the participant, (3) adding physical activity into systems that capture multiple health behaviors and outcomes, and (4) having limited resources. Although physical activity information collected by self-report questionnaires is correlated with data from motion sensors, motion sensors provide a more accurate assessment of movement. (LaPorte, Montoye, and Caspersen 1985) However, motion sensors also have limitations to consider for implementation in national and state-based physical activity surveillance systems:

1. Data from accelerometry have yet to be associated prospectively with chronic disease health outcomes. Self-report questionnaire data have been used to generate current physical activity guidelines for youth and for adults.
2. Accelerometers do not capture all aspects of physical activity such as type (e.g., walking) or context (e.g., for active transport).
3. Monitoring methodologies such as accelerometry may not currently be feasible to use in large-scale surveillance systems such as the BRFSS, which provides state-based estimates from a sample of more than 400,000 adults. Although accelerometry has been used in the 2003–2004 administration of the NHANES (Troiano et al. 2008), whether accelerometry will become a feasible method for large-scale, population-based surveillance of physical activity in the United States has yet to be determined and warrants further investigation.

STUDY QUESTIONS

1. Compare and contrast the definitions for epidemiology and for surveillance. Describe the ways they are related for the study of physical activity.
2. Describe six characteristics used to evaluate a surveillance system. How might one integrate each of these characteristics into an overall assessment of the quality of the surveillance system?

3. When is a survey not surveillance? Describe settings that are appropriate for surveys but not for surveillance.
4. Describe one U.S. surveillance system that assesses physical activity behavior and one system that assesses environmental and policy supports for physical activity. How can the information from these surveys be used to improve physical activity behaviors in the United States?
5. Describe at least three settings where physical activity surveillance data are useful to increase the prevalence of moderate- and vigorous-intensity physical activity.
6. Describe at least three challenges and three opportunities for physical activity surveillance in the twenty-first century.

REFERENCES

Blumberg, S. J., and J. V. Luke. 2009. Reevaluating the need for concern regarding noncoverage bias in landline surveys. *Am. J. Public Health* 99: 1806–1810.

Brownson, R. C., C. M. Hoehner, K. Day et al. 2009. Measuring the built environment for physical activity: State of the science. *Am. J. Prev. Med.* 36: S99–S123 e12.

Carlson, S. A., D. Densmore, J. E. Fulton et al. 2009. Differences in physical activity prevalence and trends from 3 U.S. surveillance systems: NHIS, NHANES, and BRFSS. *J. Phys. Act. Health* 6: S18–S27.

Carlson, S. A., J. E. Fulton, C. A. Schoenborn et al. 2010. Trend and prevalence estimates based on the *2008 Physical Activity Guidelines for Americans*. *Am. J. Prev. Med.* 39: 305–313.

Centers for Disease Control and Prevention. 1988. Guidelines for evaluating surveillance systems. *MMWR Morb. Mortal. Wkly. Rep.* 37(5): 1–18.

Centers for Disease Control and Prevention. 2006. School Health Policies and Programs Study (SHPPS). http://www.cdc.gov/HealthyYouth/shpps/ (accessed June 3, 2010).

Centers for Disease Control and Prevention. 2008. School Health Profiles. http://www.cdc.gov/healthyyouth/profiles (accessed June 3, 2010).

Centers for Disease Control and Prevention. 2009a. Behavioral Risk Factor Surveillance System. www.cdc.gov/brfss (accessed June 3, 2010).

Centers for Disease Control and Prevention. 2009b. Youth Risk Behavior Surveillance System. www.cdc.gov/yrbss (accessed June 3, 2010).

Centers for Disease Control and Prevention. 2010a. Physical Activity. U.S. Department of Health and Human Services. http://www.cdc.gov/physicalactivity (accessed May 24, 2011).

Centers for Disease Control and Prevention. 2010b. *State Indicator Report on Physical Activity, 2010.* Atlanta, GA: U.S. Department of Health and Human Services.

Cerin, E., B. E. Saelens, J. F. Sallis et al. 2006. Neighborhood environment walkability scale: Validity and development of a short form. *Med. Sci. Sports Exerc.* 38: 1682–1691.

Federal Highway Administration. 2009. National Household Travel Survey. http://nhts.ornl.gov/ (accessed May 23, 2011).

Galuska, D. A., and J. E. Fulton. 2009. Physical activity surveillance: Providing public health data for decision makers. *J. Phys. Act. Health* 6: S1–S2.

Guide to Community Preventive Services. 2010. Promoting physical activity: Environmental and policy approaches.

Hamilton, M. T., D. G. Hamilton, and T. W. Zderic. 2007. Role of low energy expenditure and sitting in obesity, metabolic syndrome, type 2 diabetes, and cardiovascular disease. *Diabetes* 56(11): 2655–2667.

Heath, G.W., R. C. Brownson, J. Kruger, et al. 2006. Force on community preventive services. The effectiveness of urban design and land use and transport policies and practices to increase physical activity: A systematic review. *J. Phys. Act. Health* 3(Suppl 1): S55–S76.

Kahn, E. B., L. T. Ramsey, R. C. Brownson et al. 2002. The effectiveness of interventions to increase physical activity. A systematic review. *Am. J. Prev. Med.* 22(4 Suppl): 73–107.

LaPorte, R. E., H. J. Montoye, and C. J. Caspersen. 1985. Assessment of physical activity in epidemiologic research: problems and prospects. *Public Health Rep.* 100(2): 131–146.

Last, J. M., and International Epidemiological Association. 1983. *A Dictionary of Epidemiology, Oxford Medical Publications*. Oxford: Oxford University Press.

Liao, Y., P. Tucker, C. A. Okoro et al. 2004. REACH 2010 surveillance for health status in minority communities—United States, 2001–2002. *MMWR Surveill. Summ.* 53: 1–36.

Loustalot, F., S. A. Carlson, J. E. Fulton et al. 2009. Prevalence of self-reported aerobic physical activity among U.S. States and territories—Behavioral Risk Factor Surveillance System, 2007. *J. Phys. Act. Health* 6: S9–S17.

Malina, R. M. 1996. Tracking of physical activity and physical fitness across the lifespan. *Res. Q. Exerc. Sport* 67: S48–S57.

Meyer, J., and A. A. Beimborn. 1998. Evaluation of an innovative transit pass program: The UPASS. *Transport Res. Rec.* 1618: 131–138.

National Center for Health Statistics. 2007. National Survey of Children's Health (NSCH). U.S. Department of Health and Human Services. http://www.nschdata.org (accessed June 3, 2010).

National Center for Health Statistics. 2008. National Health Interview Survey (NHIS). Centers for Disease Control and Prevention. http://www.cdc.gov/nchs/nhis (accessed June 7, 2010).

National Center for Health Statistics. 2010. Adult Physical Activity Information in the National Health Interview Survey. Centers for Disease Control and Prevention (CDC). http://www.cdc.gov/nchs/about/major/nhis/physicalactivity/physical_activity_homepage.htm. (accessed June 3, 2010).

Pate, R. R. 2009. A national physical activity plan for the United States. *J. Phys. Act. Health* 6: S157–S158.

Physical Activity Guidelines Advisory Committee. 2008. *Physical Activity Guidelines Advisory Committee Report, 2008*. Washington, DC: U.S. Department of Health and Human Services.

Resources for State and Community Programs. March 2010. CDC's Guide to Strategies for Increasing Physical Activity in the Community.

Sallis, J. F., H. R. Bowles, A. Bauman et al. 2009. Neighborhood environments and physical activity among adults in 11 countries. *Am. J. Prev. Med.* 36: 484–490.

Sallis, J. F., J. Kerr, J. A. Carlson et al. 2010. Evaluating a brief self-report measure of neighborhood environments for physical activity research and surveillance: Physical Activity Neighborhood Environment Scale (PANES). *J. Phys. Act. Health* 7: 533–540.

Schreier, P. 2010. Finding the 'science' in GIS. Scientific Computing World. http://www.scientific-computing.com/features/feature.php?feature_id=275 (accessed July 18, 2011).

Strong, W. B., R. M. Malina, C. J. Blimkie et al. 2005. Evidence based physical activity for school-age youth. *J. Pediatr.* 146: 732–737.

Task Force on Community Preventive Services. 2002. Recommendations to increase physical activity in communities. *Am. J. Prev. Med.* 224: 67–72.

Thacker, S. B., and R. L. Berkelman. 1988. Public health surveillance in the United States. *Epidemiol. Rev.* 10: 164–190.

Troiano, R. P., D. Berrigan, K. W. Dodd et al. 2008. Physical activity in the United States measured by accelerometer. *Med. Sci. Sports Exerc.* 40: 181–188.

U.S. Department of Health and Human Services. 2008. *2008 Physical Activity Guidelines for Americans*. Washington, DC: U.S. Department of Health and Human Services.

U.S. Department of Health and Human Services. 2010a. *Healthy People* 2020. http://www
.healthypeople.gov/hp2020/ (accessed December 14, 2010).
U.S. Department of Health and Human Services. 2010b. The Surgeon General's vision for a
healthy and fit nation.
Yore, M. M., S. A. Ham, B. E. Ainsworth et al. 2007. Reliability and validity of the instrument
used in BRFSS to assess physical activity. *Med. Sci. Sports Exerc.* 39: 1267–1274.

14 Physical Activity Promotion in Underserved Communities

Deborah Parra-Medina and Zenong Yin

CONTENTS

INTRODUCTION

Healthy People 2020, a set of goals and objectives (see Table 14.1) to guide U.S. health promotion and disease prevention efforts, seeks to achieve health equity, eliminate disparities, and improve health of all groups (U.S. Department of Health

TABLE 14.1
Healthy People **2020 Definitions**

Health equity	The attainment of the highest level of health for all people. Achieving health equity requires valuing everyone equally with focused and ongoing societal efforts to address avoidable inequalities, historical and contemporary injustices, and the elimination of health and healthcare disparities (U.S. Department of Health and Human Services 2010).
Health disparity	A particular type of health difference that is closely linked with social, economic, and/or environmental disadvantage. Health disparities adversely affect groups of people who have systematically experienced greater obstacles to health based on their racial or ethnic group; religion; socioeconomic status; gender; age; mental health; cognitive, sensory, or physical disability; sexual orientation or gender identity; geographic location; or other characteristics historically linked to discrimination or exclusion (U.S. Department of Health and Human Services 2010).

Source: U.S. Department of Health and Human Services, 2010.

and Human Services 2011). The physical activity objectives for *Healthy People* 2020 reflect the strong state of the science supporting the health benefits of regular physical activity among youth and adults who meet the Physical Activity Guidelines for Americans (Haskell et al. 2007). Yet, despite the known benefits of physical activity and its proven ability to protect from cardiovascular disease, type 2 diabetes, and colon cancer (U.S. Department of Health and Human Services 1996), American adults remain inactive. More than 80% of adults do not meet the guidelines for both aerobic and muscle-strengthening activities (U.S. Department of Health and Human Services 2011). Only 48% met the physical activity recommendation in *Healthy People* 2010, using data from 2007 Behavioral Risk Factor Surveillance System (Centers for Disease Control and Prevention 2008).

Physically inactive lifestyles are highest among racial/ethnic minorities, socioeconomically disadvantaged groups, women, and the elderly (Powell et al. 2006; Crespo et al. 2000; Centers for Disease Control and Prevention 2008). As a result, minorities and low-income groups suffer from higher prevalence of chronic diseases (diabetes, hypertension) that are more commonly observed among persons who are physically inactive. Historical, cultural, and socioeconomic barriers and the built environment have created challenges that make active lifestyles an unrealistic and unattainable choice for many (Taylor, Baranowski, and Young 1998; Crespo et al. 2000).

Although there is considerable progress in the scientific support for and promotion of physical activity by many national health organizations, a limited number of effective and sustainable strategies and programs are available that addresses the root causes of physical inactivity in the underserved communities (Yancey, Ory, and Davis 2006). In this chapter, we will describe disparities in participation in physical activity in underserved communities and factors contributing to these disparities. We will also recommend strategies and resources that public health professionals can use to enhance and facilitate the promotion of physical activity in these often hard-to-reach populations.

PHYSICAL ACTIVITY DISPARITIES

Data from several U.S. surveillance systems have consistently identified disparities in the rates of participation in regular moderate-to-vigorous physical activity and meeting the recommendation of physical activity in children and adults in underserved communities. Although the most frequently noted disparities in physical activity are those between racial/ethnic and population subgroups with low socioeconomic statuses (SES), it should be noted that differences in age, gender, geographic location, sexual orientation, physical ability/disability, and immigrant status also persist. The intersection of these factors leads to even greater impact on physical activity behavior.

RACE/ETHNICITY, SES, AGE, AND GENDER

People of low SES, racial/ethnic minorities, females, and the elderly are the least likely of all Americans to meet the physical activity recommendations or engage in sufficient or any leisure-time physical activity, according to national data from 2007 Behavioral Risk Factor Surveillance System (see Table 14.2) (Centers for Disease Control and Prevention 2008). These disparities are most pronounced in racial/ethnic minority groups that are low SES, older, and female (see Figures 14.1–14.3). Similar trends are reported in the analyses of the 2002–2003 National Physical Activity and Weight Loss Survey, indicating the prevalence of physical inactivity during leisure time was lowest in non-Hispanic black and Hispanic participants compared to non-Hispanic Whites, and women compared to men (Marshall et al. 2007). Higher levels of education and income were associated with lower prevalence of physical inactivity within each racial/ethnic group. A report using data from the National Health Interview Survey studied the percentage of employed adults reporting participation in leisure-time physical activity who also reported hard occupational physical activity by race/ethnicity (Centers for Disease Control and Prevention 2000). Non-Hispanic Whites had the least physical inactivity and the highest percentages of adults meeting the recommended guidelines of moderate physical activity for 30 min 5 or more days a week. Non-Hispanic Whites also had the lowest percentages of employed adults who engaged in heavy work for 5 or more hours a day. Hispanics, on the other hand, reported engaging more frequently in highly physically active jobs for 5 or more hours a day than non-Hispanic Whites or Blacks, and had the highest levels of physical inactivity during leisure time. In addition, many older African–Americans and Hispanics who performed hard physical labor throughout their lives did not view physical activity as voluntary or beneficial (Centers for Disease Control and Prevention 2000). The results of this report are consistent with the thought that occupational activity, rather than leisure-time physical activity, may explain some racial/ethnic disparities. Disparities in physical activity related to race/ethnicity, SES, and gender also have been documented for U.S. adolescents. Data from the 1996 National Longitudinal Study of Adolescent Health showed that females and

TABLE 14.2
Percent of U.S. Population Subgroups in Different Categories of Physical Activity Based on 2010 Healthy People PA Guideline Using 2007 Data from Behavioral Risk Factor Surveillance System (BRFSS)

Population Subgroups		Meeting PA Recommendation	Insufficient PA	Physically Inactive	No Leisure-Time Physical Activity
National average		49	38	14	24
Race/ethnicity	White	52	37	11	20
	Black	40	40	20	31
	Hispanic	42	37	21	36
	Other	45	39	16	24
Education	<High school	38	35	27	44
	HS graduate	46	38	16	30
	Some college	49	38	12	22
	College graduate	54	38	8	14
Age groups (years)	18–24	59	32	9	18
	25–34	53	37	10	21
	35–44	50	40	11	22
	45–64	47	40	14	25
	65+	39	37	24	33
Gender	Female	47	39	14	26
	Male	51	37	13	22

Source: Centers for Disease Control and Prevention, *Morb. Mortal. Wkly. Rep.*, 57, 1297–1300, 2008.

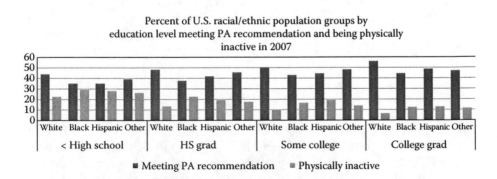

FIGURE 14.1   Percent of U.S. racial/ethnic population groups by education level meeting physical activity (PA) recommendation and being physically inactive in 2007. (Adapted from Centers for Disease Control and Prevention, *Morb. Mortal. Wkly. Rep.*, 57, 48, 1297–1300, 2008.)

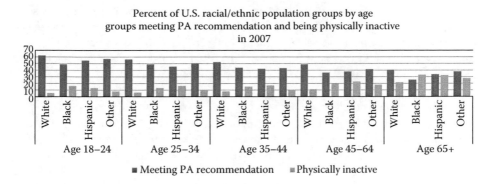

FIGURE 14.2   Percent of U.S. racial/ethnic population groups by age groups meeting PA recommendation and being physically inactive in 2007. (Adapted from Centers for Disease Control and Prevention, *Morb. Mortal. Wkly. Rep.*, 57, 48, 1297–1300, 2008.)

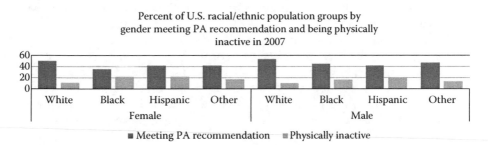

FIGURE 14.3   Percent of U.S. racial/ethnic population groups by gender meeting PA recommendation and being physically inactive in 2007. (Adapted from Centers for Disease Control and Prevention, *Morb. Mortal. Wkly. Rep.*, 57, 48, 1297–1300, 2008.)

minorities were less likely to engage in adequate physical activity compared to their male and white counterparts (Gordon-Larsen, McMurray, and Popkin 2000).

ACCULTURATION

Acculturation is the process and degree to which immigrants integrate and incorporate values, attitudes, beliefs, and practices of the host society into their lives. Acculturation may be a strong indicator influencing racial/ethnic minorities' participation in physical activity. There is some evidence that acculturated individuals are more likely to engage in leisure-time physical activity compared to their less acculturated counterparts (Hovell et al. 1991; Eyler et al. 2002; Evenson et al. 2003; Crespo et al. 2001). For example, Berrigan et al. (2006) reported that U.S. Hispanic adults were significantly more likely to engage in leisure-time physical activity with increased level of acculturation, after adjusting for age, income, education, urban residence, and body mass index. A California study found that later generation of immigration is associated with higher leisure-time physical activity in Mexican–American adults and nonleisure-time physical activity in Chinese and Filipino Americans

(Afable-Munsuz et al. 2006). Although the specific factors contributing to an increase in physical activity are not clear, possible explanations are that cultural norms and traditions play an important role in immigrants' decisions to participate in physical activity, or that acculturated immigrants may be exposed to education about the importance of physical activity and its role in prevention (Yancey, Ory, and Davis 2006; Satia et al. 2002). Some researchers suggest that education and social class may have important modifying effects on the relationship between acculturation and health (Lopez, Bryant, and McDermott 2008; Castro, Cota, and Vega 1999). Thus, acculturation is a complex process and more research is needed to further understand which aspect or aspects of acculturation are strongly related to physical inactivity.

RESIDENCE AND GEOGRAPHIC REGION

Residence in rural or inner-city areas and Southern U.S. regions is associated with limited resources and support for physical activity and higher physical inactivity compared to urban/suburban residents and Northeast, Mideast, and Western regions (Martin et al. 2005). A study of women aged 40 years and older reported that residence in the rural South was associated with being sedentary and not meeting physical activity recommendations (Wilcox et al. 2000). The link between physical inactivity and living in low-resource, high-poverty areas also was observed in children and youth. Data from the 1996 National Longitudinal Study of Adolescent Health, a sample of 17,766 adolescents enrolled in middle and high schools, showed that youth with access to recreation centers and living in low-crime areas were more likely to engage in moderate-to-vigorous physical activity (Gordon-Larsen, McMurray, and Popkin 2000). For children and adolescents, access to recreational facilities and programs are consistently related to physical activity. A study of rural children conducted in Georgia found that children who had no walking access to activity areas were four times more likely to be physically inactive compared to their peers that could walk to an activity area (Shores, Moore, and Yin 2010).

FACTORS INFLUENCING PARTICIPATION IN PHYSICAL ACTIVITY IN UNDERSERVED COMMUNITIES

Racial/ethnic minorities, low-income groups, women, the elderly, and rural residents are more likely to be inactive and, as a consequence experience, a disproportionate burden of disease and disability (U.S. Department of Health and Human Services 1996). These population subgroups are often considered "hard to reach," or underserved by public health researchers and practitioners because they do not respond to health promotion efforts targeting the general population. To ensure that public health actions are taken to increase physical activity to a level that can eliminate disparities and improve the health of all groups, as recommended by *Healthy People* 2020, it is imperative that health promotion practitioners understand facilitators of and barriers to physical activity experienced by underserved populations. To date, most physical activity research has focused on individual-level correlates of physical activity (Mier et al. 2007; Marquez and McAuley 2006; Eyler et al. 2002; Evenson et al. 2003). There is, however, an increased recognition on the importance of the social and physical environment (Sallis, Bauman, and Pratt 1998; Martinez et al. 2009; Lopez, Bryant, and McDermott 2008). It is becoming clear that physical activity among underserved populations is influenced by several social, environmental, and political factors. Ecological models are useful for understanding these complex and multilevel factors (Sallis, Bauman, and Pratt 1998), because they direct attention to influences outside the individual and to social and environmental factors, in particular, that may be root causes of the inactive lifestyles of underserved populations (Sallis et al. 2006). The ecological model focuses on intrapersonal (motivation, internal perceptions, values), interpersonal (social relationships, norms, social support), organizational (access to healthcare, preventive services), and community (safe, affordable facilities, environmental influences) resources that exist/do not exist for minority populations. Broader examination of such factors will provide a better foundation to either begin or continue a physical activity program (King et al. 2002). For example, the availability and accessibility of places to be active, such as bicycle trails, walking paths, and swimming pools, may play a role in determining the type and amount of physical activity that people engage in.

INTRAPERSONAL INDIVIDUAL FACTORS

Well-established facilitators of adult physical activity include belief in ability to exercise (self-efficacy) and expectation of benefits and enjoyment of exercise (Trost et al. 2002). Self-efficacy, the confidence in one's ability to perform a behavior, also has been consistently and positively associated with adult physical activity (Dzewaltowski 1994; Bandura 1986). Although studied less among minority populations than among the general population, self-efficacy was a consistent predictor of physical activity among more than 4000 women of diverse ethnicities in seven sites across the United States (Eyler et al. 2002).

Overall, expectations of greater positive (e.g., perceived benefits) and lower negative outcomes (e.g., perceived barriers) for physical activity are associated with higher physical activity levels (Eyler et al. 2002). The Robert Wood Johnson Foundation's Diversity Report on Physical Activity identified major barriers for participation in physical activity after getting input from community members, researchers, and related personnel who work with African Americans, Latinos, and American Indians (Robert Wood Johnson Foundation 2005). The most salient barriers to physical activity identified were: (1) not enough time; (2) not a priority; (3) level of safety in neighborhood; (4) not having the money; (5) no childcare; (6) it's tiring or not fun (lack of enjoyment); (7) others would think I'm being selfish; (8) no parks; (9) no good programs; and (10) not wanting to get sweaty (Crespo 2005). These barriers are not exclusive to underserved populations; for example, lack of time has been recognized as a major barrier for not participating in physical activity by non-Hispanic Whites also. However, there are other barriers that disproportionately affect low-income minorities, such as level of safety in the neighborhood and lack of parks or good programs. Barriers also may be defined or experienced differently within population subgroups. For example, in a study of Mexican-origin women from two distinct geographic U.S. regions, social isolation due to lack of transportation or limited English proficiency language limited their ability access physical activity resources. At both sites (Texas and South Carolina), women reported feeling isolated and having limited opportunities for regular social contact outside the home. In South Carolina, language barriers and personal experiences of discrimination contributed to generalized fear and lack of trust in others and consolidated social barriers between relatively recent Latina immigrants and the larger community. In Texas, social isolation was often related to physical distance, lack of available transportation, and social constraints on their ability to leave the home—a prevalent situation among homemakers whose husbands' migrant employment left many living home alone in isolated neighborhoods with limited access to transportation (Parra-Medina and Messias 2011).

INTERPERSONAL FACTORS

Social support from family and friends has been consistently related to physical activity, and research suggests that it may be more influential for women than men. Social support includes aid or assistance exchanged by individuals, groups, or organizations. Several types of social support relate to physical activity, such as instrumental (e.g., assist with a problem), informational (e.g., give advice), and emotional (e.g., provide encouragement). Social networks are the connections between people that may provide social support. Low levels of social support for physical activity have been associated with sedentary behavior among Caucasian, African American, Hispanic, and American Indian/Alaska Native women, whereas positive social support has been found across studies to be "an overwhelmingly positive determinant of physical activity for all groups of women" (Eyler et al. 2002). Seeing others being active is a positive influence on physical activity, and having social support during physical activity has been associated with enjoyment, and adherence to a program (Vrazel, Saunders, and Wilcox 2008). Among both African American and diverse U.S. samples of young to middle-aged women, surveys show that seeing people in the neighborhood exercise, having favorable opinions of women who exercise, and knowing people who exercise were associated with higher physical activity levels (Lopez, Bryant, and McDermott 2008; Eyler et al. 2003).

Although social support is a positive influence, social relationships and responsibilities can also present barriers to physical activity. Women of diverse backgrounds perceive family, community, and caregiving responsibilities as interfering with physical activity (Vrazel, Saunders, and Wilcox 2008; Parra-Medina and Messias 2011; Henderson and Ainsworth 2000). A review of 17 studies showed that having children and/or family responsibilities was negatively related to overall physical activity levels among African American, Caucasian, Hispanic, and American Indian women (Eyler et al. 2003). In a study of Latinas, Juarbe, Turok, and Perez-Stable (2002) noted that participants perceived little or no time for social interactions outside the home and family because of their multiple role responsibilities. Among Latinos, this perception may be the result of issues related to *familismo* (familism), the preference for maintaining a close connection to the family. Juarbe, Turok, and Perez-Stable (2002) also note that Latinas aimed to improve their roles in the context of the family, which is far more important to them than personal or individualistic gains. Similarly, Parra-Medina and Messias (2011) found that participation in leisure-time physical activity was not congruent with internalized expectation of

Mexican origin women's primary role responsibility (e.g., caring for others). Not only did women feel that they did not have the "time" for physical activity in their lives because of their family or work responsibilities, social and cultural expectations about gender roles (e.g., a woman's role is to be a good wife and mother and her place is in the home) reinforced the perception that time spent on physical activity is "selfish" or "wasted" effort (Parra-Medina and Messias 2011). Women reported being embarrassed to be seen out walking in public where others might observe them and judge them negatively because of misplaced values. Of note is that both studies were of low to moderately acculturated older Latina women; these values may differ from those that may be reported by younger and more acculturated samples of Latina women.

ORGANIZATIONAL AND COMMUNITY FACTORS

Specific organizational and community barriers to physical activity for underserved populations may vary depending on whether they live in urban, suburban, or rural areas, or in places that are predominantly low income. Low-income status disproportionately affects racial/ethnic minorities and exacerbates health disparities. Low-income populations often confront difficult organizational and community barriers to physical activity and have less means to overcome them than other income groups. Some of the most common barriers include: long distances to important daily destinations (e.g., grocery stores, work), lack of or limited public and private transportation options, unsafe neighborhood and traffic conditions, and poor access to parks and recreational facilities. Although many of these barriers also exist for other income groups, they often exist to a greater degree in low-income communities. Low-income people also are less able financially to choose more activity-friendly alternatives such as living closer to work or in a safer and cleaner neighborhood, purchasing a health club membership, paying a fee to visit the community pool or recreation center, or purchasing services that afford time for physical activity such as housecleaning or childcare.

Several studies involving self-reported perceptions have shown a positive correlation between the availability of physical activity-related facilities and settings and exercise behaviors (Sallis et al. 1990; King et al. 2000; Humpel, Owen, and Leslie 2002). Physical activity settings (e.g., sports areas, parks and green spaces, public pools and beaches, bike paths/lanes) are less available in neighborhoods with low-income and minority residents (Powell et al. 2006; Estabrooks, Lee, and Gyuresik 2003). Sallis et al. (1990) found that proximity and higher density of exercise facilities were significantly associated with increased frequency of exercise. An environmental intervention aimed at reducing barriers to physical activity (including increasing the availability of physical activity-related equipment and facilities) revealed statistically significant positive changes in overall fitness measures within the intervention community. Affordability of recreational facilities is cited as an important obstacle to physical activity by low-income respondents. Low- and medium-SES neighborhoods were found to have significantly fewer no-cost resources, but differences across low-, medium-, and high-SES census tracts were not observed for pay-for-use resources (Estabrooks, Lee, and Gyuresik 2003). Safety and access to facilities are also especially important issues that affect physical activity in underserved populations. Perceptions of neighborhood physical activity opportunity are lower in neighborhoods with more poverty (e.g., issues of crime, lack of sidewalks) and are significantly related to physical activity levels. Humpel, Owen, and Leslie (2002) found that accessibility of facilities, opportunities for programmed activities, and aesthetic attributes had significant association with physical activity. Most physical activity research to date has involved primarily middle-class, mostly white adults living in urban/suburban settings. However, environmental barriers and facilitators likely exist and vary by population characteristics and locations. Environmental barriers identified by African–American women include safety concerns or neighborhood crime; unattended dogs; distance and access to recreational facilities; cost and availability of programs; poor condition of or no sidewalks and lighting; and weather conditions (Ainsworth et al. 2003; Burroughs, Fields, and Sharpe 2004; Carter-Nolan, Adams-Campbell, and Williams 1996; Clark 1999; Eyler et al. 1998; Jones and Nies 1996; Wilbur et al. 2002; Wilcox et al. 2000, 2002; Sallis et al. 1990; King et al. 2000; Humpel, Owen, and Leslie 2002). Hispanic parents of youths aged between 9 to 13 years report more barriers to their children's physical activity than do white parents, including transportation problems, concerns about neighborhood safety, and the expense and availability of local opportunities (Duke, Huhman, and Heitzler 2003). In two largely Latino towns along the Texas–Mexico border, residents and community representatives identified similar physical conditions and environments that created barriers to leisure-time physical activity (Parra-Medina and Messias 2011). These included physical and operational barriers, such as the location of facilities (e.g., schools, parks, community centers), restricted access to tracks or walking paths (e.g., not open at convenient times or early in the morning to avoid the presence of stray animals and individuals or groups who engendered fear, such as gang members or park loiterers), and unwelcoming and unsafe physical environments (e.g., graffiti, litter, insufficient lighting, lack of sidewalks, excess motor vehicle traffic, and speeding drivers).

Although mainstream Americans associate physical activity with leisure-time recreation activities, low-income minority and immigrant populations tend to view physical activity as a form of physical labor as part of their occupational activities. Targeting or tailoring a physical activity intervention to make it appropriate for a particular priority population necessitates careful understanding of and attention to the community's cultural characteristics and the barriers the community faces. Practitioners and researchers can capitalize on this cultural knowledge, along with involvement from the community, to craft an approach for a specific community that integrates a physical activity intervention with cultural characteristics and built around community assets and resources. The goal of relating the specific community characteristics to aspects of the intervention allows the intervention to be accessible and fit the lived reality of the community.

STRATEGIES FOR PHYSICAL ACTIVITY PROMOTION IN UNDERSERVED COMMUNITIES

Health promotion is the process of enabling people to increase control over, and to improve, their health. It moves beyond a focus on individual behavior toward a wide range of social and environmental interventions. Health promotion represents a comprehensive social and political process, not only embracing actions directed at strengthening the skills and empowering the capabilities of individuals, but also actions directed toward changing social, environmental, and economic conditions, so as to alleviate their impact on public and individual health. Participation is essential to sustain health promotion action. To make "the healthy choice the easy choice," as the axiom goes, it is necessary to provide readily available, accessible, and appealing physical activity programs and settings. However, an appropriate physical activity program or message for underserved populations cannot be the same from one community to the next, or even similar to those aimed at the general population. In this regard, health promotion efforts to increase and improve levels of physical activity cannot be exactly duplicated and/or replicated across communities, and require addressing the barriers of health practice facing people living in underserved communities.

Reaching low-income minority communities remains a challenge. Interventions targeting underserved communities often take the form of a disease-specific intervention or one-time wellness event. These one-time events fail to address the needs of the community and do not provide the ongoing support needed to change behavior. Many programs use a "one-size-fits-all" approach across communities that, in practice, fits none. Community-based participatory approaches offer an opportunity to respond to the community's needs, and have been shown to successfully design and implement culturally appropriate programs and interventions that meet the needs and concerns of specific communities.

Public health practitioners and community members can combine their knowledge and assets to work together as colleagues on relevant program and policy development (Viswanathan et al. 2004). Community involvement leverages community members' diverse skills, knowledge, and expertise that can lead to: (1) enhanced and more trusting communication and relationships between public health and community partners; (2) more culturally appropriate interventions; (3) greater community interest and support; and (4) ideally, more sustainable strategies for improved health and well-being.

INVOLVEMENT OF THE COMMUNITY OF INTEREST

Programs and interventions can be more effective if they are trusted and accepted by community members. The best way for this to occur is for the programs and interventions to originate from within the community itself. Sustainability is more likely, as well, when the community feels ownership. It is important to include community individuals (e.g., persons who understand and appreciate the culture and language of the community) in planning, implementing, and evaluating interventions. This can be achieved through several means:

- Engage communities of interest by educating community partners about the overall research process, not just the intervention, including community members and organizations from initial planning stages and throughout the process.
- Hire community health workers (CHWs) and providing training and certification. CHWs are a rapidly growing public health workforce often known as "culture brokers" and "community liaisons" in underserved, hard-to-reach, and culturally and linguistically diverse communities. CHWs, which

are often referred to as lay health workers, community health advisors, *promotoras/promotores de salud*, and other titles depending on geographic region or community, are trusted community members who provide formal and informal health education and services to members of their own community (U.S. Department of Health and Human Services 1994). Major roles and responsibilities of CHWs include information dissemination, program recruitment, health education, policy and community advocacy, case management, and preventive and curative services (Swider 2002). Currently, more than 17 states have a formal program of training and/or certification of CHWs (Kash, May, and Tai-Seale 2007). Evidence based on recent systematic reviews found that CHWs can effectively increase the awareness and knowledge of disease and various health issues and induce significant long-term impacts of health behavior change, including changes in physical activity (Lewin et al. 2005; Henderson, Kendall, and See 2011).
• Learn from what others have done, but adapt approaches for local racial/ethnic minority communities, based on conversations and previous experiences within the intended community.
• Allow community members to target health problems and identify solutions.

ENGAGEMENT OF COMMUNITY STAKEHOLDERS

Leadership and active participation by community stakeholders, especially health-care providers and community and religious leaders, can strengthen the credibility of and respect for the intervention. Partnering with trusted and recognized institutions already in the community can earn valuable trust and recognition for the program. Some ways to do so are to

• Find and involve influential community members who can change perceptions from within the community or the family, which is important to program relevancy, credibility, and successful implementation.
• Collaborate with already-trusted messengers and expand on already-occurring community social groups. *Healthy People* 2020 calls for a multidisciplinary approach to promoting physical activity that brings about traditional partnerships (e.g., education and healthcare) and nontraditional partnerships (e.g., transportation, urban planning, recreation, and environmental health). Several new *Healthy People* 2020 objectives reflect this emphasis—for example, physical activity policies regarding childcare (Objective 2020-PA9) and environmental settings (Objective 2020-PA15). Involving a network of organizations allows flexibility in responding to community needs beyond the specific physical activity intervention and in ways that facilitate the building of relationships within and among community members.

DEVELOPMENT OF CULTURAL COMPETENCY IN STAFF

Strategies to reach racial/ethnic minority populations should be culturally relevant. It may be useful to provide training in cultural competency to individuals who are working with a community, so that they can learn more about the differences within and across communities and how these differences influence physical activity interventions. Cultural competency training should be ongoing and required for all staff. There is a lack of physical activity and recreational staffs or role models who reflect the racial/ethnic composition and cultural values that exist in a community. CHWs have the potential to serve as those needed role models.

TAILORING TO CULTURE

Physical activity programs and interventions tailored to reflect the culture of a population subgroup are likely to be more effective than those aimed at the general population. Some ways to do so are to

- Tailor programs, policies, and environmental changes to the community you intend to serve by addressing the community's knowledge and attitudes of physical activity and disease so as to promote relevant physical activity that is most frequently practiced in the specific community (e.g., walking, cultural dance).
- Consider characteristics such as the community's primary language, educational level, individual and family characteristics (e.g., age and age-related norms, work, complex family structures, health conditions), and available resources and infrastructures (e.g., parks, recreation centers, trails) when designing the components, materials, and messages for physical activity programs and interventions.
- Use common phrases and terms and visual imagery (e.g., photos, colors, and symbols) that represent the community and their experiences.
- Depict the family and community as primary systems of support and intervention.
- Emphasize the physical and mental health benefits of physical activity rather than focusing solely on weight loss and disease outcomes, depending on perceptions of physical activity and disease in the targeted community.
- Recognize that, in some communities, group events are preferred to individual activities to promote social support and a family-like atmosphere.
- Recognize diversity within and among groups regarding cultural norms (e.g., ideal body weight) and the complexity and differences within and across racial/ethnic minority populations.
- Recognize the importance of gender issues, such as cultural/traditional role expectations and personal expectations, when developing intervention strategies.

ADDRESSING PARTICIPANTS' NEEDS AND USING ESTABLISHED SETTINGS AND INFRASTRUCTURE

In addition, physical activity programs and interventions need to have meetings or events at convenient locations and times to address community need and maximize their participation. It may be useful to align interventions with church or community social events. Use existing infrastructures within the racial/ethnic minority community to support the intervention:

- Deliver programs through existing ethnic minority community groups and in local facilities where members of ethnic minority communities are represented on the staff of the facility and that are familiar, accessible, and affordable. A variety program and activities or menu of options will need to be offered to meet the various interests and needs of the community members (such as women-only sessions).
- Distribute messages via racial/ethnic minority publications, radio stations, and community-based minority-serving organizations, which are important sources for disseminating messages.
- Consider providing childcare and transportation to increase participation. Racial and ethnic minorities are more likely to experience poverty and cite costs as a barrier.
- Go where the people are—that is, offer programs in settings where the community frequents and has had a positive experience (e.g., schools, barbershops, churches).
- Recognize that, in some communities, barriers may need to be addressed related to time, time management, and structured activity. Encourage ways of being active that include shorter, more frequent bouts of activity rather than longer time commitments.
- Provide participants with ideas for incorporating physical activity into their daily lives (e.g., parking farther from destinations, taking the stairs, walking during breaks).

Involving local organizations and businesses can uncover existing community resources and build new infrastructures, initiatives, and community trust. For example, churches provide social, emotional, and material support in addition to religious worship, serve as a focal point for a social networking, and are well integrated into individuals' lives and communities. Trained CHWs from the faith communities could be effective intervention agents, because they are most likely to be sensitive to the community needs and to be viewed as trustworthy and well-respected individuals by potential program recipients.

ADDRESSING SAFETY CONCERNS

Safety is a strong consideration in physical activity programs and interventions. There are several types of safety to consider. For example, you might want to ensure that programmatic activity equipment is in good working order and safe for use. It is also important to consider interpersonal safety. This might include creating buddy systems so people do not have to walk alone or creating neighborhood watch programs. It is also important to ensure safety in terms of the physical environment (e.g., improvements in sidewalks and walking trails, installation of crossing aids, creation of leash laws, install traffic calming device in high traffic area, and increasing policy presence). Consider building social support within the community to address safety concerns and retain participants.

TABLE 14.3

Resources for Planning, Implementation and Evaluation of Community-Based Physical Activity Programs

Resource	Content	URL for Internet Access
2008 Physical Activity Guidelines for Americans Toolkit	Free toolkit with a User Guide and media materials for community leaders and physical activity leaders in school or state agencies to promote adults' participation in physical activity	http://www.health.gov/paguidelines/toolkit.aspx
Youth Physical Activity Guidelines Toolkit for the 2008 Activity Guidelines for Americans	Free toolkit with a User Guide and media materials for community leaders and physical activity leaders in school or state agencies to promote youth participation in physical activity	http://www.cdc.gov/healthyyouth/physicalactivity/guidelines.htm#1
The CDC's Community Guide on PA Promotion	A free resource of evidence-based programs and policies based on systematic reviews of experts, including recommendations, guides, tool kits, and supporting materials	http://www.thecommunityguide.org/pa/index.html
A Guide For Community Action Community-Based Approaches to Promoting Physical Activity	A detailed guide explaining CDC's Community Guide on PA and step-by-step guide on how to implement effective community-based strategies	http://www.cdc.gov/physicalactivity/professionals/promotion/communityguide.html
RE-AIM	Details on rationale and tools for using RE-AIM, a five-step approach to plan and evaluate large-scale community-based intervention programs	http://cancercontrol.cancer.gov/is/reaim/index.html
MAP-IT: A Guide to Using *Healthy People* 2020 in Your Community	A framework that can be used to plan and evaluate public health interventions	http://healthypeople.gov/2020/implementing/default.aspx
Community Health Worker National Education Collaborative	A detailed guidebook for training community health workers as well as identifying education partners and experts	http://www.chw-nec.org/resources.cfm

TABLE 14.4

Program Resources for Physical Activity Promotion in Underserved Communities

Resource	Content	URL for Internet Access
Y-USA's Healthier Communities Initiatives	Y's Healthier Communities Initiatives (Pioneering Healthier Communities, Statewide Pioneering Healthier Communities and ACHIEVE) promote health by addressing barriers and challenges in communities it serves	http://www.ymca.net/ healthier-communities/
STRONG WOMEN™	Low-cost, community-based exercise program for women to improve bone health and other health outcomes. Program guides and tool kits are provided	http://extension.psu.edu/ healthy-lifestyles/ strongwomen/resources
The Eat Better and Move More Program	The National Policy and Resource Center on Nutrition and Aging at Florida International University's guides and tools for a nutrition and physical activity program for older adults	http://nutritionandaging.fiu .edu/index.asp
Let's Move	A comprehensive initiative involving families, schools and communities, led by First Lady Michelle Obama, to combat U.S. childhood obesity (includes guides and tool kits)	http://www.letsmove.gov/
My Bright Future. Physical Activity and Healthy Eating: For Rural Young Women	Guides and toolkits for young women in rural areas to increase current levels of physical activity, healthy eating, and communication with their healthcare providers, and to set goals for behavioral changes (funded by U.S. Department of Health and Human Services' Health Resources And Services Administration)	http://www.ask.hrsa.gov/ detail_materials .cfm?prodid=4236
Latino/Migrant Workers by NHLBI	Resources (guides, tools) for program planners and other health professionals who work with migrant workers to promote PA and healthy eating	http://www.nhlbi.nih.gov/ health/prof/heart/latino/ lat_pro.htm
The Fruit, Vegetable, and Physical Activity Toolbox for Community Educators	Free toolbox kit (lessons, handouts, resources, evaluation tools) for community educators to promote fruit and vegetable and physical activity in low-income African–American adults	http://www.network-toolbox .net/en/index.asp

RESOURCES FOR PHYSCIAL ACTIVITY PROMOTION IN UNDERSERVED COMMUNITIES

Public health professionals often have limited support and funding to purchase tools and evidence-based programs for promotion of physical activity in underserved communities. However, many available resources for physical activity promotion exist from federal and state public health agencies, university-based research centers, or national nonprofit organizations. The sampling of resources shown in Tables 14.3 and 14.4 were selected because they are: (1) based on published research or reviews of national expert panels; (2) free or low cost; and (3) accessible via electronic media (internet and/or CD).

CONCLUSION

Statistics show that we are falling short in promoting physical activity among U.S. adults. In fact, only half meet the current recommendation for physical activity (U.S. Department of Health and Human Services 2008, 2010). Moreover, people of low SES and racial/ethnic minorities are the least likely of all Americans to meet these recommendations (U.S. Department of Health and Human Services 2008, 2010). Successful programs serving the underserved communities must bring all stakeholders to the table and address the needs of families who live in poverty, speak non-English languages, and reside in remote or resource poor communities.

STUDY QUESTIONS

1. Describe the major factors contributing to the disparities in physical activity participation in the United States.
2. What is the rationale for tailoring and targeting physical activity promotion in underserved communities, based on the discussion of the factors at different levels of the socioecological perspective?
3. Explain why it is important to take into consideration cultural norms and beliefs in designing effective physical activity intervention programs.
4. Describe three ways to culturally tailor physical activity programs and interventions.
5. Create at least two strategies to increase the community's interest and buy-in when planning and implementing physical activity promotion in underserved communities.
6. Describe the characteristics of CHWs and defend their value in delivering health promotion messages to individuals in underserved communities.

REFERENCES

Afable-Munsuz, A., A. P. Ninez, M. Rodrigues et al. 2006. Immigrant generation and physical activity among Mexican, Chinese and Filipino adults in the U.S. *Soc. Sci. Med.* 70: 1997–2005.

Ainsworth, B. E., S. Wilcox, W. W. Thompson et al. 2003. Personal, social, and physical environmental correlates of physical activity in African–American women in South Carolina. *Am. J. Prev. Med.* 25: 23–29.

Bandura, A. 1986. *Social Foundations of Thought and Action: A Social Cognitive Theory.* Englewood Cliffs, NJ: Prentice-Hall.

Berrigan, D., K. Dodd, R. P. Troiano et al. 2006. Physical activity and acculturation among adult Hispanics in the United States. *Res. Q. Exerc. Sport* 77: 147–157.

Burroughs, E., R. M. Fields, and P. A. Sharpe. 2004. Identifying walking and trail use supports and barriers through focus group research. 18th National Conference on Chronic Disease Prevention and Health Promotion. Washington, DC. Preventing Chronic Disease: Public Health Research, Practice, and Policy 1: http://www.cdc.gov/pcd/issues/2004.

Carter-Nolan, P. L., L. L. Adams-Campbell, and J. Williams. 1996. Recruitment strategies for black women at risk for noninsulin-dependent diabetes mellitus into exercise protocols: A qualitative assessment. *J. Natl. Med. Assoc.* 88: 558–562.

Castro, F. G., M. K. Cota, and S. C. Vega, 1999. Health promotion in Latino populations: A sociocultural model for program planning, development, and evaluation. In *Promoting Health in Multicultural Populations*, ed. R. M. Huff and M. V. Kline. Thousand Oaks, CA: Sage Publications.

Centers for Disease Control and Prevention (CDC). 2000. Prevalence of leisure-time and occupational physical activity among employed adults—United States, 1990. *Morb. Mortal. Wkly. Rep.* 49: 420–424.

Centers for Disease Control and Prevention (CDC). 2008. Prevalence of Self-Reported Physically Active Adults—United States, 2007. *Morb. Mortal. Wkly. Rep.* 57: 1297–1300.

Clark, D. O. 1999. Identifying psychological, physiological and environmental barriers and facilitators to exercise among older low income adults. *J. Clin. Geropsychol.* 5: 51–62.

Crespo, C. J., E. Smit, O. Carter-Pokras et al. 2001. Acculturation and leisure-time physical inactivity in Mexican American adults: results from the NHANES III, 1988–1994. *Am. J. Public Health* 91: 1254–1257.

Crespo, C. J., E. Smit, R. E. Andersen et al. 2000. Race/ethnicity, social class and their relation to physical inactivity during leisure time: Results from the Third National Health and Nutrition Examination Survey, 1988–1994. *Am. J. Prev. Med.* 18: 46–53.

Crespo, C. J. 2005. Physical activity in minority populations: Overcoming a public health challenge. In *Research Digest*, ed. C. B. Corbin, R. P. Pangrazi, and D. Young. Washington, D.C.: President's Council on Physical Fitness and Sports.

Duke, J., M. Huhman, and C. Heitzler. 2003. Physical activity levels among children aged 9–13 years—United States, 2002. *Morb. Mortal. Wkly. Rep.* 52: 785–788.

Dzewaltowski, D. A. 1994. Physical activity determinants: a social cognitive approach. *Med. Sci. Sports Exerc.* 26: 1395–1399.

Estabrooks, P. A., R. E. Lee, and N. C. Gyuresik. 2003. Resources for physical activity participation: does availability and accessibility differ by neighborhood socioeconomic status? *Ann. Behav. Med.* 25: 100–104.

Evenson, K. R., O. L. Sarmiento, K. W. Tawney et al. 2003. Personal, social, and environmental correlates of physical activity in North Carolina Latina immigrants. *Am. J. Prev. Med.* 25: 77–85.

Eyler, A. A., D. Matson-Koffman, J. R. Vest et al. 2002. Environmental, policy, and cultural factors related to physical activity in a diverse sample of women: The Women's Cardiovascular Health Network Project—summary and discussion. *Women Health* 36: 123–134.

Eyler, A. A., E. Baker, L. Cromer et al. 1998. Physical activity and minority women: A qualitative study. *Health Educ. Behav.* 25: 640–652.

Eyler, A. A., D. Matson-Koffman, D. R. Young et al. 2003. Quantitative study of correlates of physical activity in women from diverse racial/ethnic groups: The Women's Cardiovascular Health Network Project—summary and conclusions. *Am. J. Prev. Med.* 25: 93–103.

Gordon-Larsen, P., R. G. McMurray, and B. M. Popkin. 2000. Determinants of adolescent physical activity and inactivity patterns. *Pediatrics* 105: E83.

Haskell, W. L., I. M. Lee, R. R. Pate et al. 2007. Physical activity and public health: Updated recommendation for adults from the American College of Sports Medicine and the American Heart Association. *Circulation* 116: 1081–1093.

Henderson, K. A., and B. E. Ainsworth. 2000. Enablers and constraints to walking for older African American and American Indian women: The Cultural Activity Participation Study. *Res. Q. Exerc. Sport* 71: 313–321.

Henderson, S., E. Kendall, and L. See. 2011. The effectiveness of culturally appropriate interventions to manage or prevent chronic disease in culturally and linguistically diverse communities: a systematic literature review. *Health Soc. Care Community* 19: 225–249.

Hovell, M., J. Sallis, R. Hofstetter et al. 1991. Identification of correlates of physical activity among Latino adults. *J. Community Health* 16: 23–36.

Humpel, N., N. Owen, and E. Leslie. 2002. Environmental factors associated with adults' participation in physical activity: A review. *Am. J. Prev. Med.* 22: 188–199.

Jones, M., and M. A. Nies. 1996. The relationship of perceived benefits of and barriers to reported exercise in older African American women. *Public Health Nurs.* 13: 151–158.

Juarbe, T., X. P. Turok, and E. J. Perez-Stable. 2002. Perceived benefits and barriers to physical activity among older Latina women. *West. J. Nurs. Res.* 24: 868–886.

Kash, B. A., M. L. May, and M. Tai-Seale. 2007. Community health worker training and certification programs in the United States: Findings from a national survey. *Health Policy* 80: 32–42.

King, A. C., C. Castro, S. Wilcox et al. 2000. Personal and environmental factors associated with physical inactivity among different racial–ethnic groups of U.S. middle-aged and older-aged women. *Health Psychol.* 19: 354–364.

King, A. C., D. Stokols, E. Talen et al. 2002. Theoretical approaches to the promotion of physical activity: Forging a transdisciplinary paradigm. *Am. J. Prev. Med.* 23: 15–25.

Lewin, S. A., J. Dick, P. Pond et al. 2005. Lay health workers in primary and community health care. *Cochrane Database Syst. Rev.* CD004015. Review. Update in *Cochrane Database Syst. Rev.* 2010;(3):CD004015.

Lopez, I. A., C. A. Bryant, and R. J. McDermott. 2008. Influences on physical activity participation among Latinas: An ecological perspective. *Am. J. Health Behav.* 32: 627–639.

Marquez, D. X., and E. McAuley. 2006. Gender and acculturation influences on physical activity in Latino adults. *Ann. Behav. Med.* 31: 138–144.

Marshall, S. J., D. A. Jones, B. E. Ainsworth et al. 2007. Race/ethnicity, social class, and leisure-time physical inactivity. *Med. Sci. Sports Exerc.* 39: 44–51.

Martin, S. L., G. J. Kirkner, K. Mayo et al. 2005. Urban, rural, and regional variations in physical activity. *J. Rural Health* 21: 239–244.

Martinez, S. M., E. M. Arredondo, G. Perez et al. 2009. Individual, social, and environmental barriers to and facilitators of physical activity among Latinas living in San Diego County: Focus group results. *Fam. Community Health* 32: 22–33.

Mier, N., M. G. Ory, D. Zhan et al. 2007. Levels and correlates of exercise in a border Mexican American population. *Am. J. Health Behav.* 31: 159–169.

Parra-Medina, D., and D. K. H. Messias. 2011. Promotion of physical activity among Mexican-origin women in Texas and South Carolina: An examination of social, cultural, economic, and environmental factors. *Quest* 63: 100–107.

Powell, L. M., S. Slater, F. J. Chaloupka et al. 2006. Availability of physical activity-related facilities and neighborhood demographic and socioeconomic characteristics: A national study. *Am. J. Public Health* 96: 1676–1680.

Robert Wood Johnson Foundation. 2005. Active Living Diversity Project: A look at physical activity and healthy eating in African American, Latino, and Native American communities. http://www.rwjf.org/files/publications/other/PublicDiversityReport.pdf (accessed July 18, 2011).

Sallis, J. F., A. E. Bauman, and M. Pratt. 1998. Environmental and policy interventions to promote physical activity. *Am. J. Prev. Med.* 15: 379–397.

Sallis, J. F., M. F. Hovell, R. C. Hofstetter et al. 1990. Distance between homes and exercise facilities related to frequency of exercise among San Diego residents. *Public Health Rep.* 105: 179–185.

Sallis, J. F., R. B. Cervero, W. Ascher et al. 2006. An ecological approach to creating active living communities. *Annu. Rev. Public Health* 27: 297–322.

Satia, J. A., R. E. Patterson, M. L. Neuhouser et al. 2002. Dietary acculturation: applications to nutrition research and dietetics. *J. Am. Diet Assoc.* 102: 1105–1118.

Shores, K. A., J. B. Moore, and Z. Yin. 2010. An examination of triple jeopardy in rural youth physical activity participation. *J. Rural Health* 26: 352–360.

Swider, S. M. 2002. Outcome effectiveness of community health workers: An integrative literature review. *Public Health Nurs.* 19: 11–20.

Taylor, W. C., T. Baranowski, and D. R. Young. 1998. Physical activity interventions in low-income, ethnic minority, and populations with disability. *Am. J. Prev. Med.* 15: 334–343.

Trost, S. G., N. Owen, A. E. Bauman et al. 2002. Correlates of adults' participation in physical activity: Review and update. *Med. Sci. Sports Exerc.* 34: 1996–2001.

U.S. Department of Health and Human Services (USDHHS). 2011. Healthy People 2020. Available from http://healthypeople.gov/2020/# (accessed July 18, 2011).

U.S. Department of Health and Human Services (USDHHS). 1994. *Community Health Advisors: Models, Research, and Practice*, ed. Public Health Service and Centers for Disease Control and Prevention. Atlanta, GA.

U.S. Department of Health and Human Services (USDHHS). 1996. *Physical Activity and Health: A Report of the Surgeon General*. Atlanta, GA: National Center for Chronic Disease Prevention and Health Promotion, Centers for Disease Control and Prevention, U.S. Department of Health and Human Services.

U.S. Department of Health and Human Services (USDHHS). 2008. *2008 Physical Activity Guidelines for Americans*. http://www.health.gov/paguidelines (accessed July 18, 2011).

U.S. Department of Health and Human Services (USDHHS). 2010. National Partnership for Action to End Health Disparities. http://www.minorityhealth.hhs.gov/npa/templates/browse.aspx?&lvl=2&lvlid=34 (accessed July 18, 2011).

Viswanathan, M., A. Ammerman, E. Eng et al. 2004. Community-Based Participatory Research: Assessing the Evidence. http://www.mycbpr.org/CBPR-project/articles/AHRQ-cbpr-assessing-evidence.pdf (accessed July 18, 2011).

Vrazel, J., R. P. Saunders, and S. Wilcox. 2008. An overview and proposed framework of social–environmental influences on the physical-activity behavior of women. *Am. J. Health Promot.* 23: 2–12.

Wilbur, J. E., P. Chandler, B. Dancy et al. 2002. Environmental, policy, and cultural factors related to physical activity in urban, African American women. *Women Health* 36: 17–28.

Wilcox, S., C. Castro, A. C. King et al. 2000. Determinants of leisure time physical activity in rural compared with urban older and ethnically diverse women in the United States. *J. Epidemiol. Community Health* 54: 667–672.

Wilcox, S., D. L. Richter, K. A. Henderson et al. 2002. Perceptions of physical activity and personal barriers and enablers in African–American women. *Ethn. Dis.* 12: 353–362.

Yancey, A. K., M. G. Ory, and S. M. Davis. 2006. Dissemination of physical activity promotion interventions in underserved populations. *Am. Prev. Med.* 31: S82–S91.

15 Built Environmental Supports for Walking

Paula Hooper, Sarah Foster,
Andrea Nathan, and Billie Giles-Corti

CONTENTS

INTRODUCTION

In the past decade, a new field of "active living research" has emerged studying the impact of the built environment on physical activity, particularly walking. This multidisciplinary field involves not only physical activity academics, but also researchers, practitioners, and policy makers from transportation, urban planning, and geography. Collaborations of this type provide unprecedented opportunities for physical activity researchers to work in partnership with those responsible for informing how our communities are built (Bull, Giles-Corti, and Wood 2010).

This chapter presents the public health rationale for focusing on walking, defines the built environment, and introduces the theoretical underpinnings for how and why it is a key driver of walking behavior. It presents a summary of the evidence to date examining the relationship between the built environment and walking, and outlines future challenges and directions for active living research.

WALKING AS PHYSICAL ACTIVITY

The release of the U.S. Surgeon General's report in 1996 (U.S. Department of Health and Human Services 1996) heralded a shift in emphasis in physical activity research, policy, and practice toward moderate intensity lifestyle activities, such as walking, that can be accumulated throughout the day. This has since become a key strategy designed to increase global population levels of physical activity (Lee and Moudon 2004). The World Health Organization now acknowledges walking as an important health enhancing physical activity to protect against diseases associated with sedentary lifestyles (World Health Organization 2004).

Globally, walking is the most frequently engaged in and preferred type of physical activity undertaken by adults (U.S. Department of Health and Human Services 1996). Walking is a highly accessible, low-cost form of physical activity that can easily be integrated into daily routines with few barriers to participation. This makes it an appealing form of physical activity to promote, irrespective of age, gender, socioeconomic or health status, and level of fitness (Frank, Engelke, and Schmid 2003). In the past decade, physical activity researchers have turned their attention to understanding the specific correlates of walking as a form of transport, and walking for exercise or recreation. Walking for transport (or active transport) is a utilitarian behavior concerned with walking to get to and from destinations such as shops, transit stops, and work. Walking for transport is not only good for health, but has additional benefits associated with reduced car use, greenhouse gas emissions, noise pollution, and improved air quality (Frumkin, Frank, and Jackson 2004). Active transport is therefore increasingly recognized as offering cobenefits across a number of sectors beyond health, providing additional incentives to encourage walking (Giles-Corti et al. 2010a). Walking for recreation is a discretionary behavior undertaken during leisure time and involves some degree of choice (Saelens, Sallis, and Frank 2003).

THEORIES THAT UNDERPIN THE FOCUS ON THE ENVIRONMENT

Early physical activity research focused on individual determinants of behavior, such as motivation and self-efficacy. However, these models only accounted for a small amount of the variance in physical activity behaviors. As such, interest grew in exploring broader determinants of health behavior that reach beyond individual responsibility and control, such as policies and environments (McLeroy et al. 1988). This shift led to the adoption of a socioecological framework to understand physical activity, including walking. This framework considers multiple levels of influence on behavior including individual (e.g., attitudes, knowledge, and beliefs), social (e.g., friends or family), societal and cultural (e.g., social norms), and physical environmental factors (e.g., neighborhood design) (McLeroy et al. 1988; Sallis, Bauman, and Pratt 1998). Socioecologic approaches hypothesize that there is a constant interaction between individuals and their physical environment (Sallis, Bauman, and Pratt 1998). Changes to the environment have the potential to produce a shift in behavior in exposed populations, making physical activity behaviors easier or more difficult (Heath et al. 2006).

DEFINING PHYSICAL AND BUILT ENVIRONMENTS

The physical environment refers to all external surroundings and conditions in which we live. This can be further refined into the built environment and natural environment (Figure 15.1). The built environment consists of the constructed elements of the physical environment including all buildings, spaces, and products created or modified by people (Saelens and Handy 2008). Elements of the built environment can be manipulated to create more supportive natural environments (e.g., constructing trails through a forest). This chapter focuses mainly on the built environment.

THE BUILT ENVIRONMENT AND WALKING

Walking is primarily undertaken in neighborhood public spaces (Lee and Moudon 2004). In light of the popularity of walking, and its potential health benefits, understanding built environmental characteristics and neighborhood designs that support or deter walking has become a priority (Saelens and Handy 2008). This has focused attention on the urban and transportation policies that dictate the structure of our cities. A historical overview of changes to town planning that have contributed to declining levels of walking, particularly in North America and Australia, follows.

RISE AND SPRAWL OF SUBURBIA

During the mid-nineteenth century, the industrial revolution brought large influxes of people into major European and U.S. cities. The overcrowded conditions and

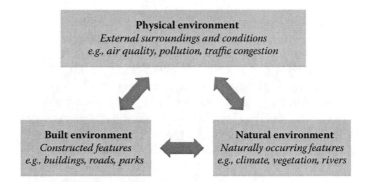

FIGURE 15.1 Conceptualizing "environments."

poor sanitation that resulted created ideal conditions for the outbreak and spread of infectious diseases (Transportation Research Board 2005). Moreover, the colocation of noxious industrial land uses alongside residential housing meant residents were exposed to environmental pollution and noise. Concerned about the impact of these environments on the health of its inhabitants, public health officials recognized the benefits of town planning as a means of lowering housing densities and separating polluting land uses from residential areas (Schilling and Linton 2005; Transportation Research Board 2005). Changes to the planning regulations of urban areas followed, with the introduction of single-use land zoning practices. This divided land into zones and specified the type of activity permitted (e.g., residential, commercial, retail, or industrial) (Transportation Research Board 2005).

Although zoning successfully separated industrial and residential land uses, and reduced communicable disease, it also segregated retail and commercial land uses, encouraging the development of isolated residential suburbs (Schilling and Linton 2005; Farr 2008). This trend toward exclusively residential suburbs escalated following the mass production of affordable motor vehicles after World War II. Private vehicles increased residents' mobility, allowing them to live greater distances from their place of work and destinations required for daily living (Giles-Corti et al. 2010b). However, the increased distances made it impractical for residents to walk or cycle to these destinations as part of their daily routine (Farr 2008; Falconer and Giles-Corti 2008). Moreover, low suburban residential densities made provision of regular transit services unviable, further fueling automobile dependency (Giles-Corti et al. 2010b; Transportation Research Board 2005). Road construction standards have since focused on moving cars long distances at high speeds at the expense of pedestrian and cycling infrastructure (Farr 2008; Duany, Plater-Zyberk, and Speck 2000).

Over the past few decades, sprawled residential suburban development (often referred to as "conventional" development) has become standard in North America and Australia, particularly on the urban fringe. This contrasts with the traditional forms of development evident throughout much of Europe, characterized by higher population densities, a good mix of destinations and a diverse range of housing (Duany, Plater-Zyberk, and Speck 2000).

Consequences of Suburban Sprawl for Walking

Technological advances that have eliminated physical exertion from most aspects of daily life, including work, household chores, travel, and leisure activities, have resulted in declining physical activity levels (Giles-Corti et al. 2010b; Transportation Research Board 2005). Postwar suburban development, as described above, has also discouraged active forms of transport and transit use (which typically involves a walking trip at each end) (MacDonald et al. 2010). There is also growing evidence suggesting that suburban sprawl is associated with increased weight (Butland et al. 2007), principally through its impact on energy expenditure by encouraging car dependence (Frank, Andresen, and Schmid 2004) and more sedentary leisure behaviors, for example, television viewing (Sugiyama et al. 2007). Indeed, in the United States and Australia, where sprawling suburban development is common-place, walking, cycling, and transit trips account for only 12% and 13% of all trips taken, respectively. In European countries, where compact development is commonplace, walking, cycling, and transit trips range from 26% to 67% of all trips (Bassett et al. 2008).

Important questions are now being asked to determine whether current suburban development patterns that emerged partly in response to nineteenth century health concerns are now contributing to twenty-first century problems related to inactivity, sedentary behavior, and obesity. These concerns have given rise to active living research, kick-started in the United States by the Robert Wood Johnson Foundation.

ACTIVE LIVING RESEARCH

The Active Living Research (ALR) program in the United States supports research to identify environmental factors and policies that influence physical activity. The program is helping to develop the field of active living research, and manages grants to assist in building the evidence base. The ALR website provides summaries of the latest research examining the relationship between environment and policy and active living and links to a wide array of tools and resources for public health practitioners and researchers. More information can be found at www.activelivingresearch.org.

CONCEPTUALIZING THE BUILT ENVIRONMENT FOR WALKING

In terms of understanding walking behaviors, research has focused on three main, interacting features of the built environment: land use patterns, transportation systems, and design features. Together, these features determine the location of destinations, facilities, and services; the ease with which they can be reached; and the pleasantness and safety of the experience (Transportation Research Board 2005) (Figure 15.2). This section describes these features in detail, their theoretical influences on walking, and compares their presence in conventional and traditional forms of development.

LAND USE PATTERNS

Land use patterns refer to the spatial distribution and mix of destinations required for all aspects of daily life and recreation (e.g., shops, work, schools, and public open space) and the density of residential dwellings (Transportation Research Board 2005). The terms "land uses" and "destinations" are generally used interchangeably. However, land use actually describes areas of land that have been zoned for specific purposes (e.g., retail or residential). Conversely, destinations refer to the specific types of businesses present (e.g., a supermarket or bank).

"Land use mix" is used to describe the diversity (or mix) of different land uses or destinations over a given area, that is, within the neighborhood (Transportation Research Board 2005). Transport theories hypothesize that walking is more likely when a variety of proximate destinations, transit stops, and areas of public open

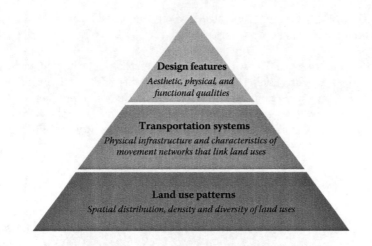

FIGURE 15.2   Aspects of the built environment that encourage walking.

space are present (i.e., mixed land uses), as these provide meaningful and convenient opportunities to walk (Duany, Plater-Zyberk, and Speck 2000).

Traditional neighborhoods tend to contain a diverse mix of destinations integrated within close proximity of a variety of residential dwelling types (i.e., apartment blocks, town houses, and detached houses). In contrast, conventional neighborhoods consist of uniform residential dwellings situated on large lots, with few (if any) destinations to walk and are instead served by large auto-oriented shopping complexes such as big-box retail parks, shopping malls, and office parks. As such, all work and leisure activities are usually undertaken outside the neighborhood.

Figure 15.3a and b illustrates land use mix in two different areas of Perth, Western Australia: an older area, located on the edge of the central business district with integrated retail and residential land uses (Figure 15.3a); and an area of conventional suburban development on the urban fringe comprising vast areas of single detached housing and large big-box retail parks (Figure 15.3b).

Measures of land use include: simple counts of different destination types or land uses; the distance (proximity) to specific destinations (measured using the road or pedestrian network); and more sophisticated methods such as entropy formulas that measure the variety and distribution of land uses over a given area (Forsyth et al. 2007; Frank et al. 2010).

"Density" is typically used as a measure of the number of people living in a given area (e.g., population density/acre) or the number of housing units present per area (e.g., residential density/acre) (Churchman 1999). In terms of walking behavior, higher population densities provide a reliable customer base for local businesses and transit, making shops and services economically viable and resulting in a greater variety of destinations within a more compact area (e.g., traditional neighborhoods). This affects walking behavior by increasing the proximity of destinations and thereby reducing the need to travel by car (Falconer and Giles-Corti 2008; Farr 2008).

Farr (2008) estimates that a minimum of 1000 households, within a 400-meter radius neighborhood (i.e., 5- to 10-min walk), are needed to support a corner store

(a)

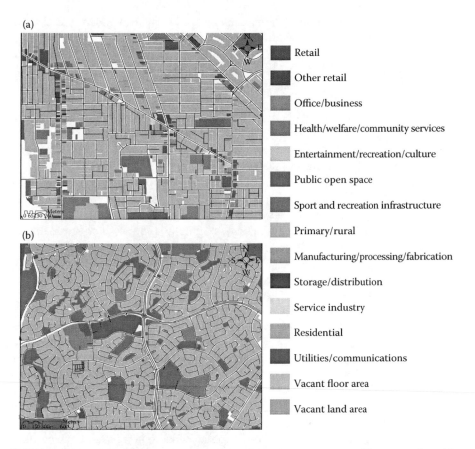

Retail

Other retail

Office/business

Health/welfare/community services

Entertainment/recreation/culture

Public open space

Sport and recreation infrastructure

Primary/rural

Manufacturing/processing/fabrication

Storage/distribution

Service industry

Residential

Utilities/communications

Vacant floor area

Vacant land area

(b)

FIGURE 15.3   (a) Typical land use mix in traditional developments. (Figure produced by Nick Middleton based on information provided by the Western Australia Land Information Authority, 2008. With permission.) (b) Typical land use mix in conventional developments. (Figure produced by Nick Middleton based on information provided by the Western Australia Land Information Authority, 2008. With permission.)

and at least 15 dwelling units per acre are needed to support a "frequent" local bus service. However, with residential densities of new U.S. developments averaging about two dwelling units per acre, the majority of conventional suburban developments fail to provide sufficient population densities to support local business and frequent transit services (Farr 2008).

TRANSPORTATION SYSTEM

The transportation system (or movement network) is the physical infrastructure that allows people to navigate between land uses or destinations. It includes the roads, sidewalks, cycle paths, and rail routes.

Connectivity—road networks. The term "connectivity" refers to the directness or ease of moving between origins (e.g., households) and destinations along the movement network (Saelens, Sallis, and Frank 2003). The proximity of destinations is also determined by how connected the street networks are en route to the destination (Transportation Research Board 2005). In terms of walking behaviors, increased connectivity reduces the distances between origins and destinations and provides a range of routes to choose from, increasing the likelihood of walking between locations (Dill 2004).

Traditionally designed neighborhoods tend to have a grid-style layout with few barriers to direct travel (e.g., dead ends and major intersecting roads), resulting in high levels of connectivity and a choice of routes (Figure 15.4a). In contrast, conventional neighborhoods are developed around a network of hierarchical roads. Curvilinear roads terminating in cul-de-sacs (i.e., lollipop-shaped dead end roads) feed from large, high-speed roads, creating low levels of connectivity (Duany, Plater-Zyberk, and Speck 2000). Residents have little or no choice of route, as often there is only one road in and out of the development, and the indirect curvilinear streets increase walking distances between destinations thereby discouraging walking (Dill 2004) (Figure 15.4b).

A wide range of measures have been used to quantify connectivity: intersection density (i.e., the number of intersections per unit area); percentage of three way intersections (i.e., T-junctions) or greater; block length or size (i.e., perimeter); and block density (i.e., the number of blocks per unit area) (Dill 2004).

Connectivity—pedestrian infrastructure. Another important consideration for recreational and transport walking is the presence and continuity of pedestrian infrastructure (i.e., sidewalks). The connectivity measures described above are typically calculated using road networks. However, this assumes that pedestrians walk via the road network, which may not accurately represent the routes available and underestimate levels of connectivity from a pedestrian perspective (Chin et al. 2008). Approaches to measuring the provision of pedestrian infrastructure include the length of sidewalks per unit area (i.e., the neighborhood); or the ratio of sidewalk

(a)   (b)

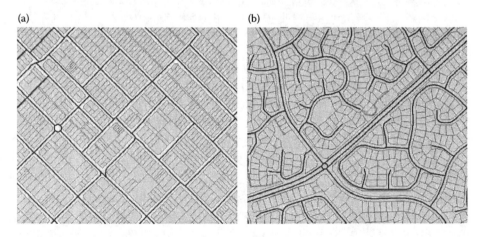

FIGURE 15.4   (a) Typical connectivity in traditional developments. (b) Typical connectivity in conventional developments.

length to road length as an indication of whether sidewalks are on one (1:1 ratio) or both sides (2:1 ratio) of the street, or less (i.e., ratio <1) (Forsyth et al. 2007).

DESIGN FEATURES

"Design features" comprise the physical qualities and aesthetics of the built environment, and relate to both land use patterns and transportation systems (Transportation Research Board 2005). Physical qualities refer to the appropriateness, condition, and maintenance of features within the built environment. Examples relevant to walking include the surface type and condition of sidewalks (i.e., free from cracks that pose trip hazards), curb heights, the provision of street furniture and lighting, and facilities provided in public open space (e.g., children's play equipment, lighting, shade, and seating). Neighborhood aesthetics determine the general appeal and presentation of the neighborhood and whether it provides a pleasant pedestrian-oriented environment (Pikora et al. 2006). It includes the diversity of the architectural design of buildings, public artworks, pleasant streetscapes, landscaping (e.g., the presence of trees or gardens), and natural vegetation (i.e., greenness). These help to create interesting scenery within the neighborhood and encourage walking (Duany, Plater-Zyberk, and Speck 2000). The maintenance and cleanliness of the neighborhood (e.g., free from graffiti and vandalism) are also important aesthetic features.

Many of these design features are thought to be important for enhancing residents' perceptions of how safe their neighborhood is for walking. For example, street lighting, smaller road widths, sidewalks, traffic slowing devices, and crossing aids help to promote personal and traffic safety (Pikora et al. 2006). Other built environment elements such as the orientation of buildings to promote natural surveillance (i.e., they front the streets or public open spaces), physical incivilities (e.g., graffiti, litter, and vandalism), and maintenance (e.g., house and garden upkeep) have important influences on actual crime and residents' perceptions of personal or crime-related safety (Foster and Giles-Corti 2008). These features are central to the field of Crime Prevention Through Environmental Design (CPTED), which seeks to deter crime by creating an environment that promotes natural surveillance, is well maintained, and signifies a sense of ownership over both private and public spaces (Crowe 1991). The design and orientation of housing in conventional suburbs can inhibit natural surveillance as houses typically have large set-backs and front yards, often with double garages or high fences fronting the property. In contrast, traditionally developed houses tend to have smaller set-backs, meaning they are closer to the sidewalk. This enables residents to monitor the street, which provides a greater sense of safety for pedestrians (Duany, Plater-Zyberk, and Speck 2000).

MEASURING THE BUILT ENVIRONMENT

The built environment can be conceptualized and studied at a number of different geographic scales, from the neighborhood or suburb level, to much larger regional, city, or country scales. Most public health and transportation research in this area is at the neighborhood level, with definitions ranging from 400- to 1600-meter distances around individuals' homes (along the street network or as the crow flies).

The impact of neighborhood size is likely to vary depending on the age of the study participants. For example, the size of the neighborhood relevant for younger children and older adults is likely to be somewhat smaller than for an able-bodied adult or adolescent. The following section provides an overview of three methods typically used to measure the built environment in physical activity and transportation research.

SELF-REPORT DATA

Early physical activity studies drew on self-report data, collected using telephone interviews or self-administered surveys, in which individuals' indicated their perceptions of the presence and quality of different features within their neighborhood. Although self-report information may not always reflect what is actually on

---

EXAMPLE OF A SELF-REPORT ENVIRONMENTAL SURVEY

Neighborhood Environment Walkability Scale (NEWS) (Saelens et al. 2003) This 98-item instrument was developed to measure residents' perceptions of local area attributes thought to be related to walking and cycling. The instrument assesses: types of residences; distance to destinations; access to services; street connectivity; walking and cycling facilities (such as sidewalks and cycle paths); neighborhood streetscapes and aesthetics; traffic safety; crime safety; and neighborhood satisfaction. It has been translated into several languages and is available at www.ipenproject.org/survey.

---

the ground, it does represent respondents' reality, and in some situations perceptions may be a more important influence on behavior than objective measures of the environment (e.g., perceived vs. objectively measured crime) (Brownson et al. 2009).

Questionnaire items that focus on fixed features, such as the presence of footpaths or cul-de-sacs, tend to have higher reliability (i.e., respondents' answers are consistent when tested at two time points) and validity (i.e., items measure what they intend to measure) than items assessing less tangible concepts or more changeable attributes (e.g., safety, neighborhood maintenance, or physical incivilities). Moreover, different items are often used to assess perceptions, and this needs to be considered when studies are compared.

ENVIRONMENTAL AUDITS

These entail the systematic observation and recording of microscale attributes that could influence walking. Trained auditors walk or drive through selected areas and complete a standardized checklist for each street segment or park (depending on the focus of the audit). Measures tend to focus on buildings and architectural characteristics (e.g., porches, visibility of house windows), pedestrian infrastructure and streetscapes (e.g., sidewalks, crossing aids, trees, lights), neighborhood maintenance and quality (e.g., garden upkeep, physical incivilities, sidewalk condition), and amenities (e.g., street furniture, signage, bins) (Brownson et al. 2009). Although audits can be time consuming, they are ideal for capturing the look and feel of an area, which cannot be readily collected through other methods. A variety of audit tools have been created to assess specific settings and population subgroups (e.g., seniors and children).

EXAMPLES OF ENVIRONMENTAL AUDIT TOOLS FOR WALKING

Systematic Pedestrian and Cycling Environmental Scan (SPACES) (Pikora et al. 2002). Developed in Australia, this 37-item audit tool covers environmental features related to functionality; safety; aesthetics; and destinations. The tool is available at www.sph.uwa.edu.au/research/cbeh/projects/?a=411954. It has also been adapted for the United States, more information can be found on the Active Living Research website (www.activelivingresearch.org/node/10641).

Public Open Space Tool (POST) (Broomhall, Giles-Corti, and Lange 2004; Giles-Corti et al. 2005). Also developed in Australia, this tool was designed for auditing public open spaces such as parks and ovals. The instrument collects data on activities; environmental quality; amenities; and safety. The POST tool is available atwww.sph.uwa.edu.au/research/cbeh/projects/post.

Numerous audit tools are now available; however, they differ in the number of features assessed, the level of detail collected, and reliability (Brownson et al. 2009). Again, fixed attributes (i.e., presence of sidewalks) usually have high interobserver reliability (i.e., different auditors rate features the same). Items that are subject to change or those requiring judgment (e.g., condition of the sidewalk) have lower reliability. It is necessary to ensure that auditors are well trained, to ensure consistent ratings are provided by different auditors.

OBJECTIVE ENVIRONMENTAL DATA (GIS)

A Geographic Information System (GIS) is a computer-based tool used to capture, analyze, and display spatially referenced information (Brownson et al. 2009). The development of GIS-based measures to quantify and describe neighborhood built environments has become increasingly widespread. Features typically measured in GIS include: road and pedestrian network connectivity; residential and population densities; land use mix and the location of destinations, parks, and transit stops.

GIS data are usually obtained from a variety of secondary sources, such as commercial or government agencies. However, these data are usually collected for land management, taxation, or advertising purposes, rather than for examining associations with walking. Also, the geographical areas for which these data are collected (e.g., by zip code) may not adequately reflect the study area of interest (i.e., the neighborhood). Thus, considerable time and effort must usually be invested to generate suitable measures that model the built environment for investigating relationships with walking behaviors (Brownson et al. 2009). Another issue, relatively unexplored to date, is the validity of the GIS data collected from various sources and how accurately the data reflect what is on the ground.

REVIEWING THE EVIDENCE: BUILT ENVIRONMENT CORRELATES OF WALKING

An expanding body of literature examining built environment correlates of walking now exists. The research on this topic has come from the transportation planning and physical activity fields. Transportation planning has focused on travel behavior and transportation demand, with walking as a mode of transport. Physical activity researchers have focused on walking as a form of physical activity, including walking for recreation and for transport (Owen et al. 2004; Saelens and Handy 2008). As researchers from both fields have collaborated, it has become clear that different built environmental features influence walking for transport or recreation (Owen et al. 2004; Saelens and Handy 2008). The importance of the built environment for walking is also acknowledged by high-level reviews and reports commissioned by government, nongovernment, and philanthropic organizations across the United States, United Kingdom, Australia, and Canada (WHO 2004; Transportation Research Board 2005; Butland et al. 2007).

Most studies have examined adults' walking behavior, with relatively less research focusing on children or adolescents (aged 5 to 18 years) and older adults (usually aged 50 to 65 years and above). This section reviews the current evidence of built environment correlates on walking for transport and walking for recreation and highlights similarities and differences in correlates for children, adults, and older adults.

WALKING FOR TRANSPORT

The most consistent land use correlate of walking for transport is population density. This has been found for children (Saelens and Handy 2008; Panter, Jones, and van Sluijs 2008) and adults (Saelens, Sallis, and Frank 2003; Owen et al. 2004; Transportation Research Board 2005; Saelens and Handy 2008), with a similar trend now emerging in the literature on older adults (Shigematsu et al. 2009). Population density is critical in mixed-use neighborhoods, providing the customers required to support local businesses, thereby increasing proximity to local destinations.

Consistently positive associations between land use patterns and walking for transport across all population groups are reported. Measures of land use mix are positively correlated with walking for transport in adults, although evidence is more inconsistent for children and older adults (Transportation Research Board 2005; Saelens and Papadopoulos 2008; Saelens and Handy 2008; Shigematsu et al. 2009).

Close proximity to neighborhood destinations is positively correlated with active transport across the life course, with specific destinations more important for different population groups. For children, distance to school is consistently associated with active commuting (Davison and Lawson 2006; Panter, Jones, and van Sluijs 2008), whereas other destination types (e.g., public open space and sports facilities or shops) appear to be more important for older children and adolescents than younger children who are less independently mobile (Panter, Jones, and van Sluijs 2008). Proximity to destinations, such as shops and parks, are positively associated with transportation walking in adults (Owen et al. 2004; Transportation Research Board 2005; Saelens and Handy 2008; Saelens and Papadopoulos 2008) and appear to be especially important for transportation walking in older adults (Shigematsu et al. 2009), possibly because of their reduced mobility.

Consistent positive associations have also been found for the presence of sidewalks and walking for transport in children (Davison and Lawson 2006; Saelens and Handy 2008) and adults (Owen et al. 2004; Transportation Research Board 2005; Saelens and Handy 2008). The evidence for older adults is mixed (Saelens and Papadopoulos 2008; Shigematsu et al. 2009).

The association between road connectivity and active transport has produced mixed results in children (Davison and Lawson 2006; Panter, Jones, and van Sluijs 2008) and adults (Saelens, Sallis, and Frank 2003; Saelens and Handy 2008). Connected road networks have been shown to be associated with more walking in older adults and children, but only when traffic-related issues are managed and the local streets are perceived to be safe (Saelens and Papadopoulos 2008). Real and perceived traffic-related safety has been associated with walking for transport in children (Davison and Lawson 2006; Saelens and Handy 2008; Panter, Jones, and van Sluijs 2008) and older adults (Saelens and Papadopoulos 2008; Shigematsu et al. 2009).

Connectivity affects walking by increasing proximity and providing more direct routes to local destinations. As identified above, access to destinations is strongly associated with walking for transport, and the presence of destinations is only possible when there is higher population density. These interactions highlight the synergistic influences of built environmental features. Researchers are therefore exploring the combined effect of connectivity, density, and land use mix on walking by using GIS to create "walkability indices" (Frank et al. 2010). Evidence from a number of countries shows positive associations between neighborhood walkability and walking for transport across the life course (Saelens and Handy 2008).

There is mixed evidence of associations between neighborhood aesthetics and walking for transport. Inconsistent associations have been identified for both children (Panter, Jones, and van Sluijs 2008) and adults (Owen et al. 2004; Transportation Research Board 2005; Saelens and Handy 2008), suggesting that land use and the transport system are much stronger predictors of transport walking than aesthetic details.

WALKING FOR RECREATION

Studies examining correlates of recreational walking focus on adult populations rather than children, who engage in active play and active transport rather than recreational walking. Positive neighborhood aesthetics are strongly associated with walking for recreation in adults (Owen et al. 2004; Saelens and Handy 2008; McCormack et al. 2004) and older adults (Shigematsu et al. 2009). There is also growing evidence that proximity to recreational destinations, particularly large, attractive public open space and beaches, is associated with adults recreational walking (McCormack et al. 2004; Giles-Corti et al. 2005).

Recreational walking is mostly undertaken in neighborhood streets, and the presence of sidewalks and other pedestrian infrastructure are consistently associated with more recreational walking in adults (Saelens and Handy 2008). Importantly, it is not simply the provision of pedestrian infrastructure that appears to be important for recreational walking, but also its quality. This may particularly relevant for older adults who are at greater risk of falls.

Some land use patterns have also been associated with recreational walking; however, the evidence is inconsistent. For instance, residential densities and land use mix appear to be associated with recreational walking in adults and older adults (Shigematsu et al. 2009; Saelens and Handy 2008; McCormack et al. 2004). However, the presence of varied land uses that create a more interesting landscape may be what encourages recreational walkers rather than the specific destinations themselves (McCormack et al. 2004).

In combination, these results highlight the importance of planning neighborhoods to provide a combination of land uses, including high-quality public open space, good accessibility, and pleasing aesthetics to encourage walking behaviors. Current research also suggests that crime-related safety may cause women and older adults to limit their walking. There is evidence that some CPTED elements such as good street lighting, neighborhood upkeep, and less physical incivilities and street features that promote safety from crime (e.g., front porches and neighborhood maintenance) can encourage walking (Foster and Giles-Corti 2008). To date, there is no clear pattern as to whether safety concerns impact more on transport or recreational walking. However, it is possible that these features may have greater impacts on discretionary behaviors where choice is involved, such as walking for recreation.

NEIGHBORHOOD COMPARISON STUDIES

The majority of the correlational evidence presented above has come from studies focusing on individual features of the built environment. However, in practice individual features are unlikely to influence walking in isolation, and the inconsistent findings highlight the need to consider the combination of neighborhood attributes that might work together to affect walking behaviors. One such method is to compare the walking behaviors of residents living in different development types. A number of recent studies have examined walking levels of those living in conventional and New Urbanist-designed developments. New Urbanism is one of a number of planning movements that have recently emerged as an alternative to current planning models responsible for suburban sprawl. It embraces traditional styles of development with the aim of creating walkable neighborhoods that encourage more active modes of transportation (Falconer and Giles-Corti 2008). Findings have shown that residents of New Urbanist neighborhoods engage in more walking for transport than those residing in conventional suburbs (Rodriguez, Khattak, and Evenson 2006) and substitute more driving trips with walking trips because of the walkable distances between residences and commercial centers, and the network of sidewalks and direct bus routes from the neighborhood to particular destinations (Khattak and Rodriguez 2005).

FUTURE DIRECTIONS IN RESEARCH AND PRACTICE RELATED TO BUILT ENVIRONMENT AND HEALTH

Amid growing concerns about physical inactivity and obesity, climate change, population growth, declining oil supplies, and their combined health, social, environmental, and economic impacts, multiple sectors are now focused on changing the built environment to increase walking, cycling, and transit use. Although active living research is a relatively new field of study, it is providing evidence to help shape policy reform to create more activity-friendly environments that encourage active lifestyles. Although enormous progress has been made in the past decade, there is still much to learn. The purpose of this section is to reflect on progress to date and future directions, and to consider the implications for policy and practice.

CRITIQUE OF THE EVIDENCE BASE

A major criticism of the evidence base to date is that most studies use cross-sectional study designs. These study designs cannot inform whether there is a causal relationship between the built environment and walking behavior. Furthermore, it also raises concerns over self-selection. It is not clear whether people who prefer to be physically active choose to live in walkable or activity-supportive neighborhoods (i.e., near shops, parks, or the beach) or whether neighborhoods themselves encourage individuals to live actively (Bull, Giles-Corti, and Wood 2010). To overcome issues related to self-selection, there have been calls for longitudinal study designs of the impact of the built environment on physical activity.

A second limitation is that much of the evidence is based on studies of able-bodied adults. Fewer studies have been conducted with children, adolescents, and older adults. There are likely to be important differences in environmental features that influence these groups that warrant investigation. For example, high walkable neighborhoods that have been shown to encourage adults to walk for transport often have more traffic, which is negatively associated with active forms of transport in children and older adults. Similarly, some studies show that men and women differ in their response to the built environment (i.e., safety). More research is required to ensure that the needs of important subgroups are fully understood and taken into account when planning neighborhoods.

FUTURE DIRECTIONS

As cities implement policies and modify environments to support active living, research opportunities to monitor the impact of these interventions will emerge. Ideally, active living researchers would adopt the gold standard for intervention research: the randomized controlled trial. However, it is impractical to randomize active living research participants to live in different (neighborhood) environments.

Evaluations of natural experiments (e.g., studying the impacts of a transport or planning policy on residents active living behaviors) provide a suitable alternative study design to inform the field (Schilling and Linton 2005; Sallis, Story, and Lou 2009). They have the potential to provide insights into how to design and produce better outcomes for communities. An example of a natural experiment evaluating a state-government policy, based on New Urbanist principles, and designed to create more "Liveable Neighborhoods" is currently in progress in Perth, Western Australia. Other recent natural experiments include evaluations of the implementation of light

THE RESIDENTIAL ENVIRONMENTS (RESIDE) PROJECT

The RESIDE project is a 5-year natural experiment designed to evaluate the impact of the "Liveable Neighborhoods Community Design Guidelines" on health and behavior. Based on the principles of New Urbanism, the guidelines aim to develop compact, well-defined and more sustainable communities with higher densities, connected street networks and mixed-use zoning that encourage more walking, cycling and public transport use (WAPC 2000; Giles-Corti et al. 2007). RESIDE participants were building homes in new housing developments, some of which were designed according to the Liveable Neighborhoods Design Guidelines. They were surveyed three times: before moving into their new home; 12 months after moving into their new home; and 3 years after moving into their new home. To read more about RESIDE, go to www.sph.uwa.edu.au/research/cbeh/projects/reside.

rail (MacDonald et al. 2010) and transport infrastructure designed to connect communities (Ogilvie et al. 2011).

Another untapped line of inquiry is research that better understands and informs policy and practice (i.e., research translation). Little is known about the barriers and facilitators to implementation of environmental interventions and policies. Barriers might include the legislative or regulatory processes (red tape), private sector funding that inhibit development approval, or funding processes and on-the-ground implementation. Understanding these barriers will assist in advancing research translation. Moreover, when policies are implemented, few (if any) published studies to date, have measured actual policy implementation (using policy specific measures monitored over time) and their impact on active living behaviors (Sallis, Bauman, and Pratt 1998). Integrating rigorous process evaluations, exploring the extent to which each component of the intervention or policy is implemented as planned is essential. Without this knowledge, it is impossible to know whether observed results (i.e., on walking behavior) are attributable to the policy or environmental intervention itself, and if no effect is found, whether it is attributable to policy failure or inadequate implementation (Dehar, Casswell, and Duignan 1993). Process evaluation information of this type will inform the development, adoption, and implementation

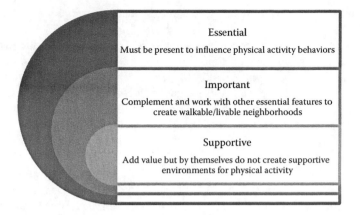

Essential

Must be present to influence physical activity behaviors

Important

Complement and work with other essential features to create walkable/livable neighborhoods

Supportive

Add value but by themselves do not create supportive environments for physical activity

FIGURE 15.5 Conceptual hierarchy of design characteristics influencing active living behaviors.

of future policies, and provide practitioners and policy-makers with examples that can be adapted elsewhere (Schilling and Linton 2005).

Collaborations are also required with economists and burden-of-disease epidemiologists to study the cobenefits across multiple sectors of urban design and transportation policies (Giles-Corti et al. 2010a). This research could extend beyond health benefits to include the economic benefits for the environment, traffic management, and property development. The latter is particularly important as a tool for engaging the private sector, which is responsible for delivering infrastructure including new housing developments.

Finally, the identification of thresholds for specific design features as well as the mix of design features required that encourage and support behavior change will be an important area of research moving forward. Given the diversity of measures currently being explored in the literature, future studies should seek to identify the relative influence of these features with a view to establishing a hierarchy of design characteristics that influence active living behaviors (see Figure 15.5). Identifying the appropriate mix of high leverage interventions (i.e., essential, important, and supportive) will assist planners, policy makers, and practitioners to prioritize specific interventions when resources are limited (Sallis, Bauman, and Pratt 1998).

IMPLICATIONS FOR POLICY AND PRACTICE

There is growing recognition that although this field is in its early stage of development, there is sufficient evidence to warrant interventions designed to increase the walkability of new and existing suburbs (Butland et al. 2007; Transportation Research Board 2005). Low-density, car-dependent, suburban sprawl is detrimental to health and the environment, and incorporating features that create livable, pedestrian-friendly communities is now required. Increasing the density of future suburban development and ensuring access to transit is critical. Moving from suburban sprawl to higher density living will require education of the general public, as well as a comprehensive advocacy campaign aimed at persuading the public, government, and the private sector of the urgent need to change the way cities are built in the future.

Finally, partnerships are needed between physical activity and health researchers and architects, urban and transport planning academics, policy makers, and practitioners (Bull, Giles-Corti, and Wood 2010). Changes to the built environment need to be informed by evidence, and any changes evaluated. Importantly, these partnerships will also ensure that physical activity researchers ask policy-relevant questions that have the potential to be translated into policy and practice.

STUDY QUESTIONS

1. Describe the important features of the built environment for walking.
2. Illustrate how you would measure the built environment for walking. What are the advantages and disadvantages of using each method listed?
3. Compare and contrast the features of the built environment that supports walking from those that promote other physical activity behaviors, such as cycling.
4. Identify built environment features in the workplace, school, and home settings that might influence physical activity behavior.
5. Think about the area in which you live, and describe how could you retrofit the neighborhood to encourage more walking.
6. Design a natural experiment to assess the impact of a new rail line on residents' walking. Consider the components of study design, sample population, measures of the built environment, and how you would evaluate the data for your experiment.

REFERENCES

Bassett, D. R., J. Pucher, R. Buehler et al. 2008. Walking, cycling and obesity rates in Europe, North America and Australia. *J. Phys. Act. Health* 5: 795–814.
Broomhall, M., B. Giles-Corti, and A. Lange. 2004. Quality of Public Open Space Tool (POST). Perth, Western Australia: School of Population Health, University of Western Australia. http://www.sph.uwa.edu.au/research/cbeh/projects/post (accessed July 18, 2011).
Brownson, R. C., C. M. Hoehner, K. Day et al. 2009. Measuring the built environment for physical activity: State of the science. *Am. J. Prev. Med.* 36: S99–S123.
Bull, F., B. Giles-Corti, and L. Wood. 2010. Active Landscapes: the methodological challenges in developing the evidence on urban environments and physical activity. In *Innovative Approaches to Researching Landscape and Health*, ed. C. Ward Thompson, P. Aspinall, and S. Bell. New York: Routledge.
Butland, B., S. Jebb, P. Kopelman et al. 2007. Foresight Tackling obesities: Future Choices— Project Report. Government Office for Science. http://www.bis.gov.uk/foresight/our-work/projects/current-projects/tackling-obesities/reports-and-publications (accessed September 30, 2010).
Chin, G. K. W., K. P. Van Niel, B. Giles-Corti et al. 2008. Accessibility and connectivity in physical activity studies: The impact of missing pedestrian data. *Prev. Med.* 46: 41–45.
Churchman, A. 1999. Disentangling the concept of density. *J. Plann. Lit.* 13: 389–411.
Crowe, T. 1991. *Crime Prevention Through Environmental Design*. Newton, MA: Butterworth-Heinemann.

Davison, K. K., and C. T. Lawson. 2006. Do attributes in the physical environment influence children's physical activity? A review of the literature. *Int. J. Behav. Nutr. Phys. Act.* 3: 19–36.

Dehar, M., S. Casswell, and P. Duignan. 1993. Formative and Process evaluation of health promotion and disease prevention programs. *Eval. Rev.* 17: 204–220.

Dill, J. 2004. Measuring Network Connectivity for Bicycling and Walking. TRB Annual Meeting. http://www.enhancements.org/download/trb/trb2004/TRB2004-001550.pdf (accessed September 30, 2010).

Duany, A., E. Plater-Zyberk, and J. Speck. 2000. *Suburban Nation: The Rise of Sprawl and the Decline of the American Dream.* New York: North Point Press.

Falconer, R., and B. Giles-Corti. 2008. Smart Development: Designing the built environment for improved access and health outcomes. In *Transitions: Pathways Towards Sustainable Urban Development in Australia,* ed. P. W. Newman. Collingwood, Victoria: CSIRO.

Farr, D. 2008. *Sustainable Urbanism: Urban Design with Nature.* Hoboken, NJ: John Wiley and Sons.

Forsyth, A., E. D'Sousa, J. Koepp et al. 2007. Twin Cities Walking Study Environment and Physical Activity: GIS protocols. University of Minnesota and Cornell. http://www.designforhealth.net/resources/gis_protocols.html (accessed September 30, 2010).

Foster, S., and B. Giles-Corti. 2008. The built environment, neighborhood crime and constrained physical activity: An exploration of inconsistent findings. *Prev. Med.* 47: 241–251.

Frank, L. D., M. A. Andresen, and T. L. Schmid. 2004. Obesity relationships with community design, physical activity and time spent in cars. *Am. J. Prev. Med.* 27: 87–96.

Frank, L. D., P. O. Engelke, and T. L. Schmid. 2003. *Health and Community Design: The Impact of the Built Environment on Physical Activity.* Washington, DC: Island Press.

Frank, L. D., J. F. Sallis, B. E. Saelens et al. 2010. The development of a walkability index: Application to the Neighborhood Quality of Life Study. *Br. J. Sports Med.* 44: 924–933.

Frumkin, H., L. Frank, and R. Jackson. 2004. *Urban Sprawl and Public Health: Designing, Planning and Building for Healthy Communities.* Washington, DC: Island Press.

Giles-Corti, B., M. H. Broomhall, M. Knuiman et al. 2005. Increasing walking: How important is distance to, attractiveness, and size of public open space? *Am. J. Prev. Med.* 28: 169–176.

Giles-Corti, B., M. Knuiman, T. J. Pikora et al. 2007. Can the impact on health of a government policy designed to create more liveable neighbourhoods be evaluated? An overview of the RESIDential Environment Project. *NSW Public Health Bull.* 18: 238–242.

Giles-Corti, B., S. Foster, T. Shilton et al. 2010a. The co-benefits for health of investing in active transportation. *NSW Public Health Bull.* 21: 122–127.

Giles-Corti, B., J. Robertson-Wilson, L. Wood et al. 2010b. The role of the changing built environment in shaping our shape. In *Geographies of Obesity: Environmental Underpinnings of the Obesity Epidemic,* ed. J. Pearce and K. Witten. Farnham: Ashgate Publishing Limited.

Heath, G. W., R. C. Brownson, J. Kruger et al. 2006. The effectiveness of urban design and land use and transport policies and practices to increase physical activity: A systematic review. *J. Phys. Act. Health* 3: S55–S76.

Khattak, A. J., and D. A. Rodriguez. 2005. Travel behaviour in neo-traditional neighborhood development: A case study in USA. *Trans. Res. Part A Policy Pract.* 39: 481–500.

Lee, C., and A. V. Moudon. 2004. Physical activity and environment research in the health field: Implications for urban and transportation planning practice and research. *J. Plann. Lit.* 19: 147–181.

MacDonald, J. M., R. J. Stokes, D. A. Cohen et al. 2010. The effect of light rail transit on body mass index and physical activity. *Am. J. Prev. Med.* 39: 105–112.

McCormack, G., B. Giles-Corti, A. Lange et al. 2004. An update of recent evidence of the relationship between objective and self-report measures of the physical environment and physical activity behaviours. *J. Sci. Med. Sport* 7: 81–92.

McLeroy, K. R., D. Bibeau, A. Steckler et al. 1988. An ecological perspective on health promotion programs. *Health Educ. Behav.* 15: 351–377.

Ogilvie, D., F. C. L. Bull, J. Powell et al. 2011. An applied ecological framework for evaluating infrastructure to promote walking and cycling: the iConnect study. *Am. J. Public Health* (Published online ahead of print January 13, 2011: e1–e9. doi:10.2105/AJPH.2010.198002).

Owen, N., N. Humpel, E. Leslie et al. 2004. Understanding environmental influences on walking: Review and research agenda. *Am. J. Prev. Med.* 27: 67–76.

Panter, J. R., A. P. Jones, and E. M. F. van Sluijs. 2008. Environmental determinants of active travel in youth: A review and framework for future research. *Int. J. Behav. Nutr. Phys. Act.* 5: 34–48.

Pikora, T. J., F. C. L. Bull, K. Jamrozik et al. 2002. Developing a reliable audit instrument to measure the physical environment for physical activity. *Am. J. Prev. Med.* 23: 187–194.

Pikora, T. J., B. Giles-Corti, M. W. Knuiman et al. 2006. Neighborhood environmental factors correlated with walking near home: Using SPACES. *Med. Sci. Sports Exerc.* 38: 708–714.

Rodriguez, D. A., A. J. Khattak, and K. R. Evenson. 2006. Can new urbanism encourage physical activity? Comparing a new urbanist neighborhood with conventional suburbs. *J. Am. Plann. Assoc.* 72: 43–54.

Saelens, B. E., and S. L. Handy. 2008. Built environment correlates of walking: A review. *Med. Sci. Sports Exerc.* 40: S550–S556.

Saelens, B. E., and C. Papadopoulos. 2008. The importance of the built environment in older adults' physical activity: A review of the literature. *Wash. State J. Public Health Pract.* 1: 13–21.

Saelens, B. E., J. F. Sallis, J. B. Black et al. 2003. Neighborhood-based differences in physical activity: An environmental scale evaluation. *Am. J. Public Health* 93: 1552–1558.

Saelens, B. E., J. F. Sallis, and L. D. Frank. 2003. Environmental correlates of walking and cycling: Findings from the transportation, urban design and planning literatures. *Ann. Behav. Med.* 25: 80–91.

Sallis, J. F., A. Bauman, and M. Pratt. 1998. Environmental and policy interventions to promote physical activity. *Am. J. Prev. Med.* 15: 379–397.

Sallis, J. F., M. Story, and D. Lou. 2009. Study designs and analytic strategies for environmental and policy research on obesity, physical activity, and diet. *Am. J. Prev. Med.* 36: S72–S77.

Schilling, J., and L. S. Linton. 2005. The public health roots of zoning: In search of active living's legal genealogy. *Am. J. Prev. Med.* 28: 96–104.

Shigematsu, R., J. F. Sallis, T. L. Conway et al. 2009. Age differences in the relation of perceived neighborhood environment to walking. *Med. Sci. Sports Exerc.* 41: 314–321.

Sugiyama, T., J. Salmon, D. W. Dunstan et al. 2007. Neighborhood walkability and TV viewing time among Australian adults. *Am. J. Prev. Med.* 33: 444–449.

Transportation Research Board. 2005. Does the Built Environment Influence Physical Activity? Examining the Evidence. Transportation Research Board Institute of Medicine. http://onlinepubs.trb.org/onlinepubs/sr/sr282.pdf (accessed September 30, 2010).

U.S. Department of Health and Human Services. 1996. Physical activity and Health: A Report of The Surgeon General. Centre for Disease Control and Prevention. http://wonder.cdc.gov/wonder/prevguid/m0042984/m0042984.asp (accessed September 30, 2010).

Western Australian Planning Commission. 2000. Liveable Neighbourhoods: A Western Australian Government Sustainable Cities Initiative (2). Western Australian Planning Commission. http://www.planning.wa.gov.au/Publications/LN_ed2.pdf?id=597 (accessed September 30, 2010).

World Health Organization. 2004. Global Strategy on Diet, Physical Activity and Health. http://www.who.int/dietphysicalactivity/strategy/eb11344/en/index.html (accessed September 30, 2010).

16 Physical Activity Promotion in Worksites

Joan Dorn and Cassandra Hoebbel

CONTENTS

INTRODUCTION

It is somewhat of a paradox that a textbook on Physical Activity and Public Health Practice includes a chapter on Physical Activity Promotion in Worksites. Why? Because many of the first studies that gave us clues to the beneficial health effects of physical activity on chronic diseases such as heart disease and cancer came from worksite cohorts. For example, it was the early work of Morris in workers of the

London Transport System that initially demonstrated the potential protective effects of physical activity on heart disease risk. Morris showed that physically active conductors of the double-decker buses had fewer incident heart attacks and sudden deaths than their sedentary colleagues who drove the buses (Morris et al. 1953). A similar beneficial effect of a physically active job on heart disease was found by Morris in studies comparing men in different job grades in the London postal service (Morris et al. 1953). In the United States, Taylor et al. (1962) and Paffenbarger et al. (1970) studied the impact of occupational activities on fatal heart disease among men who worked for the railroad and the San Francisco docks, respectively. Their findings consistently supported a lower risk of heart disease death among physically active workers compared to their sedentary counterparts.

Occupational studies have also given us an indication that active jobs may offer protection against some forms of cancer. For example, two of the first studies of physical activity and colon cancer risk were performed in occupational cohorts. Garabrant et al. (1984) showed that men with sedentary jobs were more than 1.5 times more likely to develop colon cancer compared to men in highly active jobs, and Vena et al. (1985) demonstrated that the lifetime amount and percentage of time at work in sedentary or light activities increased colon cancer risk. A Finnish study in the early 1990s compared women physical education teachers to language teachers, and evidence suggested there may be beneficial effects of increased physical activity on breast cancer risk (Vihko et al. 1992).

With increased mechanization and the technological advances in today's society, many occupationally active jobs have been eliminated. In other cases, the levels of physical activity are light, or completely sedentary. When early researchers saw this trend coming, they focused their work on leisure time activity and found similar health benefits with increasing amounts of activity (Paffenbarger, Wing, and Hyde 1978; Morris et al. 1980). Unfortunately, our current fast-paced lifestyle does not seem to include time to support daily physical activity, as evidenced by the latest estimates that 49% of Americans do not meet current national physical activity recommendations (Centers for Disease Control and Prevention 2009). Consequently, we are back to trying to incorporate opportunities to increase physical activity into the workday.

The objective of this chapter is to provide an overview of the role of the modern worksite in a public health approach to increasing the population's physical activity. The rationale for the worksite as a suitable venue for physical activity promotion is provided, along with an overview of selected tested interventions. The limitations of existing research are presented, and the chapter concludes with an example of a community-based worksite health promotion project. Information provided is restricted to studies that include physical activity, exercise, and/or fitness as the outcome. A large literature exists regarding the effectiveness of physical activity alone or as part of a comprehensive worksite health promotion program on improving health outcomes, productivity, and cost-containment but is beyond the scope of this chapter.

WHY THE WORKPLACE? WHAT IS THE RATIONALE?

The latest estimates show that approximately 140 million Americans are employed (Bureau of Labor Statistics 2010). The working population includes men and women across a wide range of age, race and ethnicity, level of education, and health risks. The typical employee spends a major portion of his/her waking hours at work. This arrangement leaves little time for structured physical activity or exercise during leisure time, while at the same time creates convenient opportunities for worksite-based intervention. Therefore, the public health implications of successful worksite interventions aimed at increasing physical activity are great, since they have the potential to reach a large, diverse segment of the population.

The worksite is its own community lending itself to a broad multilevel approach, wherein interventions can be aimed at the individual employee, groups of workers (i.e., specific unit or department), the organizational structure, and the physical workplace environment. It offers a physical and social infrastructure conducive to delivering health messages, programs, policies, and support to improve the overall health and physical activity of all employees, not just a motivated few. By providing health promotion opportunities for the workforce as a whole (population approach) as well as interventions targeting those already with risk factors or established chronic disease (high-risk), worksite programs have the capacity to impact employees across the entire spectrum of disease prevention. In other words, the worksite offers the perfect opportunity to combine individual strategies with more global strategies that include company-level interventions that make it easier for all workers to make healthy lifestyle choices. Since workers potentially stay with a job or worksite for several years, worksite initiatives could also provide opportunities for long-term, multicomponent interventions.

Another important reason the worksite is a logical venue for physical activity intervention is the potential for financial benefits to the employer. Increased physical activity as part of a comprehensive multicomponent health promotion program has the potential to improve health and reduce health risks of workers, while reducing absenteeism, improving productivity, and helping to contain stifling increases in healthcare costs (Goetzel and Ozminkowski 2008).

Along with the benefits, there are also challenges to implementing worksite physical activity promotion efforts. These include time constraints, lack of facilities, and willingness (readiness) of employees to engage in activity and utilize available resources. Despite potential financial benefits to the employer, corporate support, a vital component for success (Goetzel et al. 2007), is often insufficient or lacking altogether (Dishman et al. 1998).

The importance of worksite health promotion in general, and physical activity in particular, is recognized by many public health agencies, professional organizations, associations and societies. Examples of these are displayed in Table 16.1.

EARLY WORKSITE PHYSICAL ACTIVITY PROGRAMS

The earliest worksite interventions focused on exercise programming (Shephard 1996). The individual employee was targeted and improved fitness was the goal. This made sense at the time, because the national goal as described by the Surgeon General was to increase the number of American adults who regularly exercised vigorously (U.S. Public Health Service 1980). One of the first studies to take a "public health" approach to increasing employee exercise was published in the *Journal of the*

TABLE 16.1
Public Health Recognition of the Worksite as an Important Venue for Physical Activity Promotion

Public Health Entity	Worksite Connection
Healthy People 2010 (U.S. Department of Health and Human Services 2000)	Objective 7–5: "At least three-fourths of U.S. employers in worksites with 50 or more employees will offer a comprehensive health promotion program." Objective 7–6: "At least 88% of U.S. employees will be participating in employee sponsored health promotion activities."
Physical Activity and Health: A Report of the Surgeon General (U.S. Department of Health and Human Services 1996)	Pinpoints the worksite as an important venue for physical activity promotion
International Association for Worksite Health Promotion (IAWHP), an affiliate of the American College of Sports Medicine (ACSM)	Formed in 2008, IAWHP evolved from the American Association of Fitness Directors in Business and Industry and now provides state of the art information, resources, support and opportunities for personal and professional development as well as networking for worksite health promotion practitioners worldwide. The Association provides a website (www.acsm-IAWHP.org), and a quarterly publication, both geared specifically to the worksite health promotion practitioner
American Heart Association Policy Statement (Carnethon et al. 2009)	Endorses wellness programs at the worksite as a viable strategy for prevention of cardiovascular disease risk factors
National Institute of Occupational Safety and Health	Includes physical activity as an important component of its Worklife Initiative
National Plan to Increase Physical Activity in the U.S. (Pate 2009)	Lists business and industry together as one of eight societal factors to be included in the plan
The Surgeon General's Vision for a Healthy and Fit Nation (U.S. Department of Health and Human Services 2010)	Includes the worksite as an important setting to combat the obesity epidemic the nation is facing
The Patient Protection and Affordable Care Act (H.R. 3590) passed into law on March 23, 2010	Provides for technical assistance for employer-based wellness programs, in addition to an initiative entitled the National Worksite Health Policies and Programs Study designed to be a national evaluation of workplace health promotion and chronic disease programs and policies

American Medical Association in 1986 by Blair and colleagues. The study included more than 4000 employees at seven Johnson and Johnson companies in the United States. Employees from four of the companies received both an annual health screening and a comprehensive health promotion program. Employees from the remaining three companies received only an annual health screening. The health screening included a lifestyle questionnaire, biometric testing, and a follow-up educational session with a nurse. The health promotion program targeted exercise, as well as other important health factors such as diet, weight control, cigarette smoking, and stress, in an attempt to create an environment that supported good health. A multilayer approach aimed at increasing employee exercise included a 3-hour educational session, exercise classes at work or in the community, multimedia attempts to educate and encourage participation, and the provision of facilities for exercise on or near the worksite. Results were encouraging and showed participation in self-reported vigorous physical activity increased and measured physical fitness improved among employees in both groups. The increases were noticeably larger in the companies that offered the health promotion program in addition to the health screening, were seen in men and women with varying demographic characteristics (including age, education, socioeconomic status, job classification, race), and persisted over 2 years.

Although Blair et al.'s study demonstrated favorable results in terms of increased vigorous activity and fitness, findings reported in a review of 52 studies by Shephard (1996) and 26 studies included in a meta-analysis by Dishman and colleagues (1998) were not as encouraging. Shephard concluded that although there was some evidence worksite exercise programs can improve individual employee fitness, low participation rates in these programs limit the public health impact. Dishman et al. (1998) concluded that the existing evidence did not support significant improvements in activity levels or fitness. Both reports highlighted a number of important limitations with regard to study designs and implementation and called for more research using better scientific methods.

In 1995, new evidence-based guidelines for public health were released recommending that adults accumulate 30 minutes of at least moderate intensity level activity on most days of the week (Pate et al. 1995). With these guidelines came a shift in emphasis from vigorous exercise for fitness to physical activity for health. The new recommendations had important implications for worksite physical activity promotion, allowing interventions to expand beyond structured exercise-focused classes and programs to include activities that target incorporation of physical activity throughout the day.

In addition to the health benefits of "accumulating" regular moderate physical activity, this focus has practical benefits as well. For one, interventions can be tailored to meet the specific needs of a diverse working population. Second, the approach is amenable to a variety of multilevel interventions targeting the entire workforce, not just the interested few. Third, it offers flexibility in implementation. And finally, since it can be worked into the daily routine and does not require a change of clothes or elaborate facilities, it is a more feasible approach, especially for smaller companies with limited facilities and resources.

CONTEMPORARY WORKSITE PHYSICAL ACTIVITY INTERVENTIONS

There is no single prescription for increasing physical activity at the worksite. What works best varies from worksite to worksite, and is dependent on specific workforce needs and available resources. The diversity of the workers in terms of age, gender, race, motivational readiness, health status, and occupation must be taken into consideration. So, too, must the nature of the worksite in terms of business or industry type, size, number of locations, facilities and policies, available staff and other resources, and the degree to which upper management is committed to the effort. Substantial formative research and preparation is required to tailor any health promotion program to the needs of specific workplaces.

THEORETICAL ORIENTATION

To increase the likelihood of success, interventions aimed at changing a health behavior such as physical activity should be based on health behavior theory (Rimer and Glanz 2005). Models of health behavior emerge as theorists attempt to explain and predict behavior. Considering its complexities, it seems unlikely that any single theory could address the multiple factors that influence human behavior. However, most models of health behavior include the following key concepts (Rimer and Glanz 2005):

1. What people know and think affects how they act.
2. Knowledge is necessary for, but not sufficient, to produce most behavior changes.
3. Perceptions, motivations, skills, and the social environment are key influences on behavior.

Without going into detail regarding the many models of health behavior and health behavior change, the most widely recognized models for use in worksite physical activity programs deserve some mention and include the Stages of Change (Transtheoretical) Model and the Social Ecological Model of Health Behavior.

The Stages of Change (Transtheoretical) Model (Prochaska and DiClemente 1983) is among the most widely used model of individual health behavior change and has been applied to all major health behaviors, including physical activity. The model assumes that any attempt at behavior change will be unsuccessful if attempted when the individual is not "ready" to change. As outlined in Table 16.2, the five "stages" progress from what is called "precontemplation" to "maintenance." Individuals may move back and forth through the stages, with the ultimate goal of reaching the maintenance stage. Individuals' "stage of readiness" can be determined with varying degrees of formality and should be considered before the implementation of programs aimed at behavior change. The idea is that if individuals are not ready to change their behavior, any attempt to do so would be premature and, therefore, unlikely to succeed. In such cases, interventions should be designed to target the individual's particular stage of change with the aim of assisting the individual's progression through the stages.

In addition to individual factors addressed in the Stages of Change Model, characteristics of the environment and the interaction between the individual and his or her environment must be considered. The social ecological model of health behavior takes a broad perspective and considers the individual within the context of his or her social and physical environment (e.g., McLeroy et al. 1988). The model uses a multilevel approach to target individual-, interpersonal-, environmental-, and community-level factors. A social ecological approach could be particularly useful for worksite

TABLE 16.2

Stages of Change Model Applied to Increasing Physical Activity

Stage	Definition	Strategies
Precontemplation	Individual has no intention of increasing physical activity within the next 6 months	Increase awareness by personalizing information about the risks of physical inactivity and the benefits of increasing physical activity
Contemplation	Individual intends to increase physical activity in the next 6 months	Encourage and motivate individual to make specific plans to increase physical activity
Preparation	Individual intends to increase physical activity within the next 30 days and has taken some steps in that direction	Assist individual with setting and implementing concrete, achievable goals to increase physical activity
Action	Has increased and maintained physical activity level for less than 6 months	Provide feedback, social support, and positive reinforcement to individual
Maintenance	Has maintained an increase in physical activity for more than 6 months	Continue encouragement with reminders, feedback, positive reinforcement, and assistance in dealing with set-backs

interventions targeting physical activity because the worksite can provide social support and the physical setting conducive to increasing physical activity, covering all levels of the model. That is, worksite application of the model recognizes that there are individuals within groups inside a larger worksite community that falls within a larger geographic community.

BASELINE ASSESSMENTS

Before starting any intervention, a baseline assessment of the workforce and worksite should be conducted to determine the needs and readiness of a particular organization and its employees. Health Risk Appraisals (HRAs) are commonly used to assess the workforce by surveying individual worker health status and risk factors, personal and family health history, and lifestyle habits such as physical activity. HRA assessment of physical activity is typically limited to one or two global questions about physical activity participation, aiming to characterize workers as meeting or not meeting a given threshold of activity (e.g., current public health guidelines). Tailored individual feedback is also part of the HRA process, providing information back to the individual worker. The feedback often comes in the form of a report that highlights strengths ("what you're doing well") and areas that could be improved ("what you could do better") as well as other information on major health risk factors and lifestyle behaviors. Employers can use group results as a means to identify the risks most prevalent among their workforce and to aid in program planning. Many HRAs also include select questions designed to capture an individual's willingness and/or readiness to make changes to improve health (e.g., "In the next six months, are you planning to make any changes to increase physical activity?"). Anonymous responses to questions like these can be used to help employers and program planners determine whether the workforce is ready for programming, and if so, which programs would most likely be effective.

There are a number of commercially available HRAs that vary in mode of delivery and feedback method. HRAs can be administered by paper and pencil, online, or by phone with relatively little expense and often vary in the content and detail of questions included. Technological advances have made it possible for some employers to offer interactive Web-based HRA packages designed to evaluate each individual and provide personalized action plans. Depending on available resources, biometric measurements may be obtained to supplement the assessment. These typically include measurement of height and weight, blood pressure, lipid profiles, and fasting glucose, but more objective measures of physical activity and/or physical fitness should also be given considerable consideration.

With the increasing recognition of the significance of the worksite environment in promoting healthy behaviors, a number of instruments to assess the workplace environment have also emerged. Among the first to be developed was the "Heart Check," a 226-item interview and observational survey that focuses on workplace support for heart health promotion (Golaszewski and Fisher 2002). One of the seven subscales is devoted exclusively to physical activity and includes items probing the availability and characteristics of on-site and off-site facilities, fitness testing and programs, as well as subsidies, policies, incentives, and educational materials in place to promote and support physical activity for the entire workforce.

Other established worksite environmental assessment tools include the Checklist of Health Promotion Environments at Worksites (CHEW) (Oldenburg et al. 2002) and the Environmental Assessment Tool (EAT) (DeJoy et al. 2008), both of which include components devoted to physical activity. CHEW uses direct observation to assess the worksite in terms of its physical characteristics and features of the information environment. A third component of CHEW can be used to assess the surrounding neighborhood for facilities within view of the workplace that promote physical activity, such as local gyms or other recreational facilities. EAT builds on the strengths of Heart Check and CHEW, and uses both self-assessment techniques and direct observation to evaluate both the physical and social environment in terms of their supportiveness of good health.

An assessment tool devoted specifically to worksite physical activity support is the Workplace Physical Activity Assessment Tool (WPAAT) (Plotnikoff et al. 2005). The WPAAT was developed by a panel of experts to assist the province of Alberta, Canada, in meeting its objective to promote physical activity at the workplace. The WPAAT includes 45 items divided into three sections—preparation, program components, and procedures—and is designed to assess the supportiveness of worksite physical activity at the individual, social, organizational, community, and policy levels, and the interactions among them.

CONTEMPORARY WORKSITE INTERVENTIONS: STRATEGIES

A number of different strategies have been used in an attempt to help workers meet the latest physical activity guidelines and have been well documented (Proper et al.

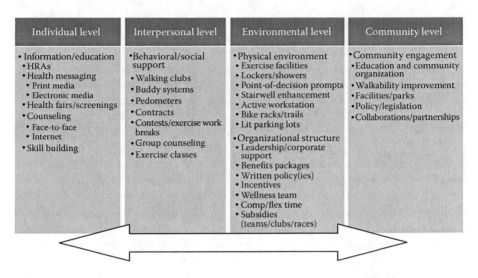

Individual level	Interpersonal level	Environmental level	Community level

• Information/education
• HRAs
• Health messaging
  • Print media
  • Electronic media
• Health fairs/screenings
• Counseling
  • Face-to-face
  • Internet
• Skill building
	•Behavioral/social support
	  • Walking clubs
	  • Buddy systems
	  • Pedometers
	• Contracts
	• Contests/exercise work breaks
	• Group counseling
	• Exercise classes
		• Physical environment
		  • Exercise facilities
		  • Lockers/showers
		  • Point-of-decision prompts
		  • Stairwell enhancement
		  • Active workstation
		  • Bike racks/trails
		  • Lit parking lots
		•Organizational structure
		  • Leadership/corporate support
		  • Benefits packages
		  • Written policy(ies)
		  • Incentives
		  • Wellness team
		  • Comp/flex time
		  • Subsidies
		    (teams/clubs/races)
			•Community engagement
			•Education and community organization
			•Walkability improvement
			•Facilities/parks
			•Policy/legislation
			•Collaborations/partnerships

FIGURE 16.1   Various levels of approach to increasing physical activity in the workplace.

2003a; Marshall 2004; Engbers et al. 2005; Conn et al. 2009; Pronk 2009). Strategies have included single and multilevel approaches and have targeted physical activity alone, or in combination with a number of other lifestyle factors including diet and tobacco use. Consistent with the social ecological approach discussed earlier in this chapter, Figure 16.1 provides an illustration of the potential levels of intervention and some specific examples of worksite interventions aimed at increasing physical activity. The arrow is intended to indicate that the various approaches are not mutually exclusive. There is often overlap and interdependence, and extensive research has highlighted the role of multicomponent interventions in successfully increasing physical activity (Kahn et al. 2002).

The specific interventions are aimed at modifying factors present within the individual, the social environment, and the physical environment in ways that facilitate and encourage physical activity. Let us take a look at a few of these.

INDIVIDUAL-LEVEL APPROACHES

The most fundamental and traditional approaches to health promotion target behavior at the individual level. Even as the field of health promotion moves toward an emphasis on multilevel interventions, individual-level interventions remain a critical element in worksite health promotion. Individual-level approaches are intended to provide education to influence individual characteristics such as knowledge and skills, as well as attitudes and beliefs.

Information and Education

Acquisition of knowledge is a necessary first step in any successful behavior change effort. The goals of educational programs and informational approaches targeting physical activity are to inform the workforce about the health benefits of an active lifestyle, increase motivation, provide the knowledge and skills to safely engage in activity, and create awareness of programs, facilities, and opportunities for physical activity. The aims of such educational programs are to facilitate a change in attitudes and/or beliefs to support the adoption and maintenance of an active lifestyle over time, while addressing barriers to physical activity and methods for overcoming them. Essentially, the hope is to encourage individuals to think differently about being physically active and to build the skills necessary for changing behaviors related to physical activity. Examples of educational programs aimed at individuals include personalized feedback from HRAs, company newsletters, posters, payroll stuffers, and e-mail messaging specific to physical activity and hands-on instruction on conditioning, intensity, proper warm-up, and other safety precautions.

Health Risk Appraisals

In addition to providing important health information and valuable feedback to employees and employers, the effectiveness of HRAs as a specific worksite intervention has recently been reviewed by the Task Force on Community Preventive Services (Soler et al. 2010). In this comprehensive review, the authors compared the use of HRAs with feedback alone to the use of HRAs with feedback as one component of a more global program that included educational sessions (with or without other interventions). Physical activity, which was assessed a variety of ways, was included as an outcome of interest across 14 studies that tested the use of HRAs with feedback alone. Overall, the findings were mixed and any favorable effects of HRAs with feedback alone were small. A number of important limitations to these studies, including frequent lack of a true comparison group and differing methods of assessing physical activity, left the authors to conclude that there was not sufficient evidence to recommend the use of HRAs with feedback alone as an effective physical activity intervention.

In contrast, the task force's findings suggested there was sufficient evidence that the use of HRAs with feedback could be effective in increasing physical activity when followed up with formal health education (with or without additional interventions). Overall, the task force concluded that HRAs with feedback have utility as an introductory intervention to comprehensive worksite wellness programs that also include formal health education sessions. The task force's findings provide further support for the use of education as an important component of effective individual-level physical activity promotion.

Health Messaging: Electronic and Print Materials

One way to educate and inform large groups of people is through the use of electronic and printed materials. The use of the Internet or e-mail to deliver health promotion information offers an opportunity to reach a large segment of the working population at little cost. It can reach those who are not interested in or unable to participate in group classes or counseling sessions, and its reach could extend to workers' families and friends. This form of communication provides information and feedback at a time convenient to the recipient and is becoming a popular way to receive health information (Plotnikoff et al. 2010). However, this method of communicating health information does have limitations, particularly when aimed at a large and diverse group. Whether electronic or printed, health messaging should, when possible, be tailored specifically to the individual's needs, interests, and readiness. Research has shown that generic health messaging targeting large groups is significantly less effective in increasing short-term physical activity than messaging tailored to specific individuals' needs and readiness (Owen 1987; Marcus et al. 1998), leading researchers to conclude that one tailored message is better than multiple standard messages.

Napolitano et al. (2003) used a Web-based physical activity intervention to target physical activity in sedentary workers recruited from multiple healthcare facilities in the United States. The intervention included a physical activity-promoting website using previously tested print materials (Marcus et al. 1998) along with 12 weekly e-mail tip sheets. The intervention provided scientific physical activity information and targeted workers' motivational readiness for physical activity. After 1 month, short-term favorable changes in readiness, participation in moderate physical activity, and walking were observed in the workers who were randomly assigned to the intervention compared to workers who did not receive the intervention. In their review of several mediated approaches for increasing physical activity (i.e., mass media, print, telephone, and website), Marshall, Owen, and Bauman (2004) suggested that no individual medium to increase physical activity should be used in isolation and that all approaches are potentially effective when used with one another or as an adjunct to wider intervention strategies aimed at increasing physical activity.

Although most of the evidence in the literature to date indicates health messaging to be effective for short-term change in physical activity, one recent study was able to demonstrate the maintenance of such changes (Plotnikoff et al. 2010). The results of this study were encouraging in that most of the positive effects in the intervention group were maintained at 6-month follow-up, and some effects actually increased over time. The intervention group received 12 weekly e-mail messages regarding physical activity, whereas the comparison group received the same information in one bulk e-mail in the 12th week. Interestingly, similar positive effects were seen in the group of participants who received the information in bulk. The results are encouraging in that small positive changes were seen in all who received the information, but questions remain as to the most effective frequency of messages.

One-on-One Counseling

Essential to the success of any behavior-change effort is for individuals to set achievable goals and to track progress over time. One-on-one counseling is one method that can be used to assist in this regard and has been found to be effective in increasing physical activity (Centers for Disease Control and Prevention 2010). Personal health counselors, also known as "health coaches," can help individuals set realistic goals to increase physical activity and can develop personalized action plans, while considering situations and barriers unique to the individual. Counselors and coaches can also serve as conduits of information, providing access or links to valuable tools and resources.

Such individualized attention can be provided face to face or by phone, and has traditionally been used in the practice of clinical medicine. This approach is gaining popularity with researchers, health plans, and practitioners interested in its effectiveness in increasing physical activity across a variety of settings.

One promising strategy shown to be effective in primary care settings is the Patient-Centered Assessment and Counseling Exercise (PACE) program (Calfas et al. 1996). This is a brief, structured program that healthcare providers can use during office visits to identify patients in terms of their current levels of physical activity and/or their "readiness" to increase physical activity. Based on the results of a brief assessment, the healthcare provider and the patient work together to develop a plan for increasing physical activity utilizing one of three counseling protocols tailored to the patient's assessment results.

The brevity of the assessment and tailored counseling protocols make this program attractive to employers who have limited time and resources to devote to one-on-one health counseling for employees. Proper et al. (2003a) adapted the PACE protocol to the worksite with mixed results. Although no effects were found for the proportion of participants meeting the public health recommendation for moderate physical activity, positive effects were found on select indicators of physical activity, such as total energy expenditure, physical activity during sports, and cardiorespiratory fitness.

Unfortunately, individualized face-to-face counseling is often not feasible or even desirable for every member of the workforce. More recent technological developments, such as customized digital health coaching/counseling, offer innovative approaches to individualized interventions that offer many of the same benefits as human counselors with more convenience and greater confidentiality.

Interpersonal Level Approaches

As has become apparent, most worksite health promotion programs do not rely exclusively on individual-level interventions. Interpersonal level approaches aim to provide opportunities for coworker and supervisory support through team-based interactive physical activities. In their review of existing research, the Task Force on Community Preventive Services reported that time spent in physical activity, knowledge of physical activity, and confidence in ability to become physically active all increased when individuals were supported by those around them (Kahn et al. 2002). Based on this evidence, the task force recommends the use of social support to promote health behaviors in community settings such as workplaces. Interventions involving coworker support are primarily designed to help change behavior within the context of the social setting (sometimes called the "culture") of the workplace. This approach relies largely on preexisting social networks wherein coworkers provide and receive support while increasing physical activity (Kahn et al. 2002). Typically, such interventions include "buddy" systems where partners plan activities of their own design and agree to be accountable to one another. Other interactive activities designed to increase awareness while building and maintaining supportive social networks could include walking clubs, challenges, and other team activities focused on changing physical activity behavior.

Group Counseling/Classes
Counseling and educational sessions on skill-building and physical activity behavior change have been used to provide information to groups of workers while offering

the opportunity for social interaction and support. Formal and informal support sessions offered in group settings, via the Internet or telephone can be used to facilitate discussion about perceptions of physical activity and barriers to participating in physical activity. This approach has been used in a variety of settings, including the workplace, and has been shown to be effective in increasing both the frequency and duration of physical activity (Kahn et al. 2002). Offering on-site regularly scheduled exercise classes accessible to all employees is another way to build social support into physical activity worksite interventions.

All of these and other activities can be incorporated into competitive team-based physical activity programs where employees can earn participation "points" that can be accumulated and exchanged for predetermined rewards. Rewards can include anything of value to the employee population from cash to paid time off and can be used to increase motivation and incentivize participation. The Centers for Disease Control and Prevention (CDC) refers employers to the President's Challenge (www.presidentschallenge.org) as an approach to encouraging and incentivizing employee participation in team-based sports challenges.

It is important to note that the options listed above are examples of approaches to worksite wellness, and the list is not exhaustive. Some of the approaches could be appropriate to any working population, whereas others should be tailored to each workforce's needs, interests, resources, and readiness.

ENVIRONMENTAL LEVEL INTERVENTIONS

When thinking about the worksite environment's influence on health in general, and physical activity in particular, it is important to consider both the physical structure and facilities, as well as the organization's policies and services available to support healthy behaviors in and around the workplace. Environmental interventions are designed to impact the entire workforce and do not require individual employees to volunteer for specific programs or activities. By decreasing barriers and making healthy choices more readily available, an environmental approach makes it easier for everyone to incorporate physical activity into their day.

Physical Environment Interventions: The Built Environment

As shown in Figure 16.1, facilities to promote physical activity and exercise at the worksite can include anything from fully staffed and equipped on-site fitness centers to the provision of showers, locker rooms, and bike racks to facilitate active commuting. The thought is that access to safe and convenient facilities makes it easier for all workers to increase their physical activity during the working day. Unfortunately, on-site facilities are often used by a small number of employees, and generally by those who are already regularly physically active (Marshall 2004; Shephard 1996). Furthermore, there is evidence that increased spending on equipment and facilities does not necessarily result in proportional increases in participation in physical activity programs among employees (Shephard 1996). Since even the best-designed interventions will not succeed in the absence of a physical environment that supports increased activity, arrangements for adequate facilities do need to be in place before other interventions are initiated. However, health promotion professionals should be aware that access to adequate facilities is necessary but not sufficient to increase employee daily physical activity levels.

Point-of-Decision Prompts

Point-of-decision prompts generally take the form of signs, posters, or banners that provide health information or motivational messages that encourage the use of stairs. As their name implies, they are typically placed in a location where the decision to be physically active or not actually takes place, such as entrances to staircases, escalators, or elevator doors. Prompts can be used alone, or accompanied by stairwell enhancements such as artwork or music. Stair use provides workers an opportunity to accumulate physical activity by adding short sessions to daily routines. Although climbing individual flights of stairs amount to small increases in energy expenditure, the intensity level is greater than riding elevators or escalators, and accumulation of activity over time can be significant. In addition, if the prompts encourage a large percentage of a given workforce to take the stairs, even small increases in individual energy expenditure could have meaningful population health benefits.

Point-of-decision prompts have been shown to be effective at increasing stair use when placed in community locations such as shopping malls (Kerr, Eves, and Carroll 2001a), commuter stations (Blamey, Mutrie, and Aitchison 1995), and airports (Coleman and Gonzalez 2001). Unfortunately, according to a review by Eves and Web (2006), evidence for the success of point-of-decision prompts in the worksite is less convincing. Among studies that have shown favorable effects on increased stair use the increases are generally small and short term (Marshall et al. 2002; Kerr et al. 2004), whereas other studies have reported no significant increases at all (Adams and White 2002).

For example, small, short-term increases in stairwell use were observed when motivational signs along with footprints directing staff and visitors to the stairs were displayed in a healthcare facility (Marshall et al. 2002). The signs and footprints were put in place twice, for 2 weeks, with a 2-week period in between when the signs were removed. During the first phase of the intervention, the overall percentage of stair users increased above preintervention levels, but only by 1%. When the signs and prints were removed stair use reverted toward the baseline level, and no increases were noted when the intervention was put in place the second time.

Point-of-Decision Prompts with Stairwell Enhancements

The impact of signs combined with environmental stairwell enhancements in worksites has also been examined (Kerr et al. 2004; Boutelle et al. 2001). In a study of more than 600 CDC employees in the United States, paint and carpeting were first used to improve stairwell appeal followed by artwork, motivational signs, and music in sequence (Kerr et al. 2004). Signs and music only were associated with significant stair use increases. Since the intervention involved multiple components added sequentially, the authors were unable to determine the specific effects of one or more of the components.

The potential benefits of adding stairwell enhancements to point-of-decision signs to increase stair use were also studied at the University of Minnesota School of Public Health (Boutelle et al. 2001). The signs alone did not result in increased stair use; however, when music and artwork were added, the daily percentage of people who used the stairs increased significantly from 11.1% at baseline to 15.5% at follow-up. Four weeks after the intervention, daily stair use declined somewhat (to 13.8%), but remained higher than baseline levels. It is noteworthy that in this study, stairwell users were more likely to exit via the stairwells than enter by them, suggesting that the intervention was more successful at encouraging stair use on the way down than on the way up. Preference for descending over climbing was also demonstrated by others (Kerr, Eves, and Carroll 2001b). Although any use of the stairs increases activity above that of an elevator or escalator ride, this finding has important implications for worksite physical activity promotion since stair climbing requires nearly three times the energy of descending (Ainsworth et al. 2000).

Explanations for the differing effects of point-of-decision prompts in public and community locations compared to worksites remain unclear. There is some evidence that as the number of floors in a workplace increases, the number of employees taking the stairs decreases (Eves and Web 2006). The floor on which one works may also influence stair use, with employees who work on lower floors more likely to use the stairs than those who work on higher floors, with approximately four flights being the limit (Kerr, Eves, and Carroll 2001b). Visibility and the location of the stairs in relation to the elevators or building entrances can also impact stair use (Nicholl 2007). In public places such as malls and airports, stairs are often located next to escalators, whereas in worksites elevators are more likely used than escalators and may be located at a considerable distance from stairwells and from the building entrances. Other potential barriers to stair use in worksites include employee dress (particularly in office buildings) and the need to carry briefcases, backpacks, or other loads. In regards to the interventions themselves, the short-term effects observed in workplaces as well as studies showing a second round of the intervention has little or no impact suggest that in the workplace, people may get accustomed to the prompts and they lose their impact. In public places, passersby are less frequently exposed to the prompts so they notice them and are perhaps more likely to heed their informative and motivational messages.

It is clear that more research is needed to explore why point-of-decision prompts have shown more consistent increases in stair use in public places than in worksites. In the meantime, encouraging stair use as a way of increasing workers' daily physical activity offers a relatively low-cost opportunity to target the entire workforce. Stairs are required in buildings with multiple floors, and even modest daily increases can add up over time. Given the number of employed persons worldwide, engaging a substantial percentage of the workforce in increased stair use would have important implications for public health.

Active Workstations

Spurred by increasing obesity trends and the fact that a large segment of the working population works at computer stations, novel approaches to increasing energy expenditure at the worksite include replacing standard office chairs with therapy balls, standing desks, and walking treadmills (Levine and Miller 2007; Beers et al. 2008). Research has shown that sitting on a therapy ball or working at a standing desk results in significantly more energy expenditure than sitting in a standard office chair (Beers et al. 2008). When asked, both men and women reported that they liked sitting on the therapy ball as much as the office chair, and more than standing. Although these office adaptations do not increase physical activity per se, they have been shown to result in passive energy expenditure (Beers et al. 2008), that over time may help combat progressive age-associated increases in body weight.

Walking workstations provide yet another alternative to increasing physical activity during the workday. Levine and Miller (2007) developed a vertical workstation that included an adjustable desk that could be used while sitting, standing, or walking on a treadmill. Research conducted at the Mayo Clinic Research Center using the vertical workstation in sedentary, obese computer-based workers showed significant increases in energy expenditure during routine computer tasks performed while walking on the treadmill when compared to doing the same tasks while seated in a typical office chair (Levine and Miller 2007). The study participants tolerated the treadmill well, selected their own speed, reported no falls or injuries, and expressed enthusiasm in continuing use of the workstation beyond the study period. The authors speculated that workers using the vertical workstation for even half of the working day could increase energy expenditure by approximately 500 kcal/day.

Further studies have demonstrated that although fine motor skills, such as computer mouse speed, may be slightly affected, reading comprehension, selective attention, and overall processing speed of worked performed at active workstations is similar to that performed at traditional workstations (Dinesh et al. 2009).

Active Commuting

Since resources vary across worksites and it is not possible for all worksites to offer on-site physical activity programming or facilities, less organized approaches to increasing physical activity throughout the workday may hold potential for affecting the overall workforce (Marshall 2004). One such approach includes promoting active commuting to work. Employees from organizations that encourage active commuting have been shown to be less likely to drive to work than those from non-encouraging work environments (Wen, Kites, and Rissel 2010). Increases in daily physical activity associated with interventions aimed at promoting active commuting can be substantial. Mutrie et al. (2002) conducted a randomized controlled trial among Finnish workers using a "readiness" tailored self-help intervention packet to promote walking and biking to work. After 6 months, among employees who did not walk to work but were thinking about it at baseline, those who received the packets reported spending an average of 125 min/week walking to work. This increase was significantly greater than the average of 61 min/week reported by similar readiness-stage controls. Among workers who were irregularly active commuters at baseline, those who received the intervention packets also increased the amount of time they walked to work more than controls (27 vs. 10 min/week). Active commuting has also been shown to be positively received by workers and can be sufficient to improve fitness (Vuori, Oja, and Paronen 1994). Therefore, promoting active commuting offers a relatively inexpensive opportunity to increase physical activity in the workforce.

In addition to encouraging the use of stairs, providing active work stations, and promoting active commuting, employers can help workers to incorporate physical activity into their daily work lives by promoting "walk and talk" meetings, active breaks, and other lifestyle activities, at the same time discouraging overuse of e-mail and telephone communication when feasible. Although many of these approaches have been less empirically tested than others, they appear to have the potential to provide low-cost options to promote physical activity for worksites with limited budgets.

Organizational Policies

In addition to the physical environment, changes in the organizational structure of the workplace environment can help to promote physical activity among workers. When it is difficult or impossible to work formal interventions directly into the workplace, policies that offer discounts or subsidies for home fitness equipment and/or local gym memberships for employees and their families should be explored.

Other written policies that allow "flex-time" for workers to engage in physical activity during their usual work shift could reduce barriers for workers with limited time. In addition to reducing some of the barriers that employees face when attempting to increase physical activity, such written policies can provide more evidence of corporate support for the health of the workforce.

Added benefits such as discounted health insurance, additional life insurance, days off, cash payments, or other bonuses or rewards can also be offered by employers to encourage physical activity within the workforce (Golaszewski and Fisher 2002).

It is always important for policy makers and program planners to know what is most valuable to workers (e.g., time, money) and understand that this might vary between and within workforces. At the same time, it is critical that incentives that reward behavior such as increased physical activity, do not undermine the individual's intrinsic motivation to engage in the activity because as the tangible rewards become less important or pertinent to the individual, the behavior is likely to decrease (Marcus et al. 2006).

Although research into the effectiveness of using incentives to increase physical activity is still evolving, early research has demonstrated some positive effects (e.g., Herman et al. 2006). One study specific to physical activity was designed to examine the effectiveness of introducing cash incentives to an existing online physical activity intervention and found that enrollment in the program increased by 300% when incentives were offered. However, it is important to note that the program attracted a greater proportion of individuals who were already at low health risk and were more likely to be physically active (Herman et al. 2006).

COMMUNITY-LEVEL APPROACHES

Although the worksite represents its own small community, it is also part of the larger community in which it resides. Community-level approaches aim to engage the worksite with the larger community to facilitate social, physical, and policy changes that support or regulate healthy actions such as physical activity. Partnerships and collaborations outside of the workplace can provide benefits for the company and its employees as well as the residents of surrounding neighborhoods. For example, subsidizing memberships to off-site gyms or recreational facilities offers workers a place for physical activity and at the same time supports local businesses. Company-sponsored "community clean up" days can go a long way toward improving walking trails, bike paths, and parks, ultimately providing not only employees but all members of the community access to desirable places to be more physically active.

Partnerships with local public health agencies, healthcare providers, health maintenance organizations, and universities may provide valuable resources, facilities, and
expertise that may be particularly helpful for small worksites with limited resources.
And finally, partnerships with political leaders and governmental agencies may help
to create policies that can support healthy lifestyles for workers, their families, and
the overall community.

WESTERN NEW YORK WELLNESS WORKS

An example of a community-based collaboration is the Western New York Wellness
Works (WNYWW) initiative. WNYWW is a unique partnership among the
University at Buffalo School of Public Health and Health Professions, diverse worksites throughout the Western New York (WNY) region, major health insurers in
WNY, and the State Department of Health. Funding that came from the state of New
York and was made possible by a local state senator. The collaboration drew on the
expertise of researchers at the university to develop a regional partnership and design
a community-based study designed to improve the health and wellness of workers
and companies in WNY.

To generate community and corporate support, identify working subcommittees,
develop partnerships, share experiences, and provide input regarding important corporate outcomes, an advisory board of community members with a wide range of
expertise was assembled. Worksites submitted a proposal describing plans for a self-
directed wellness intervention specific to their needs. The maximum funding available for any one company was $50,000, and a minimum of one-to-one matching of
funds was required to double available resources for the projects while establishing
a strong employer commitment.

Twenty-six organizations, representing 35,235 employees, submitted proposals.
Thirteen applicants representing 12,601 employees from three WNY counties were
selected for participation (Figure 16.2).

The selected companies ranged in size from 42 to 3900 employees, and one
to 100+ worksites. Industries represented included education, manufacturing,

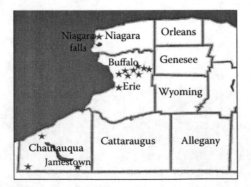

FIGURE 16.2   Location of WNYWW participating worksites.

professional services, health and human services, and automobile dealerships. The amount requested ranged from $3000 to $50,000 over 2 years. Most companies proposed a multifaceted wellness program incorporating traditional health promotion activities in conjunction with environmental improvements.

Program focus and methods of delivery were as diverse as the worksites themselves. Interventions targeting physical activity were among the most popular, but a number of other interventions such as weight management, nutrition education, stress reduction, and smoking cessation were included. Some worksites assigned a full-time in-house employee to the project, whereas others depended on third-party vendors, such as Weight Watchers® and local YMCA/YWCAs. Modes of program delivery included structured classes and seminars, face-to-face counseling, print and electronic materials, and subsidized fitness memberships. A number of different incentives were used including token gifts (e.g., T-shirts, pedometers, sporting event tickets, gift certificates) or policies such as flexible scheduling or compensation time for physical activity or participation in health promotion classes.

To standardize the evaluation of the project, all participating worksites were required to implement the same HRA (UM-HMRC) and the Heart Check (Golaszewski and Fisher 2002) environmental assessment tool at baseline and follow-up. A culture questionnaire (Allen 2002) was also administered to ascertain individual employee's perceptions of the worksite culture as it relates to physical activity and the maintenance of an overall healthy lifestyle.

At the end of the nearly 2-year intervention period, three of the original 13 organizations dropped out; two because of failure to meet study requirements and the third because the evolving automobile industry crisis pushed wellness to the back burner, unfortunately at the time when it was likely needed most. Among the 10 remaining organizations, significant improvements in the environmental health of the worksites were observed (Table 16.3). At baseline, the overall health of the companies received

TABLE 16.3
Specific Component and Overall Environmental Health of Worksites: WNYWW Project

Component	Baseline Score (%)	Follow-up Score (%)
Smoking	36.5	63.7**
Nutrition	34.7	70.8**
Physical activity	31.0	59.8**
Stress	49.2	63.2
Screening	33.8	78.7**
Administrative support	37.6	68.7***
Organizational Foundations	48.2	62.8**
Overall Environmental Health	37.6	66.3***

Note: Results are for companies that have completed both baseline and follow-up Heart Check ($n = 10$);
$**p < 0.01, ***p < 0.001$.

a score of 37.6% but improved to 66.3% (scale of 0% to 100%) at the end of the study. Scores of the physical activity component nearly doubled, indicating that the companies were successful in making environmental changes to support increased physical activity.

There was evidence that the culture of the workplaces shifted more toward health as the scores on the culture questionnaire were improved in almost every category, including getting regular exercise, maintaining a healthy weight, eating nutritious foods, and avoiding fat and sugar. In regards to cultural items pertaining to physical activity, at baseline 37.2% of employees indicated their coworkers expected each other to exercise regularly. By the end of the project, that percentage increased to 44.1%, and was significantly higher than at baseline ($p < 0.001$).

More than 2500 individual workers completed HRAs at baseline, and 1721 completed them at follow-up. From these two cross-sectional surveys, employees were more knowledgeable at follow-up about two important health risk factors: blood pressure and cholesterol. However, only a small nonsignificant increase in the percentage of employees who reported doing regular physical activity at least three times per week was observed (Table 16.4). Among employees who completed both surveys, no increase in the percentage of those who met this goal was noted at follow-up.

The results above represent totals for the entire WNYWW participating workforce and document the intervention from the overall public health perspective of such an initiative. Below are findings from a single company in the project that specifically focused on increasing employee physical activity. Led by intensive efforts of the occupational health nurse, the program included educational sessions, tailored goal-setting walking programs, sponsorship of YWCA memberships, and provision of numerous incentives including pedometers and gift certificates to purchase exercise clothing or equipment.

The results of this intense and focused effort offer optimism that it is possible for worksites to increase employee physical activity. As seen in Table 16.5, the program resulted in improvements in the worksite environment to promote physical activity, the culture was more supportive, and there was a 53% significant increase in the percentage of employees who reported being physically active three or more times a week.

The successes of the overall WNYWW initiative are many, including the establishment of a multilevel community-based partnership working together to improve

---

TABLE 16.4

Individual Employee Health Risks in WNYWW Employees at Baseline and Follow-Up

HRA Item	Baseline ($n = 2567$)	Follow-up ($n = 1721$)
Know their BP (%)	47.7%	61.8%***
Know their cholesterol (%)	35.0%	50.0%***
Physically active (3+ times/week) (%)	55.6%	57.7%

***$p < 0.001$.

TABLE 16.5

Results of a Single WNYWW Company's Multilevel Physical Activity Intervention

Physical Activity-Related Measure	Baseline (%)	Follow-up (%)
Heart Check: Environmental PA component	34	52
Culture Question:	26.2	44.4*
Coworkers expect each other to exercise regularly		
HRA: % Physically active (3+ times/week)	41.9	64.2**

$*p < 0.05, **p < 0.01.$

the health of the regional workforce. The incorporation of standardized measurements across the sites for individual and worksite health and culture is an important strength and shows that health improvements were made in the environment, culture, and employee's knowledge. The results also provide confirmation of the challenges of changing behavior and lifestyle, particularly physical activity among a large segment of the working population. These results are similar to others in the literature, and continue to indicate more intense interventions are required to see favorable changes in individual behaviors such as increasing physical activity.

SUMMARY AND CONCLUSIONS

Since the introduction of the evidence-based physical activity guidelines in 1995 and earlier reviews on the effectiveness of worksite interventions on increasing physical activity and exercise were published, a number of new studies have been conducted and are summarized in more recent reviews (Proper et al. 2003b; Marshall 2004; Engbers et al. 2005) and a meta-analysis (Conn et al. 2009). The quality and focus of the studies vary across a wide range of worksites and target populations. The overall evidence in support of worksite interventions to increase employee physical activity remains mixed, although findings from the highest quality studies have been somewhat more promising. One review that included only the most scientifically rigorous studies and a primary focus of increasing physical activity or fitness (Proper et al. 2003b) suggested that there was strong evidence to support their effectiveness in increasing employee physical activity. In contrast, however, Marshall (2004) concluded that studies conducted since the 1998 review by Dishman et al. (1998) continued to show little overall evidence that physical activity programs at the worksite were effective at improving long-term physical activity levels of the workforce. Some individual-specific successes were noted, although they tended to be in groups of volunteers with high levels of motivation. Similar to the Proper review (Proper et al. 2003b), studies whose primary focus was on increasing physical activity appeared to be more effective than those targeting multiple risk factors. In a review of three controlled trials of worksite health promotion interventions with environmental improvements, Engbers et al. (2005) described evidence of their effectiveness as inconclusive, since one study showed no changes in employee exercise with the addition of an on-site walking track, another showed significant increases in exercise behavior when space and equipment for exercise were modified, and the third demonstrated efforts to increase stair use resulted in self-reported exercise in the control group and the intervention group. Most recently, Conn and colleagues (2009) used meta-analytic techniques in an attempt to synthesize and quantify the results of physical activity interventions studies conducted in more than 100 diverse worksites between 1969 and 2007. Although the results were widely variable, with some programs showing more effectiveness than others, overall physical activity behavior and physical fitness were found to be modestly increased by worksite physical activity interventions (Conn et al. 2009).

Although the existing evidence in support of the worksite as a venue for increasing daily physical activity is disappointing and understandably leaves the health promotion specialist confused about what to do, there are some consistencies in the literature worth pointing out. First, behavior change is difficult. The studies that have shown improvements are often limited to workers who are already healthy, active, and motivated. From the public health point of view, the challenge is to recruit a significant proportion of the workforce, particularly employees who are less motivated, to participate in formal exercise programs. Interventions aimed at the worksite environment such as point-of-decision prompts have the potential to encourage incidental activity throughout the day in a large segment of the workforce. Second, providing facilities and equipment is not enough. Supplemental efforts aimed at education, skill training, behavior modification, etc., are necessary to effect any change in behavior. Third, the strongest evidence supports programs that are theory-based and individually tailored to employee interests, abilities, and readiness to adopt physical activity into their lifestyle. Fourth, single risk factor interventions targeting physical activity may be more successful than those that include physical activity interventions as part of a multi-risk factor health promotion program. Fifth, since even in the best case, the observed improvements in physical activity levels tend to be short term, more must be done to make achieving the established public health physical activity goals part of the worksite culture, rather than merely the focus of a short-term intervention.

There is also the need for more research in this area. Many of the studies to date have been limited by less-than-ideal research designs and methods. Despite the challenges of conducting randomized controlled trials in worksites, efforts should be made to test interventions of interest using this valuable design. Future studies should strive to recruit a larger percentage of the workforce, particularly those less motivated than typical volunteers and to include diverse populations in order to improve generalizability of the findings. There is also the need to use more objective measures of physical activity than self-report and to follow participants over a longer period. Formal testing of novel interventions particularly those aimed at reducing time spent sitting is lacking, as are studies of comprehensive multilevel interventions that are woven into the overall workplace culture. And last, but not least, researchers and health promotion specialists must weigh the impact of these interventions on cost-containment in terms of employee productivity and escalating healthcare costs. In the spirit of challenging economic climates, without convincing evidence of a favorable cost–benefit ratio for the employer, programs such as these are likely to be cut at a time when they are needed most.

Physical inactivity continues to be a major public health concern. Since it is unlikely we will ever revert to the times studied by Morris, Taylor, and Paffenbarger, it is imperative we continue to explore ways to help all members of the workforce incorporate physical activity in their working day. Even small increases in activity levels in a large segment of the population can have important positive public health implications.

So . . . get to work!

STUDY QUESTIONS

1. Discuss the benefits of providing worksite physical activity promotion opportunities.
2. Compare how worksite physical activity programs have changed over time, and identify key components of current worksite health promotion programs.
3. Provide an example of various strategies for worksite physical activity programs within each level of the socioecological model. In your opinion, what types of programs have the best success to improve physical activity in worksite settings and why?
4. Assume you are a staff in a state or county public health department and are charged to develop programs to increase physical activity in worksites for state and county employees. Describe the type of strategies you would use to engage employees that involves free choice and incentives to be more physically active.
5. Assume you are a CEO for a worksite and you wish to reduce healthcare costs by starting a health promotion program. Describe the components of your program and the pros and cons of conducting health risk appraisals as part of the program.

REFERENCES

Adams, J., and M. A. White. 2002. A systematic approach to the development and evaluation of an intervention promoting stair use. *Health Educ. J.* 61: 272–286.

Ainsworth, B. E., W. L. Haskell, M. C. Whitt et al. 2000. Compendium of physical activities: an update of activity codes and MET intensities. *Med. Sci. Sports Exerc.* 32: S409–S516.

Allen, J. R. 2002. Building supportive cultural environments. In *Health Promotion in the Workplace*, 3rd edn., ed. M. O'Donnell, 202–217. Albany, NY: Delmar.

Beers, E. A., J. N. Roemmich, L. H. Epstein et al. 2008. Increasing passive energy expenditure during clerical work. *Eur. J. Appl. Physiol.* 103: 353–360.

Blair, S. N., P. V. Piserchia, C. S. Wilbur et al. 1986. A public health intervention model for work-site health promotion. Impact on exercise and physical fitness in a health promotion plan after 24 months. *JAMA* 255: 921–926.

Blamey, A., N. Mutrie, and T. Aitchison. 1995. Health promotion by encouraged use of stairs. *Br. Med. J.* 311: 289–290.

Boutelle, K. N., R. W. Jeffery, D. M. Murray et al. 2001. Using signs, artwork, and music to promote stair use in a public building. *Am. J. Public Health* 91: 2004–2006, 10.2105/AJPH.91.12.2004.

Bureau of Labor Statistics, U.S. Department of Labor. 2010. Labor Force Statistics from the Current Population Survey. http://www.bls.gov/cps/cpsatabs.htm (last modified October 6, 2010).

Calfas, K. J., B. J. Long, J. F. Sallis et al. 1996. A controlled trial of physician counseling to promote the adoption of physical activity. *Prev. Med.* 25: 225–233.

Carnethon, M., L. P. Whitsel, B. A. Franklin et al. 2009. Worksite wellness programs for cardiovascular disease prevention. A policy statement from the American Heart Association. *Circulation* 120: 1725–1741.

Centers for Disease Control and Prevention. 2009. Behavioral Risk Factor Surveillance System Survey Data. http://apps.nccd.cdc.gov/brfss/list.asp?cat=PA&yr=2009&qkey=4418&state=All (accessed October 6, 2010).

Centers for Disease Control and Prevention. 2010. Worksite Health Promotion. http://www.cdc.gov/workplacehealthpromotion/implementation/topics/physical-activity.html (last updated March 11, 2010).

Coleman, K. J., and E. C. Gonzalez. 2001. Promoting stair use in a U.S.–Mexico Border Community. *Am. J. Public Health* 91: 2007–2009.

Conn, V. S., A. R. Hafdahl, P. S. Cooper et al. 2009. Meta-analysis of workplace physical activity interventions. *Am. J. Prev. Med.* 37: 330–3309.

DeJoy, D. M., M. G. Wilson, R. Z. Goetzel et al. 2008. Development of the Environmental Assessment Tool (EAT) to measure organizational physical and social support for worksite obesity prevention programs. *J. Occup. Environ. Med.* 50: 126–137.

Dinesh, J., D. Bassett, D. Thompson et al. 2009. Effect of using a treadmill work station on performance of simulated office work tasks. *J. Phys. Act. Health* 6: 617–624.

Dishman, R. K., B. Oldenburg, H. O'Neal et al. 1998. Worksite physical activity interventions. *Am. J. Prev. Med.* 15: 344–361.

Engbers, L. H., M. N. M. van Poppel, A. Chin, et al. 2005. Worksite health promotion programs with environmental changes. A systematic review. *Am. J. Prev. Med.* 29: 61–70.

Eves, F. F., and O. J. Web. 2006. Worksite interventions to increase stair climbing: Reasons for caution. *Prev. Med.* 43: 4–7.

Garabrant, D. H., J. M. Peters, T. M. Mack et al. 1984. Job activity and colon cancer risk. *Am. J. Epidemiol.* 119: 1005–1014.

Goetzel, R. Z., D. Shechter, R. J. Ozminkowski et al. 2007. Promising practices in employer health and productivity management efforts: Findings from a benchmarking study. *JOEM* 49(2): 111–130. doi:10.1097/JOM.0b013e31802ec6a3.

Goetzel, R. Z., and R. J. Ozminkowski. 2008. The health and cost benefits of worksite health-promotion programs. *Annu. Rev. Public Health* 29: 303–323.

Golaszewski, T., and B. Fisher. 2002. Heart check: The development and evolution of an organizational heart health assessment. *Am. J. Health Promot.* 17: 132–153.

Herman, C. W., S. Musich, C. Lu et al. 2006. Effectiveness of an incentive-based online physical activity intervention on employee health status. *J. Occup. Environ. Med.* 48: 889–895.

Kahn, E. B., L. T. Ramsey, R. C. Brownson et al. 2002. The effectiveness of interventions to increase physical activity: A systematic review. *Am. J. Prev. Med.* 22: 73–107.

Kerr, J., F. Eves, and D. Carroll. 2001a. Six-month observational study of prompted stair climbing. *Prev. Med.* 33: 422–427.

Kerr, J., F. Eves, and D. Carroll. 2001b. Can posters prompt stair use in a worksite environment? *J. Occup. Health* 43: 205–207.

Kerr, N. A., M. A. Yore, S. A. Ham et al. 2004. Increasing stair use in a worksite through environmental changes. *Am. J. Health Promot.* 18: 312–315.

Levine, J. A., and J. M. Miller. 2007. The energy expenditure of using a "walk-and-work" desk for office workers with obesity. *Br. J. Sport Med.* 41: 558–561.

Marcus, B. H., B. C. Bock, B. M. Pinto et al. 1998. Efficacy of an individualized, motivationally tailored physical activity intervention. *Ann. Behav. Med.* 20: 174–180.

Marcus, B. H., D. M. Williams, P. M. Dubbert et al. 2006. Physical activity intervention studies. What we know and what we need to know. A scientific statement from the American Heart Association Council on Nutrition, Physical Activity, and Metabolism (Subcommittee on Physical Activity); Council on Cardiovascular Disease in the Young; and the Interdisciplinary Working Group on Quality of Care and Outcomes Research. *Circulation* 114: 2739–2752.

Marshall, A. L. 2004. Challenges and opportunities for promoting physical activity in the workplace. *J. Sci. Med. Sport* 7: 60–66.

Marshall, A. L., A. E. Bauman, C. Patch et al. 2002. Can motivational signs prompt increases in incidental physical activity in an Australian health-care facility? *Health Educ. Res.* 17: 743–749.

Marshall, A. L., N. Owen, and A. E. Bauman. 2004. Mediated approaches for influencing physical activity: Update of the evidence on mass media, print, telephone and Website delivery of interventions. *J. Sci. Med. Sport* 7: s74–s80.

McLeroy, K. R., D. Bibeau, A. Steckler et al. 1988. An ecological perspective on health promotion programs. *Health Educ. Q.* 15: 351–378.

Morris, J. N., J. A. Heady, P. A. B. Raffle et al. 1953. Coronary heart disease and physical activity of work. *Lancet* 265(6795):1053–1057, and 265(6796): 1111–1120.

Morris, J. N., R. Pollard, M. G. Everitt et al. 1980. Vigorous exercise in leisure time: Protection against coronary heart disease. *Lancet* 2(8206): 1207–1210.

Mutrie, N., C. Carney, A. Blamey et al. 2002. "Walk in to Work Out" a randomised controlled trial of a self help intervention to promote active commuting. *J. Epidemiol. Community Health* 56: 407–412.

Napolitano, M. A., M. Fotheringham, D. Tate et al. 2003. Evaluation of an internet-based physical activity intervention: A preliminary investigation. *Ann. Behav. Med.* 25: 92–99.

Nicholl, G. 2007. Spatial measures associated with stair use. *Am. J. Health Promot.* 21: 346–352.

Oldenburg, B., J. F. Sallis, D. Harris et al. 2002. Checklist of Health Promotion Environments at Worksites (CHEW): Development and measurement characteristics. *Am. J. Health Promot.* 16: 288–299.

Owen, N., C. Lee, L. Naccarella et al. 1987. Exercise by mail: A mediated behavior-change program for aerobic exercise. *J. Sport Psychol.* 9: 346–357.

Paffenbarger, R. S. Jr., M. E. Laughlin, A. S. Gima et al. 1970. Work activity of longshoreman as related to death from coronary heart disease and stroke. *N. Engl. J. Med.* 282: 1109–1114.

Paffenbarger, R. S. Jr., A. L. Wing, and R. T. Hyde. 1978. Physical activity as an index of heart attack risk in college alumni. *Am. J. Epidemiol.* 108: 161–175.

Pate, R. R. 2009. A National Physical Activity Plan for the United States. *J. Phys. Act. Health* 6: S157–S158.

Pate, R. R., M. Pratt, S. N. Blair et al. 1995. Physical activity and public health. A recommendation from the Centers for Disease Control and Prevention and the American College of Sports Medicine. *JAMA* 273: 402–407.

Plotnikoff, R. C., M. A. Pickering, L. J. McCargar et al. 2010. Six-month follow-up and participant use and satisfaction of an electronic mail intervention promoting physical activity and nutrition. *Am. J. Health Promot.* 24: 255–259.

Plotnikoff, R. C., T. R. Prodaniuk, A. J. Fein et al. 2005. Development of an ecological assessment tool for a workplace physical activity program standard. *Health Promot. Pract.* 6: 453–463.

Prochaska, J. O., and C. C. DiClemente. 1983. Stages and processes of self-change of smoking: Toward an integrative model of change. *J. Consult. Clin. Psychol.* 51: 390–395.

Pronk, N. P. 2009. *ACSM's Worksite Health Handbook. A Guide to Building Healthy and Productive Companies*, 2nd edn. United States: Human Kinetics.

Proper, K. I., V. H. Hildebrandt, A. J. Van der Beek et al. 2003a. Effect of individual counseling on physical activity fitness and health: A randomized controlled trial in a workplace setting. *Am. J. Prev. Med.* 24: 218–226.

Proper, K. I., M. Koning, A. J. van der Beek et al. 2003b. The effectiveness of worksite physical activity programs on physical activity, physical fitness, and health. *Clin. J. Sport Med.* 13: 106–117.

Rimer, B. K., and K. Glanz. 2005. *Theory at a Glance: A Guide for Health Promotion and Practice*, 2nd edn. Washington, DC: U.S. Department of Health and Human Services and National Cancer Institute.

Shephard, R. J. 1996. Worksite fitness and exercise programs: A review of methodology and health impact. *Am. J. Health Promot.* 10: 436–452.

Soler, R. E., K. D. Leeks, S. Razi et al. 2010. A systematic review of selected interventions for worksite health promotion. The assessment of health risks with feedback. *Am. J. Prev. Med.* 38: S237–S262.

Taylor, H. v L., E. Klepetar, A. Keys et al. 1962. Death rates among physically active and sedentary employees of the railroad industry. *Am. J. Public Health* 52: 1697–1707.

U.S. Department of Health and Human Services. 1996. *Physical Activity and Health: A Report of the Surgeon General*. Atlanta, GA: U.S. Department of Health and Human Services, Centers for Disease Control and Prevention, National Center for Chronic Disease Prevention and Health Promotion.

U.S. Department of Health and Human Services. 2000. Healthy people 2010. *Understanding and Improving Health and Objectives for Improving Health*, 2 vols. Washington, DC: U.S. Government Printing Office, 76.

U.S. Department of Health and Human Services. 2010. *The Surgeon General's Vision for a Healthy and Fit Nation*. Rockville, MD: U.S. Department of Health and Human Services, Office of the Surgeon General, January 2010.

U.S. Public Health Service. 1980. *Promoting Health/Preventing Disease: Objectives for the Nation*. Washington, D.C.: U.S. Government Printing Office.

Vena, J. E., S. Graham, M. Zielezny et al. 1985. Lifetime occupational exercise and colon cancer. *Am. J. Epidemiol.* 122: 357–365.

Vihko, V. J., D. L. Apter, E. L. Pukkala et al. 1992. Risk of breast cancer among female teachers of physical education and languages. *Acta Oncol.* 31: 201–204.

Vuori, I. M., P. Oja, and O. Paronen. 1994. Physically active commuting to work-testing its potential for exercise promotion. *Med. Sci. Sports Exerc.* 26: 844–850.

Wen, L. M., J. Kites, and C. Rissel. 2010. Is there a role for workplaces in reducing employees' driving to work? Findings from a cross-sectional survey from inner-west Sydney, Australia. *BMC Public Health* 10: 50. http://www.biomedcentral.com/1471-2458/10/50.

17 Promotion of Physical Activity in Schools

Dianne Stanton Ward and Christopher Ford

CONTENTS

INTRODUCTION

No organization has greater potential to affect physical activity in children and adolescents than schools. Schools enroll more than 95% of all children, and young people spend a high proportion of their days in school: on average, about 6.6 h/day and approximately 178.5 days/year (U.S. Department of Education 2007). This makes school second only to home as the most influential setting to affect physical activity. However, the school day currently is, for the most part, a sedentary period in a young person's daily routine. In the traditional classroom, a high priority is given to order and quiet. With the exception of physical education (PE) classes, recess, or other break times such as lunch and transitions between classrooms, students are expected to remain seated and focused on learning. However, each of these opportunities for physical activity has been reduced, limited, and threatened in recent years. PE requirements in many schools have been cut, and concerns have been raised that the amount of physical activity provided in many PE classes is insufficient. In addition, many schools have reduced or eliminated recess in an effort to increase classroom instruction time in response to high-stakes testing. Despite these disquieting trends, it is possible for all students to be more physically active during the school day, and for many students, through after-school programs, club sports, and interscholastic participation.

Informational and educational approaches are often used to promote healthy behavioral changes. Such methods are designed to motivate young people to make the right choice (be active) and modify their behavior through volitional effort (personal responsibility). However, such approaches may be inadequate because youth are in various stages of development and many are unable to appreciate the long-term benefits of regular physical activity. In contrast to efforts that rely on personal responsibility, public health strategies support physical activity in youth by creating social and physical environments that enable positive behavior change. Often called "upstream" efforts, they are considered to be more population-focused rather than individually focused, and have a greater likelihood of influencing the physical activity behavior of many children. "Downstream" strategies, those that focus more on individual factors that influence behavior, require the target individuals to be more motivated and to make decisions for behavior change.

Many important influences, or determinants, of physical activity in children and adolescents have been identified by behavioral experts (Sallis, Prochaska, and Taylor 2000; Van Der Horst et al. 2007), and these are both "downstream" and "upstream" factors. For example, development of motor skills and goal-setting behaviors are individual-level factors, and social support for physical activity from friends or family members is an interpersonal factor. "Upstream" factors are environment and policy changes that affect many children and adolescents, such as creating engaging outdoor playgrounds at school, providing play equipment, or requiring daily PE classes. An ecological model emphasizes the importance of considering multiple levels of influence and the relationship between the environment and behavior. Some environments are not conducive to physical activity, whereas other environments have been designed to encourage activity. These "downstream" and "upstream" influences exist within school settings, and can be organized into levels using an ecological model (McLeroy et al. 1988).

COORDINATED SCHOOL HEALTH MODEL

Using multicomponent approaches to encourage physical activity at school can be organized in two categories: comprehensive and coordinated. *Comprehensive* school programs promote physical activity in multiple school settings, for example, a program that promotes more physical activity during PE class, provides before- and during-lunch activities opportunities, and creates a walk-to-school program. *Coordinated* programs in school settings are also comprehensive, but place a greater emphasis on coordination at the school level. Therefore, a coordinated program will have an oversight committee or team composed of teachers, school officials, parents, and other community members. An example of a coordinated model that can be used in support of physical activity at school is the Center for Disease Control and Prevention's (CDC) Coordinated School Health Program (CSHP) model, which is composed of eight interactive components, and illustrates the importance of involving educators, families, communities, religious organizations, and medical professionals in addressing the country's health problems. Further explanation of each of

the eight components can be found on the CDC's website at: http://www.cdc.gov/
HealthyYouth/CSHP/components.htmhttp://www.cdc.gov/HealthyYouth/CSHP/.
CSHPs are particularly useful for promoting physical activity because they target
multiple levels of impact (personal, social, and environmental)—an approach more
likely to create behavior change in the school environment. Another advantage of the
CHSP model is that it emphasizes the use of existing school resources and programs,
rather than creating new structures or programs. Using multiple components within
the school provides the opportunity for reinforcement of health messages through
multiple approaches and channels.

In the next section, we review a variety of school-based research programs and
interventions that have resulted in an increase in physical activity in children and
adolescents. These programs have yielded varying degrees of success, have been
implemented at all levels (elementary, middle, high school), and can be replicated in
other schools. Although cost and timing may present significant barriers to implementing such programs, the cost of failure to act at this juncture will likely exceed
such barriers to action. As national rates of overweight and obesity in youth reach
epic proportions, increasing physical activity has the potential to slow or eliminate
the epidemic.

SPECIFIC SCHOOL-BASED APPROACHES

PHYSICAL EDUCATION

PE is the paramount approach to achieving adequate amounts of physical activity among children. Based on a systematic review of existing research, the U.S.
Preventive Service study group concluded that there was strong evidence in favor of
the effectiveness of school-based PE (Kahn et al. 2002). In a review of 16 interventions, researchers found that children's physical activity was positively affected by
the amount of time children spent in PE classes. Several studies clearly show that
children who regularly receive PE obtain significantly greater amounts of physical
activity than children who do not receive such educational programming (Gordon-
Larsen, McMurray, and Popkin 2000; Cawley, Meyerhoefer, and Newhouse 2007;
Durant et al. 2009).

Gordon-Larsen and colleagues surveyed 17,766 U.S. middle and high school students and found that participation in school-based PE was positively related to high
levels of moderate to vigorous physical activity (MVPA) (Gordon-Larsen, McMurray,
and Popkin 2000). These authors also showed that students who reported having
PE classes five times per week were significantly more likely to report engaging
in 25 h or more of MVPA physical activity per week (Gordon-Larsen, McMurray,
and Popkin 2000). Similarly, in a survey of 8th, 9th, and 12th grade girls, Pate et al.
(2007a) found that PE enrollment was positively associated with levels of physical
activity. Eighth, 9th and 12th grade girls enrolled in PE participated in 12, 30, and
39 min more of MVPA, respectively, than those not enrolled in PE class (Pate et al.
2007b). These findings were supported by Durant et al. (2009), whose survey of 165
twelve- to 18-year-olds showed a positive relationship between the number of PE
classes per week and overall levels of physical activity. Cawley, Meyerhoefer, and

Newhouse (2007) demonstrated the importance of having a binding requirement for PE, with a positive relationship observed between time spent in PE class and the amount of vigorous exercise among 15- to 18-year-olds, especially girls.

Just as the *amount* of PE is of critical importance, the *quality* of PE instruction is an integral component of physical activity in children. PE programs that include the use of standardized curricula, goals for active classes, and instructors with PE-specific training, result in children who are more physically active (Luepker et al. 1996; McKenzie et al. 1996; Sallis et al. 1997). In The Child and Adolescent Trial for Cardiovascular Health, students attending the intervention schools followed a standardized PE curriculum composed of three 30-min lessons weekly, skill and fitness instruction, goals for active class time, and staff development (Luepker et al. 1996). Students in the intervention group engaged in 12.1 min more of vigorous physical activity (VPA) than students in the control group (Luepker et al. 1996; McKenzie et al. 1996). Results from the Sports, Play, and Active Recreation for Kids (SPARK) study supported these findings. In SPARK, fourth and fifth grade students across seven schools received three PE sessions per week, each consisting of 15 min of health-fitness activities and 15 min of skill-fitness activities (Sallis et al. 1997). Schools were randomly assigned to one of three groups: a group led by non-PE teachers who had received brief training in PE; a PE specialist-led group; and a self-management group in which students received triweekly instruction in self-management skills to facilitate physical activity outside of school (Sallis et al. 1997). Students who received instruction from a PE specialist engaged in significantly more MVPA (7.5 min/week) than students who received instruction from non-PE teachers (Sallis et al. 1997).

Goal-setting, self-monitoring, and enlisting family support through PE classes may further increase amounts of physical activity among young people (Young et al. 2006). In a randomized control trial, 221 ninth grade African American girls attended a standard PE class or a Social Action Theory (SAT)-based PE class for an 8-month period (Young et al. 2006). The SAT-based PE instruction focused on goal setting, self-monitoring, problem-solving, and family support. Students in the SAT-based PE group spent significantly more time in MVPA (46.9% vs. 30.5% of class time) than students in the standard PE class (Young et al. 2006).

CLASSROOM ACTIVITY BREAKS

The regular academic classroom, where children spend the majority of their time engaged in sedentary behaviors, may present a significant barrier to physical activity (DuBose et al. 2008). A positive relationship between physical activity and academic performance has been well described (DuBose et al. 2008; Dwyer et al. 2001; Field, Diego, and Sanders 2001; Nelson and Gordon-Larsen 2006; Pate et al. 1996; Sigfusdottir, Kristjansson, and Allegrante 2007; Trudeau and Shephard 2008). However, if part of a "regular" class's time is used for physical activity, how will the students' academic work be affected? In fact, evidence shows that incorporating physical activity into classroom time does not negatively affect academic performance (Carlson et al. 2008), but rather the opposite is observed (Donnelly et al. 2009; DuBose et al. 2008).

Mahar et al. (2006) showed that regular exercise breaks improved on-task class-room behavior among third and fourth grade students. Children who participated in 10-min, teacher-led physical activity breaks called Energizers, once a week for 12 weeks, obtained more physical activity (about 1000 additional steps) and showed a significant improvement in on-task classroom behavior (Mahar et al. 2006). Similarly, Donnelly et al. (2009) observed that elementary children who participated in 40 min of daily aerobic exercise scored higher in executive functioning than students who did not participate in the exercise. In a subsample of students who wore accelerom-eters for 4 days, students obtained an additional 26 min of MVPA—more than one-third more than students who did not participate in classroom breaks (Donnelly et al. 2009). Furthermore, elementary children who attended schools participating in a 3-year intervention to integrate 90–100 min of weekly physical activity into class-room instruction (Physical Activity Across the Curriculum) saw greater improve-ments in composite, reading, math, and spelling scores (Donnelly et al. 2009; DuBose et al. 2008). Thus, the current body of evidence suggests that incorporating physical activity into the "regular" classroom not only increases levels of physical activity, but may also improve academic performance.

RECESS

Recess is an important time for children to engage in active play and constitutes as much as 42% of the available opportunity for physical activity for some children (Robert Wood Johnson Foundation 2007). Yet, in many schools recess time may be limited to favor more academic classroom time (Zygmunt-Fillwalk and Bilello 2005). In 2000, only 4.1% of the states required elementary schools to regularly offer recess (Department of Health and Human Services 2006), prompting the National Association for Sport and Physical Education (NASPE) and other organizations to call for elementary schools to provide daily recess (National Association for Sport and Physical Education 2001). In 2006, the NASPE strengthened this recommenda-tion by calling for all elementary schools to provide at least 20 min of daily recess (National Association for Sport and Physical Education 2006). The number of states requiring regular recess has more than doubled since 2000, yet only 11.8% of states required elementary schools to provide regular recess in 2006 (Kann, Telljohann, and Wooley 2007).

As policy changes and national recommendations continue to yield gradual improvements in the state of recess, many schools may benefit from specific strate-gies to optimize recess time. In schools that use techniques to enhance physical activ-ity during playtime, recess may constitute nearly one-third of the MVPA required for children each day (Ridgers, Stratton, and Fairclough 2006). Without such strate-gies, however, recess time may constitute as little as 5% of the recommended daily physical activity for children (Ridgers, Stratton, and Fairclough 2006). In addition to providing ample time for recess, helpful strategies include supplying play equip-ment, decorating play areas and designating space, and providing appropriate super-vision. Schools that use these strategies tend to have more physically active students (Ridgers et al. 2007; Stratton and Mullan 2005; Verstraete et al. 2006; Willenberg et al. 2010).

Access to play equipment may be positively related to the amount of physical activity children engage in during recess (Verstraete et al. 2006; Willenberg et al. 2010). In a randomized trial among fifth and sixth graders at seven schools, 122 children received a set of game equipment as well as activity cards that described the ways in which that equipment might be used (Verstraete et al. 2006). The children's physical activity levels were measured using accelerometers at baseline and the 3-month follow-up. Results showed that MVPA increased significantly among children who received the game equipment, and decreased among children in the comparison group (Verstraete et al. 2006). Among the children who received the game equipment, the proportion of time spent in MVPA increased by 13%, whereas MVPA among children in the comparison group fell by 10% over the same period (Verstraete et al. 2006).

Although portable play equipment may increase physical activity levels *in all* children, low-income youth may especially benefit from access to such equipment. In Melbourne, Australia, researchers observed 3006 students in 12 primary schools (U.S. equivalent of grades 1–7) to determine how elements of the playground environment influence levels of physical activity during playtime. Direct observations were conducted using the System for Observing Play and Leisure Activity in Youth (SOPLAY), a method that uses left-to-right scanning of an area at predetermined intervals to quantify the number of children who are engaged in sedentary, walking, or very active physical activities (Willenberg et al. 2010). The observations, conducted before school, during recess, and after school, revealed that more students participated in VPA when portable play equipment was provided (60% vs. 52%) (Willenberg et al. 2010).

Playground decoration and designation of specific play areas with colorful markings are additional ways to increase children's physical activity levels, especially among low-income youths. At four schools in northeast Wales, researchers measured the activity levels of 30 randomly selected children, aged between 4 to 11 years, before and after their playgrounds were painted according to school preference. Playgrounds were decorated with bright fluorescent colors, and markings were used to designate specific play areas (Stratton and Mullan 2005). Physical activity was measured using heart rate telemetry, and children in schools with marked playgrounds were compared to children in schools with unmarked play areas (Stratton and Mullan 2005). Children's physical activity levels were collected during the 4 weeks before the playground modifications and then again during the 4 weeks after the modifications. MVPA physical activity increased by 13.6% among children whose playgrounds had been marked, whereas MVPA decreased by 6.5% among children in the comparison group (Stratton and Mullan 2005). Ridgers and colleagues (2007) supported these findings in a study that examined the effect of playground markings among students at 26 elementary schools in economically deprived neighborhoods from one large English city. Fifteen schools were provided funds for playground redesign that included color-coded designation of three specific play areas: red for sports, blue for multiple activities, and yellow for quiet play (Ridgers et al. 2007). Students in the intervention schools were compared to students in schools whose playgrounds were not remodeled (Ridgers et al. 2007). Physical activity levels were assessed, using heart rate telemetry and accelerometry, 6 weeks before playground modification, and again 6 months after modification (Ridgers et al. 2007). Students whose playgrounds had been remodeled engaged in more MVPA and VPA than students in the comparison schools (Ridgers et al. 2007).

SCHOOL FACILITIES AND JOINT-USE AGREEMENTS

For many youths, opportunities for active play may be delimited to the school environment. Therefore, it is important that schools provide variety of indoor and outdoor spaces for children to engage in physical activity both during and after school hours. Furthermore, ample availability and accessibility of physical environments within and around schools are essential for optimizing physical activity in children and adolescents. Evidence indicates that youth who attend schools with a variety of accessible spaces for active play participate in greater amounts of physical activity (Nichol, Pickett, and Janssen 2009; Sallis et al. 2001; Haug et al. 2010).

Researchers in Canada found that adolescents in grades 6 and 10 were more active both during and after school in school settings with a greater number of recreational features (Nichol, Pickett, and Janssen 2009). Nichol, Pickett, and Janssen analyzed data from the 2005–2006 Canadian Health Behaviour in School-Aged Children Survey obtained from 7638 students in 154 public schools across all Canadian provinces and territories. Children were asked about physical activity levels at school and after school. Principals or vice principals completed an administrator survey of school characteristics, including physical facilities and policies to increase physical activity and provision of sports teams. In schools with more recreational facilities and greater opportunities for activity, students reported more in-school and out-of-school physical activity (Nichol, Pickett, and Janssen 2009). High school boys in schools with more recreational facilities reported about 50% more in-school activity than boys in schools with fewer facilities, whereas high school girls' free-time physical activity was greater for schools with more facilities (Nichol, Pickett, and Janssen 2009).

Sallis and colleagues (2001) saw a similar relationship between facilities and physical activity in 24 middle schools in San Diego. Researchers collected observational data of physical activity levels at a number of potential physical activity areas at 24 schools. Environmental variables included area type (e.g., court, open field, indoor facilities), area size (in square meters), and permanent improvements (e.g., courts, diamonds, hoops/goals). Physical activity was assessed by observation using SOPLAY during three periods: before school, during lunch, and after school. Results indicated that improvements in school facilities and provision of supervision explained more than 40% of the variance in girls' and nearly 60% of boys' non-PE physical activity (Sallis et al. 2001).

The relationship between access to school facilities and youth physical activity has been observed for outdoor facilities even in regions with extremely cold climates. Researchers in Norway obtained data from 16,471 students attending 130 schools in grades 4 through 10 (Haug et al. 2010). Students completed a brief survey reporting on physical activity during school classes, transportation to school, and recess activity. Principals completed a questionnaire on school policies, environmental, and organizational structures related to physical activity opportunities. Multiple logistic regression models demonstrated that boys at secondary schools with more available facilities were more than 2.7 times as likely to be active at recess as boys in schools with fewer facilities (Haug et al. 2010). Girls were even more likely to be active (2.9 times) during recess in schools with more facilities compared to girls enrolled in schools with fewer facilities (Haug et al. 2010).

Even when facilities are present, adolescents may have difficulties accessing them during nonschool hours. Unfortunately, many schools limit access after school due to a variety of reasons, many related to liability for potential injuries that might occur. An illustration of this issue was highlighted by the work of Scott et al. (2007). Researchers visited schools and parks near the residences of adolescent girls in six states and found that schools represented nearly half (44%) of the available sites for physical activity for these girls (Scott et al. 2007). Yet on the day of observation, a third of the schools were locked (Scott et al. 2007).

Recently, the concept of "joint-use agreements" has been identified as a potential strategy for increasing physical activity opportunities after school and on weekends by providing children with access to play spaces (Maddock et al. 2008). Such arrangements may be more important in areas where nonschool options for active play are reduced, such as low-income, inner-city, or rural settings. Schoolchildren, as well as other community residents, can become and remain more physically active when schools and communities enter into joint-use agreements that allow for the use of school property and equipment outside of school hours. An example of a successful joint-use agreement occurred between an urban high school and the city of Honolulu that allowed the creation of a recreational program that increased physical activity for students, teachers, and staff, as well as community residents (Maddock et al. 2008). Results from a pilot study in a low-income, African American inner-city neighborhood in New Orleans further illustrate the importance of the availability of the schoolyard for free play (Farley et al. 2007). In two low-income neighborhoods in New Orleans, researchers opened a schoolyard after school and on weekends over a 2-year period. Using the system for observing fitness instruction time (SOFIT) instrument, they observed the children's activity levels on five randomly selected weekend days and four randomly selected weekend days, 4 weeks before the opening of the schoolyards and each quarter throughout the intervention period. Researchers found that opening schoolyards after school and on weekends resulted in an 84% increase in the number of children who were outdoors and active compared to those in a comparison school where the play areas were unavailable (Farley et al. 2007). These studies underscore the importance of providing access to school facilities after-school and on weekends, which may be of special importance to youths in lower income communities with fewer options for activity.

ACTIVE SCHOOL TRAVEL

Active travel has been positively associated with higher daily levels of physical activity (Rosenberg et al. 2006; Cooper et al. 2006) and higher cardiorespiratory fitness (Andersen et al. 2009; Voss and Sandercock 2010). Albeit 30 years ago more than half of all U.S. children walked or biked to school, the number of youth who now use active transportation to get to school has declined significantly (McDonald 2007).

Still, one program in the United States that holds promise for promoting active school travel is the *Safe Routes to School* program. Safe Routes to School initiatives, which are generally supported by U.S. federal highway funds, include physical infrastructure changes (such as improvements in sideways or bikeways), as well as educational, promotional, and policy activities. Safe Routes to School (formerly referred to as Walk to School [WTS]), an international movement that has been embraced in communities throughout many countries, is designed to increase the number of children who walk or bicycle to school by supporting projects that remove barriers and promote the use of active transportation to school (National Center for Safe Routes to School 2010).

Although efforts to increase children's use of active transportation to school require community involvement, walk-to-school programs are also an important component of a comprehensive and coordinated effort to increase children's activity levels. School personnel can work in concert with community members to facilitate meaningful changes that support children's activity. A recent evaluation of the WTS program found that a quarter of WTS coordinators reported policy changes resulting from program efforts (Vaughn et al. 2009). The most common changes included modified automobile drop-off/pick-up policies (51.5%) or locations, and availability of crossing guards (42.4%) (Vaughn et al. 2009). Another 28.3% reported "other" policy changes that included the addition of signage, increased supervision, and modification of traffic patterns (Vaughn et al. 2009). More than a third of coordinators reported physical environment changes such as painted or marked crosswalks (43.6%) and repaired or cleared sidewalks (Vaughn et al. 2009). Another 35.2% indicated that "other" physical changes had been made, including improvements in communication strategies, modification of walking routes, and increased adult supervision (Vaughn et al. 2009). Although a few evaluation studies of the WTS efforts to promote active school travel have been undertaken, further evaluation of these programs in which children's individual physical activity levels are measured is an important next step.

AFTER-SCHOOL PROGRAMS

After school programs may offer additional opportunities for children to obtain physical activity beyond what they get during school hours, but more research is needed. After school programs consist of a variety of different opportunities including after-school childcare, special programs, and youth sports. In two review papers, Beets et al. (2009) and Pate and O'Neill (2009) note that research evidence on after-school physical activity is mixed; however, after-school programs have good potential for increasing physical activity in children. The reviews also call for more research with better methodology and greater attention to theories and levels of implementation (Beets et al. 2004; Pate and O'Neill 2009). Furthermore, there remains a need for research examining the impact of school sports (e.g., intramural, club-level, or interscholastic) on physical activity in children and adolescents. Although after-school programming has strong potential for increasing physical activity in youth, in the absence of further study, the relative value of this strategy to increase physical activity in youth remains unclear.

In a study of seven after-school programs in Kansas, Trost, Rosenkranz, and Dzewaltowski (2008) found that boys and girls received about 20 min of MVPA in after-school programs, with boys receiving more activity than girls. However, more than 40% of the children's time was spent in sedentary activities (Trost, Rosenkranz, and Dzewaltowski 2008). These findings demonstrate that after-school programs may provide untapped opportunities for increasing children's physical activity.

A recent study from Georgia on the potential of after-school programs to increase physical activity in youth is encouraging (Gutin et al. 2008). Georgia Fitkids involved children from 18 schools in an afternoon program that included academic enrichment activities (homework and school reinforcement), healthy snacks, and MVPA. During the program, third through fifth grade children participated in more than 1 h of physical activity each day, half of which was at a vigorous intensity (Gutin et al. 2008). Analysis of youth who remained in the same schools for the 3-year period (measured at all six time points) and who attended at least 40% of the sessions in each of the 3 years, showed that children in intervention schools improved in fitness and percentage body fat during the school years (Gutin et al. 2008).

Low-active individuals may reap the greatest benefit from after-school programs. Secondary students in three schools in Australia participated in a study to compare two types of after-school programs (Lubans and Morgan 2008). A group of 116 students was assigned to one of two after-school programs. The "Learning to Enjoy Activity with Friends" program involved structured exercise activities along with behavioral strategies such as activity monitoring using pedometers and goal setting. Students in the comparison group were offered only structured exercises. Low-active adolescents in the intervention group increased their physical activity level by more than 30%, or approximately 25 min/day, whereas activity levels of the students in the comparison group did not change (Lubans and Morgan 2008).

Whole School Programs

Multicomponent, or *whole school*, programs provide opportunities for physical activity across the school day and supplement the contribution of PE classes. Whole school programs use other classes and other time periods—such as recess, in-class breaks, and after-school events—to increase children's physical activity. In a systematic review, van Sluijs, McMinn, and Griffin (2007) reviewed 57 studies of interventions designed to promote physical activity in children and adolescents, including school-based programs with multiple components. The authors found "strong evidence" in support of multicomponent interventions to increase physical activity in adolescents. Both U.S. and international studies have shown that children are much more physically active if they attend schools that schedule, promote, and supervise more school-based opportunities beyond those provided by PE classes (van Sluijs, McMinn, and Griffin 2007).

Whole school efforts to increase students' physical activity have been consistently shown to work and have been effectively implemented at all school levels. In some cases, whole school programs address physical activity only, but may also include a focus on other health behaviors aimed at obesity prevention. Some programs have had greater impact on the activity levels of boys, whereas others have been more successful with girls. Thus, both boys and girls should be considered when whole school programs are designed and implemented.

Action schools! BC (AS!BC) is an example of a whole school program implemented at the elementary school level. Ten schools were randomly assigned to one
of three approaches: (1) External Liaison School: person outside of the school staff
who provided teachers with weekly contact, training, and resources; (2) Champion
School: facilitator identified within the school who, with appropriate training, served
to implement the model; and (3) Usual Practice School: schools received no active
intervention. Similar to other whole school programs, AS!BC targeted increased
physical activity across six "zones": school environment, PE, classroom activities,
family and community, extracurricular, and school spirit (fundraisers and assem-
blies). The intervention was implemented over an 11-month period. Although results
were modest (about 10 additional min per day compared to control), the program was
well received by staff, students, and the community, and demonstrated the feasibility
of the whole-school approach (Naylor et al. 2006).

Middle-School Physical Activity and Nutrition (MSPAN) program is an example
of a whole school intervention at the middle school level. In addition to focusing
on nutrition, MSPAN included a physical activity component that incorporated an
enhanced PE curriculum, more efficient use of PE equipment and space, and training
for PE staff. At the end of the 2-year intervention, students spent an average of 2.6
more min in MVPA per PE lesson than controls or 13 min more of physical activity
per week (McKenzie et al. 2004). Physical activity levels for boys in the program
increased more than three times that of boys in the nonintervention classes; however,
the program was less effective for girls (McKenzie et al. 2004).

High school girls benefited from exposure to a whole-school physical activity program in the Lifestyle Education for Activity Program (LEAP) intervention (Pate et al.
2005). Twenty-four schools and approximately 3000 eighth grade girls were recruited
and randomized into intervention and control groups. The LEAP intervention used the
Coordinated School Health model (described above) and focused on six of the components: PE, health education, school environment, school health services, faculty/staff
health promotion, and family/community involvement. Intervention schools identified a
Program Champion (an individual within the organization who assumes leadership and
is a strong advocate for the physical activity program) and organized a school LEAP
Team composed of school personnel. Accelerometer data showed that girls in the intervention schools had higher levels of VPA compared to controls (Pate et al. 2005). For
schools that fully implemented the LEAP program, intervention effects were still measurable at the 4-year follow-up, thereby suggesting that a whole-school physical activity
program can encourage long-term VPA in high school girls (Pate et al. 2007a).

A number of whole-school programs have been implemented in European school
settings. Two examples are JUMP-in and ICASPS. JUMP-in was a comprehensive, theory-based intervention conducted in Amsterdam that included environmental changes to increase physical activity in early adolescent students (Jurg et
al. 2006). In addition to educational activities conducted during school, additional
school sports activities, parent information, and periodic parent–child activities
at local sports clubs were provided. JUMP-in had an impact on physical activity
participation; sixth-grade children in the intervention group maintained their preintervention activity levels, whereas activity levels of children in the control group
decreased (Jurg et al. 2006). ICAPS (Intervention Centered on Adolescents' Physical

Activity and Sedentary Behavior) was a multicomponent intervention implemented in eight middle schools in France that used a more coordinated approach (Simon et al. 2004). The intervention aimed to improve physical activity knowledge, attitudes, and motivation, as well as social, environmental, structural, and institutional support for physical activity. The intervention created many partnerships with school and community organizations (such as parks and recreation, medical staff, and transportation officials). Environmental changes included providing additional physical activity opportunities during and after school, and requesting that policy makers provide a supportive environment for physical activity. ICAPS resulted in a significant increase in the number of youth who engaged in supervised physical activity outside of PE, as well as a significant reduction in time spent in sedentary activities (Simon et al. 2004).

FEDERAL AND STATE-LEVEL POLICIES

State-level policies requiring that children receive a specific amount of physical activity each day are an effective strategy, with the potential to increase physical activity in large numbers of children. State efforts to create laws or make policies requiring schools to provide children with a minimum amount of physical activity (such as 30 min daily) have resulted in good implementation and increased amounts of physical activity in children (Kelder et al. 2009; Barroso et al. 2009; Evenson et al. 2009). In 2001, the Texas legislature passed a law requiring that students in public elementary schools engage in 30 min of physical activity daily, or 135 min/week (Kelder et al. 2009). In 2007, the Texas legislature passed an additional law that recommended coordinated school health programs and provided implementation training in approved programs (Kelder et al. 2009). Four studies that assessed the effectiveness of school physical activity policy changes to increase physical activity showed favorable results. In one study, a probability sample of 171 elementary schools representative of Texas and individual public health regions was conducted a two time points 1 year apart (2004–2005 and 2005–2006). A second study examined implementation of the policy in schools on the Texas–Mexico border where obesity levels are very high. After implementation of the law, researchers found that administrators had a high level of overall awareness of the law for coordinated school health program and the 30 min of daily physical activity policy (96–97%), and that children participated in 30% more than the required amount of physical activity, or 179 min/week (Kelder et al. 2009). In a similar evaluation study in Texas conducted at the middle school level, an even stronger effect was observed. Adolescents participated in PE 4 days per week and 58 min per class, compared to 2 days of participation before implementation (Barroso et al. 2009). Similar policy change in North Carolina K–8 schools also showed favorable outcomes in implementation (Evenson et al. 2009).

In contrast to state policy changes, efforts to improve physical activity at the national level in the United States have had limited success. The Child Nutrition and WIC Reauthorization Act of 2004 required school districts to develop local wellness policies in an effort to create healthier school environments. In an evaluation of the implementation of this policy, researchers found that most districts mentioned physical activity in their local school wellness policies, but few outlined specific physical activity requirements (Robert Wood Johnson Foundation 2009). It is likely that a tendency for states to set weak standards may have resulted in the poor outcomes. Accordingly, more rigorous policies are needed, along with additional financial resources, to increase physical activity opportunities for children in schools.

CONCLUSION

School-based approaches are the key to increasing physical activity in youth and adolescents. In fact, an Institute of Medicine report on the prevention of obesity in children and youth recommends that schools ensure that children and youth partici-pate in at least 30 min of MVPA during the school day. In this chapter, we presented a number of different strategies for increasing physical activity at school that address individual, interpersonal, environmental, and policies levels (see Table 17.1).

Based on several studies, PE classes may be the most important strategy for pro-viding physical activity during schools. Studies demonstrated the importance of a having a binding requirement, supporting a quality PE program, and providing trained teachers—keys to increased physical activity. Classroom time can also be used to increase physical activity in children and adolescents, and research suggests that regular physical activity breaks may improve classroom performance. Recess time, a quintessential period for active play and socialization, can also be optimized to promote physical activity in children and adolescents. Ensuring that children have ample weekly recess time, access to portable play equipment, and attractively designed play areas with designated spaces, are just a few ways in which recess time can be enhanced to promote physical activity. Still, access to recreational facilities during school hours may be insufficient for many students and extending access beyond school hours through joint-use agreements can increase opportunities for active play among children in their communities. Transportation to and from school can also be used to promote physical activity in children. Although programs like Safe Routes to School have been successful, further efforts are needed to extend their reach. Some evidence suggests that after school programs may be another means to increase opportunities for physical activity in youth; however, further studies are needed to determine which children will benefit most from this approach. Perhaps the most effective school-based approaches to increase physical activity in youth are whole school programs that involve specific strategies at multiple levels of influence. Whole school programs that are coordinated through strong leadership groups and program champions within the school and combine efforts from both community members and school staff have a greater likelihood to result in greater physical activ-ity levels in children and adolescents.

An important key to increasing physical activity in schools is policy decisions. As noted above, requirements for PE, standards for curricula, and use of trained teachers result in more physical activity than when these strategies are not in place. Policymakers must create these standards and requirements. When schools or school districts make policies or pass laws that specify how much physical activity children must obtain each day, there is greater likelihood that they will obtain more activity. A greater reach can be achieved through specific policies (e.g., children must obtain 30 min of physical activity each day) at the state and federal level, and such policies

TABLE 17.1

Strategies for Increasing Physical Activity at School

School-Based Strategy	Important Characteristics
Physical education	• Need for binding requirements, potentially daily PE • Quality PE programs have set curricula, have active classes (at least 50% MVPA), and staff development • Trained PE specialists provide the best classroom leadership, but if classroom teachers are used, training should be provided
Classroom activity breaks	• Classroom breaks offered in academic classes in elementary schools consistently result in more activity for children • Additional benefits of classroom breaks include better on-task behavior and other improvements in academic performance
Recess	• Recess adds additional activity time for children during the school day • Access to portable play equipment during recess time results in children receiving more activity during recess • The addition of colorful playgroup markings can attract children to play areas during recess and result in greater activity levels
School facilities and Joint-use agreements	• Schools with more physical facilities have more active students • Access to facilities increases their use, especially during after-school periods • Joint-use agreements can result in school facilities being open to children and families after school and on weekends
Active school transportation	• Interventions to support children walking to school require both school and community participation • Infrastructure changes need the addition of educational programming to increase children's active travel to school
Whole-school programs	• Whole-school programs add additional activity levels beyond that provided by PE classes • Activity programs that address multiple school areas can create a synergism that enhances activity for children and adolescents • Attention should be paid to both boys and girls in program design; not all interventions are equally effective • Focusing on coordinated, comprehensive approaches requires leadership from multiple school personnel and community involvement
After-school programs	• After-school programs offer opportunities for youth to obtain additional physical activity • Research findings are mixed as to the effectiveness of after-school programs to contribute consistently to children's physical activity levels
Federal and state-level policies	• State laws and/or recommendations that specify a specific amount of daily physical activity (e.g., 30 min) is an effective approach for assuring minimal levels of physical activity in children and adolescents • Requirements need to be specific and should have mechanisms for enforcement

are key to ensuring that physical activity is a priority for schools, even in the face of budget shortfalls. To date, some evidence has shown policy efforts to be successful in promoting physical activity. Still, additional efforts are needed to create policies, and to ensure that policies are enforced. In the future, each of the strategies outlined in this chapter will play an important role in public health endeavors to promote physical activity in youth. Combined, these strategies represent perhaps the greatest promise of improving the health of children and adolescents, and slowing (or even reversing) the trends in overweight and obesity.

STUDY QUESTIONS

1. Evaluate how schools can be important settings for promoting physical activity.
2. The social–ecologic model posits that there are multiple levels of influence on human behavior. What components of the school structure correspond to individual, interpersonal, environmental, and policy factors that have the potential to influence physical activity?
3. Describe how physical education programs could be modified to increase the amount of physical activity children and adolescents currently obtain at school.
4. Identify physical activity promotion strategies that would be considered curricular and those that would be considered noncurricular.
5. Defend your choices for the most important school policies to implement to increase physical activity. Which of the policies are "downstream" and "upstream" policies?
6. Explain how the costs of implementing the school-based strategies described in this chapter might compare to the healthcare costs of increases in obesity and being overweight. How might the healthcare costs be reduced or prevented by these school-based strategies?

REFERENCES

Andersen, L. B., D. A. Lawlor, A. R. Cooper et al. 2009. Physical fitness in relation to transport to school in adolescents: The Danish youth and sports study. *Scand. J. Med. Sci. Sports* 19: 406–411.

Barroso, C. S., S. H. Kelder, A. E. Springer et al. 2009. Senate Bill 42: Implementation and impact on physical activity in middle schools. *J. Adolesc. Health* 45: S82–S90.

Beets, M.W., A. Beighle, H. E. Erwin, and J. L. Huberty. 2009. After-school program impact on physical activity and fitness: A meta-analysis. *Am. J. Prev. Med.* 36: 527–537.

Carlson, S. A., J. E. Fulton, S. M. Lee et al. 2008. Physical education and academic achievement in elementary school: data from the early childhood longitudinal study. *Am. J. Public Health* 98: 721–727.

Cawley, J., C. Meyerhoefer, and D. Newhouse. 2007. The impact of state physical education requirements on youth physical activity and overweight. *Health Econ.* 16: 1287–1301.

Cooper, A. R., N. Wedderkopp, H. Wang et al. 2006. Active travel to school and cardiovascular fitness in Danish children and adolescents. *Med. Sci. Sports Exerc.* 38: 1724–1731.

Department of Health and Human Services. 2006. School Health Policies and Programs Study. Centers for Disease Control and Prevention.

Donnelly, J. E., J. L. Greene, C. A. Gibson et al. 2009. Physical Activity Across the Curriculum (PAAC): A randomized controlled trial to promote physical activity and diminish overweight and obesity in elementary school children. *Prev. Med.* 49: 336–341.

DuBose, K. D., M. S. Mayo, C. A. Gibson et al. 2008. Physical activity across the curriculum (PAAC): Rationale and design. *Contemp. Clin. Trials* 29: 83–93.

Durant, N., S. K. Harris, S. Doyle et al. 2009. Relation of school environment and policy to adolescent physical activity. *J. Sch. Health* 79: 153–159; quiz 205–206.

Dwyer, T., J. F. Sallis, L. Blizzard et al. 2001. Relation of academic performance to physical activity and fitness in children. *Pediatr. Exerc. Sci.* 13: 225–238.

Evenson, K. R., K. Ballard, G. Lee et al. 2009. Implementation of a school-based state policy to increase physical activity. *J. Sch. Health* 79: 231–238, quiz 244–246.

Farley, T. A., R. A. Meriwether, E. T. Baker et al. 2007. Safe play spaces to promote physical activity in inner-city children: Results from a pilot study of an environmental intervention. *Am. J. Public Health* 97: 1625–1631.

Field, T., M. Diego, and C. E. Sanders. 2001. Exercise is positively related to adolescents' relationships and academics. *Adolescence* 36: 105–110.

Gordon-Larsen, P., R. G. McMurray, and B. M. Popkin. 2000. Determinants of adolescent physical activity and inactivity patterns. *Pediatrics* 105: E83.

Gutin, B., Z. Yin, M. Johnson, and P. Barbeau. 2008. Preliminary findings of the effect of a 3-year after-school physical activity intervention on fitness and body fat: The Medical College of Georgia Fitkid Project. *Int. J. Pediatr. Obes.* 3: 3–9.

Haug, E., T. Torsheim, J. F. Sallis et al. 2010. The characteristics of the outdoor school environment associated with physical activity. *Health Educ. Res.* 25: 248–256.

Jurg, M. E., S. P. Kremers, M. J. Candel et al. 2006. A controlled trial of a school-based environmental intervention to improve physical activity in Dutch children: JUMP-in, kids in motion. *Health Promot. Int.* 21: 320–330.

Kahn, E. B., L. T. Ramsey, R. C. Brownson et al. 2002. The effectiveness of interventions to increase physical activity. A systematic review. *Am. J. Prev. Med.* 22: 73–107.

Kann, L., S. K. Telljohann, and S. F. Wooley. 2007. Health education: Results from the School Health Policies and Programs Study 2006. *J. Sch. Health* 77: 408–434.

Kelder, S. H., A. S. Springer, C. S. Barroso et al. 2009. Implementation of Texas Senate Bill 19 to increase physical activity in elementary schools. *J. Public Health Policy* 30: S221–S247.

Lubans, D., and P. Morgan. 2008. Evaluation of an extra-curricular school sport programme promoting lifestyle and lifetime activity for adolescents. *J. Sports Sci.* 26: 519–529.

Luepker, R. V., C. L. Perry, S. M. McKinlay et al. 1996. Outcomes of a field trial to improve children's dietary patterns and physical activity. The Child and Adolescent Trial for Cardiovascular Health. CATCH collaborative group. *JAMA* 275: 768–776.

Maddock, J., L. B. Choy, B. Nett et al. 2008. Increasing access to places for physical activity through a joint use agreement: A case study in urban Honolulu. *Prev. Chronic Dis.* 5: A91.

Mahar, M. T., S. K. Murphy, D. A. Rowe et al. 2006. Effects of a classroom-based program on physical activity and on-task behavior. *Med. Sci. Sports Exerc.* 38: 2086–2094.

McDonald, N. C. 2007. Active transportation to school: Trends among U.S. schoolchildren, 1969–2001. *Am. J. Prev. Med.* 32: 509–516.

McKenzie, T. L., P. R. Nader, P. K. Strikmiller et al. 1996. School physical education: Effect of the child and adolescent trial for cardiovascular health. *Prev. Med.* 25: 423–431.

McKenzie, T. L., J. F. Sallis, J. J. Prochaska et al. 2004. Evaluation of a two-year middle-school physical education intervention: M-SPAN. *Med. Sci. Sports Exerc.* 36: 1382–1388.

McLeroy, K. R., D. Bibeau, A. Steckler et al. 1988. An ecological perspective on health promotion programs. *Health Educ. Q.* 15:351–377.

National Association for Sport and Physical Education. 2001. Recess in elementary schools. Reston, VA.

National Association for Sport and Physical Education. 2006. Recess for elementary school students. Reston, VA.

National Center for Safe Routes to School. 2010. Safe Routes. Available at: http://www.saferoutesinfo.org/ (accessed January 31, 2010).

Naylor, P. J., H. M. Macdonald, J. A. Zebedee et al. 2006. Lessons learned from Action Schools! BC—an "active school" model to promote physical activity in elementary schools. *J. Sci. Med. Sport* 9: 413–423.

Nelson, M. C., and P. Gordon-Larsen. 2006. Physical activity and sedentary behavior patterns are associated with selected adolescent health risk behaviors. *Pediatrics* 117: 1281–1290.

Nichol, M. E., W. Pickett, and I. Janssen. 2009. Associations between school recreational environments and physical activity. *J. Sch. Health* 79: 247–254.

Pate, R. R., G. W. Heath, M. Dowda et al. 1996. Associations between physical activity and other health behaviors in a representative sample of U.S. adolescents. *Am. J. Public Health* 86: 1577–1581.

Pate, R. R., and J. R. O'Neill. 2009. After-school interventions to increase physical activity among youth. *Br. J. Sports Med.* 43: 14–18.

Pate, R. R., R. Saunders, R. K. Dishman et al. 2007a. Long-term effects of a physical activity intervention in high school girls. *Am. J. Prev. Med.* 33: 276–280.

Pate, R. R., D. S. Ward, J. R. O'Neill et al. 2007b. Enrollment in physical education is associated with overall physical activity in adolescent girls. *Res. Q. Exerc. Sport* 78: 265–270.

Pate, R. R., D. S. Ward, R. P. Saunders et al. 2005. Promotion of physical activity among high-school girls: a randomized controlled trial. *Am. J. Public Health* 95: 1582–1587.

Ridgers, N. D., G. Stratton, and S. J. Fairclough. 2006. Physical activity levels of children during school playtime. *Sports Med.* 36: 359–371.

Ridgers, N. D., G. Stratton, S. J. Fairclough et al. 2007. Long-term effects of a playground markings and physical structures on children's recess physical activity levels. *Prev. Med.* 44: 393–397.

Robert Wood Johnson Foundation. 2007. Recess rules: Why the undervalued playtime may be America's best investment for healthy kids and schools. Princeton, NJ.

Robert Wood Johnson Foundation. 2009. Local school wellness policies: How are schools implementing the congressional mandate? In *Research Brief*.

Rosenberg, D. E., J. F. Sallis, T. L. Conway et al. 2006. Active transportation to school over 2 years in relation to weight status and physical activity. *Obesity (Silver Spring)* 14: 1771–1776.

Sallis, J. F., T. L. Conway, J. J. Prochaska et al. 2001. The association of school environments with youth physical activity. *Am. J. Public Health* 91: 618–620.

Sallis, J. F., T. L. McKenzie, J. F. Alcaraz et al. 1997. The effects of a 2-year physical education program (SPARK) on physical activity and fitness in elementary school students. Sports, Play and Active Recreation for Kids. *Am. J. Public Health* 87: 1328–1334.

Sallis, J. F., J. J. Prochaska, and W. C. Taylor. 2000. A review of correlates of physical activity of children and adolescents. *Med. Sci. Sports Exerc.* 32: 963–975.

Scott, M. M., D. A. Cohen, K. R. Evenson et al. 2007. Weekend schoolyard accessibility, physical activity, and obesity: The Trial of Activity in Adolescent Girls (TAAG) study. *Prev. Med.* 44: 398–403.

Sigfusdottir, I. D., A. L. Kristjansson, and J. P. Allegrante. 2007. Health behaviour and academic achievement in Icelandic school children. *Health Educ. Res.* 22: 70–80.

Simon, C., A. Wagner, C. DiVita et al. 2004. Intervention centred on adolescents' physical activity and sedentary behaviour (ICAPS): Concept and 6-month results. *Int. J. Obes. Relat. Metab. Disord.* 28: S96–S103.

Stratton, G., and E. Mullan. 2005. The effect of multicolor playground markings on children's physical activity level during recess. *Prev. Med.* 41: 828–833.

Trost, S. G., R. R. Rosenkranz, and D. Dzewaltowski. 2008. Physical activity levels among children attending after-school programs. *Med. Sci. Sports Exerc.* 40: 622–629.

Trudeau, F., and R. J. Shephard. 2008. Physical education, school physical activity, school sports and academic performance. *Int. J. Behav. Nutr. Phys. Act.* 5: 10.

U.S. Department of Education. 2007. *Digest of Education Statistics.* National Center for Education Statistics. Available at http://nces.ed.gov/programs/digest/d09/tables/dt09_033 .asp (accessed January 8, 2011).

Van Der Horst, K., M. J. Paw, J. W. Twisk et al. 2007. A brief review on correlates of physical activity and sedentariness in youth. *Med. Sci. Sports Exerc.* 39: 1241–1250.

van Sluijs, E. M., A. M. McMinn, and S. J. Griffin. 2007. Effectiveness of interventions to promote physical activity in children and adolescents: Systematic review of controlled trials. *BMJ* 335: 703.

Vaughn, A. E., S. C. Ball, L. A. Linnan et al. 2009. Promotion of walking for transportation: a report from the Walk to School day registry. *J. Phys. Act. Health* 6: 281–288.

Verstraete, S. J., G. M. Cardon, D. L. De Clercq et al. 2006. Increasing children's physical activity levels during recess periods in elementary schools: The effects of providing game equipment. *Eur. J. Public Health* 16: 415–419.

Voss, C., and G. Sandercock. 2010. Aerobic fitness and mode of travel to school in English schoolchildren. *Med. Sci. Sports Exerc.* 42: 281–287.

Willenberg, L. J., R. Ashbolt, D. Holland et al. 2010. Increasing school playground physical activity: A mixed methods study combining environmental measures and children's perspectives. *J. Sci. Med. Sport* 13: 210–216.

Young, D. R., J. A. Phillips, T. Yu et al. 2006. Effects of a life skills intervention for increasing physical activity in adolescent girls. *Arch. Pediatr. Adolesc. Med.* 160: 1255–1261.

Zygmunt-Fillwalk, E., and T. E. Bilello. 2005. Parents' victory in reclaiming recess for their children. *Childhood Educ.* 82:19(5). Available at FindArticles.com. 19 July 2011. http://findarticles.com/p/articles/mi_qa3614/is_200510/ai_n15715573/ (accessed July 19, 2011).

18 Policy for Physical Activity Promotion

Kelly R. Evenson and Semra A. Aytur

CONTENTS

INTRODUCTION

Recent history shows that policy can have a remarkable impact on population health (Brownson, Chriqui, and Stamatakis 2009). Many of the 10 major public health achievements of the twentieth century were attributable, at least in part, to policy changes (Centers for Disease Control and Prevention 1999). These include school policies requiring vaccinations, seatbelt laws to improve motor vehicle safety, and policies and regulations to create safer workplaces. This chapter considers the power of policy as a tool to promote physical activity.

Although most people realize that physical activity is good for their health, many do not attain the current recommended levels of physical activity (U.S. Department of Health and Human Services 2008). What makes integrating physical activity into daily routines so difficult? Researchers and public health practitioners recognize that many interrelated factors influence physical activity. The ecological framework of

TABLE 18.1
Five Levels of Ecological Framework, with Definitions and Examples

Level	Definition	Examples
1. Intrapersonal (individual)	Genetics, physiology, motivation, skill	Your genetic makeup, your ability to perform an activity (e.g., knowing how to swim), your intentions and motivation to make time for physical activity
2. Interpersonal, social, or cultural factors	Social or cultural factors, which include formal and informal social networks and support systems including family and friends	Having friends to exercise with, living in a family that exercises together, living in a culture that supports physical activity for both men and women
3. Institutional or organizational factors	The social and physical environment of workplaces, schools, government institutions, hospitals, and other organizations	Having gym facilities available at work or at school
4. Policy	Laws, regulations, ordinances, formal and informal rules, and agreements that can be developed either by government or by the private sector (e.g., worksites, hospitals)	Having a job that gives you a free gym membership (workplace policy), living in a city has a zoning ordinance to prevent low density development or protects open space for parks (city government policy), living in a state that allocates a percentage of transportation funds to support infrastructure for walking and bicycling (state government policy)
5. Community factors	The social and physical environment of neighborhoods and cities	Having sidewalks in your neighborhood, having bicycle paths connecting your neighborhood to your school, having safe and accessible parks and trials in your city/town

health behavior provides a way to understand these connections between people's behaviors and their environments.

The ecological framework has five general levels of influence (McLeroy et al. 1988; Sallis and Owen 1997). These five levels are described in Table 18.1 and shown in Figure 18.1; they include intrapersonal, interpersonal, institutional or organizational, policy, and community or environmental. The policy level is critical because policies can help produce behavior changes that individuals are unlikely to achieve by themselves. However, changing policy is challenging, and may require action by several decision makers, including those in private and public (governmental) sectors spanning local, state, and federal jurisdictions.

A person's choice to engage in physical activity may be influenced by a number of factors. These factors may work independently or together, across many levels of the ecologic framework, such that their effects accumulate or "add up." For example, a person who does not know how to swim lacks skills (intrapersonal), but this may have been influenced by having siblings who did not swim (interpersonal), living in a town without a public pool (community), or not having affordable swimming lessons (policy). All of these factors "add up" to create barriers to physical activity.

Policy interventions, especially when used along with community (environmental), interpersonal, and intrapersonal interventions, are promising strategies for increasing population levels of physical activity (Kahn et al. 2002; Heath et al. 2006; U.S. Department of Health and Human Services 2008). Yet, policy remains one of the least studied levels of the ecological framework (Schmid, Pratt, and Witmer 2006; Sallis and Owen 1997). This chapter will help you to understand how to harness the power of policy to promote physical activity.

SEDENTARY BEHAVIOR

Although the focus of this chapter is on physical activity behavior, it is important to note that policies may also directly target reducing sedentary behavior. Sedentary behavior includes activities such as sitting, lying down while watching television, or reading. A person who is physically active may or may not have high levels of sedentary behavior as well.

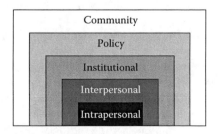

FIGURE 18.1   Five levels of the ecological framework.

DEFINING A PHYSICAL ACTIVITY POLICY

Policies can be defined as laws, regulations, formal and informal rules, codes, standards, and understandings or agreements that are adopted to guide both individual and group behavior (Schmid, Pratt, and Witmer 2006). Laws are made by legislative bodies, typically at the federal or state level. Regulations, rules, codes, and standards are usually made by local or state agencies responsible for carrying out the laws. Regulations and rules may also be drafted in the private sector for places such as worksites and hospitals. Informal understandings or agreements can occur anywhere.

Policies that affect physical activity can be grouped into three broad categories (Schmid, Pratt, and Witmer 2006):

1. The first category includes formal written laws, codes, or regulations bearing legal authority, such as a state law that affects the development of trails.
2. The second category includes standards that guide choices. Implementation of the policy may be accompanied by a written statement, explanation, or decision about the policy. Examples of written standards include a local (such as a city) pedestrian plan, bicycle plan, greenway or trail plan, or a system-wide park plan. Each of these plans can guide local decisions about policies, infrastructure, and programming, in turn affecting physical activities, such as walking or bicycling.
3. A third category includes social norms. Social norms are unwritten rules that guide appropriate and inappropriate attitudes, beliefs, values, and behaviors. For example, a workplace policy on using break time for physical activity may not be written in any documents, but norms may dictate whether walking outside during that time is acceptable or unacceptable workplace practice.

Policies that promote physical activity can be administered through many sectors, such as the workplace, school, or neighborhood, and also at different scales, such as in local, regional, state, or national domains (Schmid, Pratt, and Witmer 2006; Sallis et al. 2006). Table 18.2 provides some examples of policies operating through different sectors and scales to affect physical activity. The variety of sectors and scales demonstrates a wide range of settings outside of traditional health settings that may impact physical activity behavior. The population impact, as opposed to the impact on a single individual, of a change in policy on physical activity could vary depending on the sector and scale, such as a workplace, city, or county.

Policies may influence physical activity directly or indirectly. For example, requiring physical education in schools should have a direct or immediate effect on physical activity of children taking physical education classes. In contrast, a more indirect effect may result from a change to a state law such as "recreational user statutes" that allow the general public to use school facilities. By clarifying and reducing the liability risk for schools that allow use of their property for physical activity after hours, the law could assist more schools in providing access and ultimately increasing physical activity in the community.

TABLE 18.2

Examples of Policies Affecting Physical Activity by Sector and Scale

Sector	Scale	Examples
Health	Local	A local health department adopts a policy that all staff will be trained to conduct health impact assessments, and that equity will be considered in all decisions affecting health and the built environment
	Regional or State	State health departments and transportation departments agree to create a new staff position that will serve as a liaison between health and transportation planning
	National	The federal government mandates that health impact assessments be used for all major infrastructure decisions (e.g., highway or bridge expansions, new housing projects)
Recreation, parks, and public spaces	Local	A park master plan, designed to provide a vision and goals for the future of park planning in a local community
	Regional or State	Policies regarding coordination of park development when a large park exists in more than one county or municipality
	National	Money allocated from the federal government to support parks
School	Local	A school or school district changes their joint use policy to allow use of the grounds before or after school and on weekends for physical activity by community members
	Regional or State	Legislation to protect schools from liability when providing joint use of schools for physical activity
	National	National standards for physical education in public schools
Transportation	Local	Pedestrian plan, designed to provide a vision and goals for the future of walking in a local community
	Regional or State	Subsidy on transit passes
	National	Allocation of funding of pedestrian and bicycle projects
Worksite	Local	Norms regarding walking on work breaks
	Regional or State	State policy allowing physical activity during work breaks for governmental positions
	National	Federal workplace standards on building design that might impact physical activity, such as stair placement
Home	Local	Subdivision policy requiring developers to provide sidewalks in new developments
	Regional or State	Change in land use codes to allow for mixed use development
	National	National physical activity plan

PROMOTING PHYSICAL ACTIVITY THROUGH POLICIES

Policies that promote or inhibit physical activity can be grouped into at least four categories (Dunton, Cousineau, and Reynolds 2010):

1. Policies can promote or inhibit physical activity by increasing or decreasing opportunities. For example, following guidance from a bicycle and

pedestrian plan, retrofitting a road to include bicycle lanes and sidewalks could enhance bicycling and walking. In contrast, retrofitting a road to move vehicles more quickly would inhibit opportunities for bicycling and walking. City governments use certain policies that allow them to build sidewalks and bicycle paths. For example, a policy called a "zoning ordinance" specifies where a bicycle path can be built and how land can be used (Schilling and Linton 2005). Policies also include allocating money through government agencies for specific purposes (e.g., setting aside money from the city transportation budget that can be used to build the bicycle path).

2. Policies can promote or inhibit physical activity by offering incentives or disincentives for the behavior. As an example, worksites may have a policy to offer free passes for public transportation, which encourages walking from the transit stop to the worksite. In contrast, a policy to provide free parking to workers may be viewed as a disincentive to walk or bicycle to work or to use public transportation.

3. Policies can promote or inhibit physical activity by regulating what types of behavior are allowed in certain places. Examples include pedestrian-oriented streets and Ciclovía programs that close streets or lanes to vehicles on certain days to allow walking and bicycling (Sarmiento et al. 2010). Policy decisions usually are made to help make the necessary changes to the streets and to allow street closures when the Ciclovía program occurs. An example of a policy that prohibits physical activity would be one that closes schools after hours, prohibiting physical activity on school grounds.

4. Policies can promote physical activity by providing information about the behavior. For example, a health curriculum at a school might be changed to provide more education about the benefits of lifetime physical activity.

The process of bringing together citizens to tackle a policy issue, can be health promoting (Brisson and Roll 2008). Partnerships and bonds formed can build ties in the community and enhance the capacity of community members to address health problems, such as lack of physical activity.

Lessons learned from other countries can be especially helpful when considering promotion of physical activity through policy change. For example, researchers found that Germany and the Netherlands have markedly reduced the number of pedestrian and bicyclist deaths over the past 25 years by implementing a wide range of policies to improve safety (Pucher and Dijkstra 2003). In these countries, policy was used to create autofree zones that cover much of the city center, provide well-lit sidewalks on both sides of the street, expand a network of bicycle paths in both urban and rural areas, provide pedestrian refuge islands for crossing streets, and install pedestrian-activated crossing signals. Additionally, these countries are increasing the number of "bicycle streets," where cars are permitted but cyclists have strict right-of-way over the entire breadth of the roadway.

PUBLIC HEALTH PRACTITIONERS

Public health practitioners are engaging more with people in other disciplines, to address physical activity policy and seek ways to accomplish overlapping goals. For example, both public health professionals and urban planners are interested in walking and bicycling, the latter typically with a focus on health promotion and the former from a transportation perspective (Evenson et al. 2011). Working together, the two professions can identify overlapping goals and develop interdisciplinary, creative solutions. The National Society for Physical Activity Practitioners in Public Health is a professional organization that can help practitioners in this process (Newkirk 2010). This organization is dedicated to growing the capacity of physical activity practitioners in public health, which include professionals from health promotion and education, public health, exercise science and exercise physiology, and physical education (website: http://www.nspapph.org).

UNDERSTANDING THE POLICY PROCESS

Policy making to promote physical activity can be a complicated process. Tools from the field of policy analysis will help better explain the process. Policy analysis has been explained as determining what decision-makers do, why they do it, and what difference it makes (Dye 1976). There are many different approaches to policy analysis (Coveney 2010; Sabatier and Jenkins-Smith 1993; Bacchi 1999), with overlapping concepts between the approaches. Two policy analysis approaches are highlighted.

MULTIPLE STREAMS FRAMEWORK

One approach focuses on the timing of critical events around the policy process. For example, Kingdon's (2003) multiple streams framework focuses on the timing of policy actions. Kingdon's framework underscores the existence of three distinct, but complementary, processes, or "streams," in policy making, known as the "problem," "policy," and "political" streams.

Problem Stream

In this stream, a given situation has to be publicly recognized as a "problem" before it can be addressed through policy. Conversely, a situation not defined as a problem, and for which alternatives are never proposed, will not be converted into a policy issue.

Policy Stream

This stream focuses on how an issue rises or falls on the political agenda. It includes the formulation of different policy options (policy alternatives) and proposals to develop solutions to the problem.

Political Stream

This stream focuses on the willingness of various political decision-makers to place an issue on the agenda, so that action may be taken. Political events, such as an impending election or a change in government, can affect the presence of a given topic or policy on the agenda.

Kingdon (2003) proposes that the convergence of these streams creates a "window of opportunity," at a given time and in a given context, for a particular issue to become policy. This framework aims to explain why some issues and problems make it onto the policy agenda and are eventually translated into policies, whereas others do not.

In one example of how to use the policy analysis process, researchers considered the three streams—problem, policy, and political—to better understand how the adoption of a policy affected daily physical activity in schools in Alberta, Canada (Gladwin, Church, and Plotnikoff 2008). Higher levels of obesity and lack of physical activity were recognized as a "problem." Support came from scientific evidence that linked daily physical activity to favorable educational outcomes (Active Living Research 2009) and from many teachers. They favored the policy change because aspects of the implementation were left up to the individual teacher and no rigid requirements were imposed on them. A physician who took office as the Minister of Learning supported the policy change and framed the issue as highly important, emphasizing the need for increased physical activity in the school setting. He was able to take advantage of the "window of opportunity" to succeed in changing policy by proposing an educational sector solution.

STAGES OF THE POLICY PROCESS

Another approach to policy analysis is the stage approach, which focuses more specifically on different stages of the policy process, rather than on the timing of the three streams. Policy scholars have developed several different "staged" frameworks, each with specific ways of conceptualizing the stages (Brownson et al. 2006; Laswell 1971; Bridgman and Davis 2002; Clark 2002). For example, a six-stage framework on the policy process is summarized in Figure 18.2 (Anderson 2006; Brownson et al. 2010). These stages are explored in more detail next. Because there is overlap between these stages and the "streams" highlighted in Kingdon's (2003) approach, terms from both approaches will be used.

Step 1: Policy Agenda Setting

The first step is to identify an issue that is a problem worthy of placing on the policy agenda. What policy that affects physical activity will be the focus for change? This is similar to Kingdon's multiple streams framework (Kingdon 2003), in which agenda setting is viewed as a political, competitive process among different interest groups to gain the attention of the media, the public, and policymakers.

To help make the case for why a problem merits attention, public health practitioners can present data on the scope of a problem. Public health surveillance data (such as the Behavioral Risk Factor Surveillance System in the United States; http://www.cdc.gov/brfss/) on physical activity will help indicate population groups who

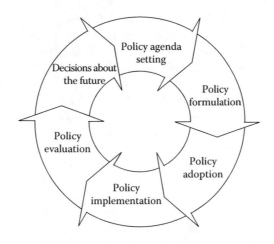

FIGURE 18.2 A six-stage framework on the policy process. (From Anderson, J., *Public Policymaking*, 6th ed, Houghton Mifflin Company, Boston, 2006; Brownson, R. C. et al., *Ann. Epidemiol.*, 20, 436–444, 2010. With permission.)

are less active. Clinical and epidemiologic studies can identify the reasons why it is important to be active, and intervention studies can indicate the best strategies to focus on when making a change in policy. As the needs of policy makers change over time, the supporting studies and evidence may change as well (Bauman et al. 2006).

Step 2: Policy Formulation

The second step in the policy process is to determine and consider alternative policies, called "policy formulation." In this stage, the development of the policy should consider the evidence, guidelines, or scientific studies to formulate a policy that is based on the best available evidence. In public health, evidence includes both quantitative data (e.g., statistical) and qualitative information (e.g., stories, narrative accounts, and case studies). Data that support legislative change often include the level of public support for a particular issue, relevance at the local (such as voting district) level, and anecdotal data that personalize an issue through compelling stories about how lives are affected. Scientists and policymakers may disagree about which types of evidence are considered most relevant. Scientists generally favor numerical data, whereas policymakers often prefer stories and visual images.

Step 3: Policy Adoption

The third step in the policy process is "policy adoption," or getting the policy enacted or "passed" by an authoritative body (such as the legislature). Factors such as public opinion, organized political forces (e.g., interest groups, lobbyists), changes in governmental participants such as legislative or administrative turnover, election results, jurisdictional boundaries between governmental agencies, and the necessity of compromise all affect policy adoption (McGinnis 2001; Kingdon 2003). The following examples illustrate this point.

In the United States, researchers examined factors associated with state-level childhood obesity prevention legislation from 2003 to 2005, which included legislation on physical activity and nutrition. Topics included physical education, health education, safe routes to school, walking and bicycle paths, nutrition and vending machine standards, menu labeling, and soda and snack tax (Boehmer et al. 2008). The factors associated with an increased likelihood of state policy adoption included: having multiple bipartisan sponsors (supported by both major political parties) versus a single sponsor, having budget proposals (examples include line items designating funds for walking or bicycling trails), being introduced in the state Senate (versus the House), and having content areas related to safe routes to school, walking/biking trails, model school policies (such as those that propose changes to state curriculum requirements for nutrition, health, or physical education classes), and statewide initiatives (such as the establishment of school wellness councils). At the state level, political factors related to policy adoption included having 2-year legislative sessions (rather than single-year sessions) and Democratic control of both the House and the Senate. Researchers also examined factors that enabled and impeded state-level childhood obesity prevention legislation from 2005 to 2006 (Dodson et al. 2009). Factors that positively influenced the passage of legislation included gaining the support of key individuals or groups, including parents, physicians, and schools, national media exposure, and introduction of the policy by senior legislators. Factors that negatively influenced passing of obesity-related state legislation included powerful lobbyists, program costs, and misconceptions about legislating foods at schools.

Step 4: Policy Implementation

The fourth step in the policy process is "policy implementation." Implementation is the process of carrying out the policy and enforcing it in places such as cities, towns, schools, daycare centers, worksites, or parks. Often, the implementers of a policy are not the same groups as those who adopted or authorized the policy. For example, a state legislature may adopt a policy mandating that physical activity is to be integrated into school curricula. It is up to the schools to implement the policy, meaning that school boards, principles, teachers, parents, and students all have roles in implementation. Little is known about which policy approach provides the greatest physical activity benefit and when it should be implemented, regardless of the sector of interest.

One study conducted in Montgomery County, Maryland, identified a variety of factors related to the successful implementation of local physical activity policies (Salvesen et al. 2008). The findings suggested that knowledge and awareness, commitment of staff, funding, intergovernmental coordination, the presence of an advocate or champion, and conflict influence physical activity policy implementation at the local level.

Research suggests that a federal act passed in 2004 to require wellness policy development was implemented differently across states. The U.S. Department of Agriculture Child Nutrition and WIC (Women, Infants, and Children) Reauthorization Act (public law 108-265) required schools participating in federal school meal programs to develop a local wellness policy that would include goals for physical activity, nutrition education, and other school-based activities designed to promote student wellness and establish a plan for measuring implementation of the local wellness policy, beginning in 2006 and 2007. This federal policy resulted in most public school systems in the country having such a policy "on the books," but these policies are not being equally implemented and enforced (Chriqui et al. 2009, 2010).

Step 5: Policy Evaluation

The fifth step in the process involves an assessment or appraisal of how the policy is being implemented and whether it is achieving its purpose. This stage is called "policy evaluation." Evaluation of policies that affect physical activity is very important. For example, policymakers often need data to show their constituents (those they represent) that a policy is worth the time and money spent on it, because resources are generally limited. If policy change is to be embraced by key decision-makers, such as those making the policies, convincing data can help show that a policy will impact physical activity. Evaluation can provide feedback to determine which policies are working and thus whether they should be supported in a given setting. Combined with economic tools, it can also help determine the most cost-effective policy.

Creating a healthy environment, which makes the healthy choice the easier choice, often requires a complex set of activities in many different sectors. Because many forces influence whether a policy is adopted, implemented, and sustained, it can be difficult to measure or evaluate whether policies are really working. It can be even more difficult to evaluate why they are or are not working.

There are two broad types of evaluation to consider in assessing physical activity policy change. The first is process evaluation, which focuses on the quality and implementation of ongoing activities and interventions. This type of evaluation includes documenting the components of the intervention and assessing whether the planned intervention activities match what actually happens. It documents all aspects of implementation so that adjustments can be made if needed. Process evaluation addresses questions such as

- Is the policy being implemented as intended? Is it reaching the target audience?
- Are we on track with time and resources?
- Are partnerships supporting the policy change working together effectively?
- What is working well and why? What is not working well and why?
- Should we be doing anything differently?

The second is outcome evaluation, which concentrates on assessing whether the policy achieved its purpose or intent by focusing on short-, intermediate-, or long-term outcomes or goals. Outcome evaluation should build on the process evaluation. Outcome evaluation addresses questions such as

- Did the policy change impact physical activity behavior or other outcome indicators?
- Were there any unintended effects of the policy change?
- What outside influences could have enhanced or hindered the expected outcomes?
- Is the policy change more effective than alternative policy changes (including doing nothing) on the outcomes of interest?

Depending on which stage of the policy process is of primary interest, and the resources available, it may be necessary to focus on process evaluation or outcome evaluation, or both.

An example of outcome evaluation applied to physical activity policy comes from a U.S. nationwide study (Cawley, Meyerhoefer, and Newhouse 2007) that examined the impact of state physical education requirements (the policy of focus) on several outcomes of interest, including physical activity during physical education. Researchers found that high school students living in states with a binding physical education requirement reported an average of 31 additional minutes per week being physically active in physical education classes as compared to high school students living in states without the requirement.

Although the goal in policy change may be to increase physical activity, it is important to consider the unintended consequences of a policy change. Policy evaluation can help highlight these unintended consequences. As an example, new sidewalks may be built in wealthier neighborhoods where residents are organized and politically active, but in a less timely way in lower-income neighborhoods that may not have as much influence. Thus, policy evaluation should be sensitive to possible differential effects on population subgroups, such as whether policy changes maintain, increase, or decrease health disparities.

There are often challenges to successful process and outcome evaluation, two of which are highlighted here. First, evaluation costs money and may take away money that could be spent on other aspects of the policy process. Sometimes outcome evaluation is not conducted or instead is conducted on short-term indicators that might be easier and cheaper to collect than the long-term indicator or goal that various parties are trying to change. Second, evaluation should be planned earlier rather than later in the process. To fully understand the process and impact of policy change on physical activity, data collection could start as the policy is designed and continue through its implementation.

To better understand these terms, we apply them to a hypothetical project that is intended to favorably impact physical activity. The project is to change joint use policies at schools that allow community members to use the schools after hours, and to promote the changes among residents who live near the schools. The process indicator includes documentation of changes in joint use policies during the intervention period. For the outcome evaluation, the project might conduct a random survey of people who live near the school to determine if they used the school property for physical activity, and if their levels of physical activity changed as a result of the policy. However, this may prove to be expensive and time consuming for the project. Alternatively, short-term outcome indicators could be assessed, such as observations of outdoor physical activity among community members on the school property both before and after the policy changes. These short-term indicators are expected to precede changes in resident levels of physical activity.

In addition to numerous challenges to successful evaluation, there may be times when sufficient evaluation evidence is not available to make a decision. When this happens, one of the considerations is the lost opportunity to do something different with that effort and money, called opportunity cost (Brownson et al. 2010). The opportunity cost can be critical in policy discussions and certainly applies to physical activity policy.

Step 6: Decisions about the Future

The sixth and final step in the policy process is to decide if the policy should continue based on the evaluation evidence. In some cases, it may make sense to modify or terminate the policy if physical activity or some other indicator of success has not improved. In other cases, the evidence might indicate that the policy should continue. This illustrates the need to regularly reevaluate the policy agenda and consider alternative policies.

The stages in the policy process are cyclical, but the policy process can be subject to competing demands and shifting priorities. Although Figure 18.2 indicates that each stage progresses into the next stage, the reality is that there are times when stages are skipped, the process ends early and must start over, or stages have to be repeated several times before progress is made. Public health professionals have many choices of policy analysis frameworks to apply to physical activity policy, several of which were highlighted in this section. Often, the specific context and the aspects of policy that are of particular interest will guide the choice.

TOOLS FOR TAKING ACTION

Public health professionals have many choices of policy analysis frameworks to apply to physical activity policy, several of which were highlighted in this section: the community action model, which helps to consider how policy works together with other factors to influence healthy behavior; the RE-AIM framework (Reach, Effectiveness, Adoption, Implementation, Maintenance), which helps to consider how a policy change will reach different groups of people and whom it is likely to benefit the most; and health impact assessment (HIA), which also considers the potential health impacts of a proposed policy on different groups of people (even if the policy is in a "nonmedical" sector like transportation or agriculture). Often, the specific context and the aspects of policy that are of particular interest will guide the choice of which approach to use.

COMMUNITY ACTION MODEL

When considering changing policy to promote physical activity, it is important to consider how the process works, and what factors might enhance success. The community action model describes five strategies to influence change in communities around physical activity (Bors et al. 2009). Known as the "5 Ps," these include not only policy, but also preparation, promotions, programs, and physical projects. The five Ps (Jilcott et al. 2007; Glasgow et al. 2006) are defined in Table 18.3. Preparation includes taking the time to gather information and plan for the physical activity initiative. Promotions include the development of messages and materials to educate the general public and key decision makers and leaders around the physical activity topic. Programs involve organized activities to increase physical activity and physical projects, create opportunities for, or remove barriers to physical activity.

These five Ps provide direction to interventions that address factors influencing physical activity across multiple levels of the ecologic framework (McLeroy et al. 1988; Sallis and Owen 1997). In working with the five Ps, the effect of using all of

TABLE 18.3

Community Action Model: Defining the Five Strategies and Providing a Walk to School Example

Strategies	Definition	Walk to School Example
Preparation	The time deliberately taken to lay the groundwork for an initiative and to strategize ways to reinforce plans for action	Gathering information and materials, planning promotional messages, garnering support for the project
Promotions	Include the development of messages and materials through the media and are an important way to educate the public, as well as to gain buy-in from community leaders, key decision makers, and the public	News media coverage, notification of changes through an automated calling system to parents, pedestrian, and bicycle safety activities
Programs	Involve organized activities that either directly or indirectly engage individuals in physical activity	Participating in Walk to School Day, walking program
Physical projects	Create opportunities for or remove barriers to physical activity	Sidewalks added on routes that lead to the school, bicycle racks installed at the school
Policies	Laws, regulations, ordinances, formal and informal rules and agreements that can be developed either by government or by the private sector	Implementing no transport zone policies and safety policies, funding

them simultaneously is expected to be greater than using one or a few of the strategies. Focusing only on policy change, while ignoring the necessary preparation and the opportunities for promotions, programs, and physical projects, is probably a less effective means of intervening on physical activity.

A case study tested this assumption by comparing the success of walk to school initiatives at two different elementary schools (Fesperman et al. 2008). Examples of the different strategies according to the five Ps can be found in Table 18.3. Both schools used similar strategies including promotions, policies, and physical projects; however, only one of the elementary schools used all five strategies. The scope and duration of these strategies varied by school and ultimately influenced their success. The application of the community action model suggested intervention efforts were maximized when multiple strategies were used rather than just focusing on one strategy, such as policy.

RE-AIM FRAMEWORK

Various frameworks have been used to conceptualize the impact of public health interventions, including policy interventions to increase physical activity. The RE-AIM framework provides guidance on evaluating interventions (Glasgow et al. 2006) and has been specifically applied for policy and environmental evaluation (Jilcott et al. 2007; King, Glasgow, and Leeman-Castillo 2010). The definitions and an example are provided in Table 18.4. To use the RE-AIM framework, four questions could be answered: (1) Whose health is to be improved as a result of the policy? (2) What organization or governing body is responsible for passing or adopting the policy? (3) Who is responsible for adhering to or complying with the policy? (4) What organization, institution, or governing body is responsible for enforcing the policy?

TABLE 18.4
RE-AIM Framework Applied to Physical Activity Policy

Framework Component	Definition Applied to Policy	Example
Reach	The number, proportion, and representativeness of people who are willing to participate or are affected by a policy	A city government allocates money to build a bicycle path from a downtown neighborhood to a nearby office complex. Who would have access to the bicycle path? Although the path might benefit the office workers, would it reach other persons who may be at higher risk of lack of physical activity?
Effectiveness	Measures of impact on outcomes and unintended consequences of the policy	To measure the effectiveness of the new bicycle path, one could measure whether higher percentages of office workers commute by bike after the path is built compared to before. The percentage of the population bicycling in the surrounding lower-income neighborhoods could also be measured. Consider that even if the rate of bicycling in lower income neighborhoods remains unchanged, but bicycling increases among the office workers, health disparities would actually have gotten worse (unintended consequence).
Adoption	The number, proportion, and representativeness of settings that adopt the policy	In this example, the city adopted the policy by allocating funds and distributing infrastructure; the wealthier neighborhood and the office complex benefit from the policy.
Implementation	The extent to which the policy change is implemented as intended and the time and cost	Imagine that halfway through the project, city funds ran low and the cost of completing the project were higher than anticipated, resulting in only half of the bicycle path being paved. This is an example of a policy that was not fully implemented.
Maintenance	The extent to which the policy becomes institutionalized or part of routine practice and policy	If the bicycle path was built, how will it be maintained over time? Did the city allocate money for maintenance? If the new bike path did result in more office workers riding their bikes to work after the path was built, are those behavior changes sustained over many years?

HEALTH IMPACT ASSESSMENT

HIA is another framework that can bring an equity focus to policy decisions (Dannenberg et al. 2008). HIA is set of procedures, methods, and tools by which a policy, program, or project may be judged as to its potential effects on the health of a population and the distribution of those effects within the population (http://www.cdc.gov/healthyplaces/hia.htm). HIA can be used to assess the potential health effects of a policy or project before it is implemented. For example, in Humboldt County, California, HIA was used to update a rural county's General Plan (a planning document that guides future growth and building in the community; more information at http://www.humpal.org) (Harris et al. 2009). As a rural area, Humboldt County was considering three different development plans to accommodate future population growth, ranging from limiting growth in urban areas to sprawl. The HIA process successfully identified and analyzed potential health outcomes associated with each development plan, including the impact on transportation modes such as walking and bicycling. The HIA process raised awareness of health impacts related to planning decisions among county agencies, project decision-makers, participating community members, and the public. As this example illustrates, potential public health impacts can be brought into the decision-making process for plans, projects, and policies that might impact physical activity that fall outside of traditional public health arenas, including transportation, land use, and housing.

POLICY DISSEMINATION

According to the Institute of Medicine (Institute of Medicine 1997), the goals of dissemination are to inform the public about health-related matters and to provide information regarding effective prevention programs (and in this case policies) to health officials and community leaders. Currently, there is very little research on the dissemination of evidence-based physical activity interventions, especially those targeting policy (Bauman et al. 2006) and underserved populations (Yancey, Ory, and Davis 2006). However, we can learn from other types of public health interventions. For example, efforts aimed at reducing tobacco use in the United States over the past half century have been successful. Tobacco-control activities began with efforts to influence individual smokers (intrapersonal level), primarily through education and counteradvertising. Over time, awareness grew about the addictive properties of tobacco. Public health and legal strategies increasingly focused on exposing the industry's efforts to manipulate and conceal information regarding the harmful effects of nicotine, the dangers of second-hand smoke, and their marketing to youth. As social norms changed, the public supported additional policy changes to include community interventions, legal actions, and sanctions against the tobacco industry (Green et al. 2006).

Researchers have identified several steps in the dissemination of public health interventions (Cuijpers, de Graaf, and Bohlmeijer 2005). These steps include (1) identification of potentially effective interventions (through systematic literature searches or reviews); (2) assessing the levels of evidence and using appropriate criteria to determine which interventions or policies should be recommended for adoption; and

(3) deciding whether the intervention or policy can be successfully implemented in other contexts, with diverse populations. For example, a policy that is very effective in one state may not be politically or economically feasible in another. Successful dissemination requires a delicate balance between being sensitive to local values, while simultaneously recognizing that there may be a range of different opinions within a given community about any policy issue (Yancey, Ory, and Davis 2006).

POLICY COMMUNICATION

Dissemination requires the use of a variety of communication channels to reach different groups of people. For example, public health professionals may receive information through presentations at national conferences, peer-reviewed publications, and websites. Community members may receive information through town meetings or special training sessions. Both community members and policy makers may prefer concise summaries in the form of policy briefs that can convey a message succinctly. Stories or narratives are often used to affect legislator decision-making as well (Stamatakis, McBride, and Brownson 2010). More recently, photos of the environment, using a technique called photovoice, have been used effectively to change decisions about policies and environments related to physical activity (Kramer et al. 2010).

When thinking about who to communicate with about a policy concern, consider who has the authority to change policy. The first people that may come to mind are local, regional, state, or national policy makers and their staff. However, consider the sector (e.g., health, parks and recreation, schools, transportation, worksite, home) where the focus will be. Other people to target could include principals, school board members, worksite managers, or park and recreation directors, depending on the sector.

If the focus is on policy makers and their staff, consider the danger of information overload while they try to become experts in a topic area. It may be your role to provide them with clear, brief summaries of what is known regarding the particular physical activity policy you are trying to change or sustain. Moreover, the data presented will often be more compelling if it can match the target area and include maps, pictures, or stories. For example, if the focus is on a county-level policy change, then providing county-related health statistics would be most useful, especially in comparison to other neighboring counties.

CONCLUSION

Physical activity is a complex, multifaceted behavior that impacts a wide range of health outcomes. Physical activity may be favorably or unfavorably impacted by policies, both written and unwritten. Considering the ecologic framework, policy remains one of the least studied levels, yet perhaps one of the most influential on physical activity. This chapter offered tools for analyzing policy and for understanding different stages of the policy process. Evaluating policy changes that affect physical activity is important, so that the evidence base can be improved and interventions can be more successful. Public health professionals have many opportunities to become involved in policy, and a public health voice is increasingly sought in diverse policy decisions ranging from transportation to housing. Understanding how physical activity is influenced by policy can lead to more effective strategies to promote physical activity, with the ultimate goal of improving the health of all people.

STUDY QUESTIONS

1. Choose one sector as shown in Table 18.2 and describe new examples of policies that might affect physical activity at the local, regional, and national levels.
2. Choose a different sector as shown in Table 18.2 and generate examples that describe the four categories of policies that can be used to promote physical activity. For more information, review the "Promoting Physical Activity through Policies" section of this chapter.
3. Repeat the exercise in question no. 2 for policies to reduce sedentary behaviors.
4. Imagine that you are the public health director of a local health department in a low-income, rural county. Use the community action model's five Ps (preparation, promotions, programs, physical projects, and policy) as shown in Table 18.3 to develop a comprehensive strategy to increase physical activity in the county over the next 5 years. Consider that the county has no public transportation system, one small park littered with trash, five elementary schools, one high school, one hospital, and one community health center. There are no bicycle paths, and only a few poorly maintained sidewalks in the downtown area. There is no public swimming pool, but there is a pool in one of the high schools. A large number of retired people live in the county. There is also a growing population of immigrants who have recently settled in the county; many of them have young children. As you develop your strategy, think about how you will address the needs of these different groups of people, at multiple levels of the ecological framework. Since resources are limited, you may have to make difficult decisions about what to prioritize. What process will you use to make these decisions? For additional readings on the Community Action Model, see Bors et al. (2009) and Fesperman et al. (2008).
5. Choose a policy that affects a physical activity behavior that you would like to change. Identify the decision-makers who can change the policy. Describe the pros and cons to changing the policy. Consider whether the policy change might have unintended consequences.
6. Imagine that you are working in a local health department, and you have been asked to talk with a local high school about adopting a joint-use policy that would allow community residents to use the school track and sports facilities during nonschool hours. Your supervisor has told you to use a policy analysis framework to guide your discussion and to inform future activities if the policy is adopted. Using the six-stage framework outlined in this chapter, apply it following the steps from beginning to end. In addition, use the RE-AIM to develop your evaluation plan as shown in Table 18.4. For additional reading on the six-stage framework, see Brownson et al. (2010). For additional readings on RE-AIM, see Glasgow et al. (2006), Jilcott et al. (2007), and King, Glasgow, and Leeman-Castillo (2010).

7. Consider the choices you made today about whether to engage in physical activity. Describe how policy may have affected your choice, either directly or indirectly. For example, did you go to a gym or athletic center on campus? Did you pay to use the gym? Did you play on an intramural sports team or club? *Hint*: If you are a student at a university, a policy was probably created that allowed the use of the athletic facilities for intramural sports, which includes paying staff to keep the facility open and being willing to take on the insurance risk that some students might get hurt while playing sports. How did you travel to classes? Did you walk, ride a bike, take a bus, drive, or use a combination of these? Why did you make that choice? Do you have safety concerns about walking or riding your bike from your residence to your classroom? *Hint*: Policies determine where sidewalks are built and how they are maintained, as well as whether safety officers patrol the area.

8. There may be times when sufficient evaluation evidence is not available to make a public health related decision. Provide an example, using the physical activity literature as a guide, of a situation where the "opportunity cost" would need to be considered.

ACKNOWLEDGMENTS

We thank Sara Satinsky and Drs. Barbara Ainsworth, Carol Macera, and Ross Brownson for helpful comments on earlier drafts of this chapter.

REFERENCES

Active Living Research. 2009. Active education: physical education, physical activity and academic performance. San Diego, CA. Available at: http://www.activelivingresearch .org/files/Active_Ed_Summer2009.pdf., Robert Wood Johnson Foundation (accessed October 25, 2010).

Anderson, J. 2006. *Public Policymaking*, 6th ed. Boston: Houghton Mifflin Company.

Bacchi, C. 1999. *Women, Policy, and Politics: The Construction of Policy Problems*. Thousand Oaks, CA: Sage.

Bauman, A. E., D. E. Nelson, M. Pratt et al. 2006. Dissemination of physical activity evidence, programs, policies, and surveillance in the international public health arena. *Am. J. Prev. Med.* 31: S57–S65.

Boehmer, T. K., D. A. Luke, D. L. Haire-Joshu et al. 2008. Preventing childhood obesity through state policy. Predictors of bill enactment. *Am. J. Prev. Med.* 34: 333–340.

Bors, P., M. Dessauer, R. Bell et al. 2009. The Active Living by Design national program: Community initiatives and lessons learned. *Am. J. Prev. Med.* 37: S313–S321.

Bridgman, P., and G. Davis. 2002. *The Australian Policy Handbook*. Crows Nest, Australia: Allen and Unwin.

Brisson, D., and S. Roll. 2008. An adult education model of resident participation: Building community capacity and strengthening neighborhood-based activities in a comprehensive community initiative. *Adv. Soc. Work* 9: 157–175.

Brownson, R. C., J. F. Chriqui, C. R. Burgeson et al. 2010. Translating epidemiology into policy to prevent childhood obesity: The case for promoting physical activity in school settings. *Ann. Epidemiol.* 20: 436–444.

Brownson, R. C., C. Royer, R. Ewing et al. 2006. Researchers and policymakers: Travelers in parallel universes. *Am. J. Prev. Med.* 30: 164–172.

Brownson, R. C., J. F. Chriqui, and K. A. Stamatakis. 2009. Policy, politics, and collective action: Understanding evidence-based public health policy. *Am. J. Public Health* 99: 1576–1583.

Cawley, J., C. Meyerhoefer, and D. Newhouse. 2007. The impact of state physical education requirements on youth physical activity and overweight. *Health Econ.* 16: 1287–1301.

Centers for Disease Control and Prevention. 1999. Ten great public health achievements— United States, 1900–1999. *MMWR Morb. Mortal. Wkly. Rep.* 48: 1141–1147.

Chriqui, J. F., L. Schneider, F. J. Chaloupka et al. 2010. *School District Wellness Policies: Evaluating Progress and Potential for Improving Children's Health Three Years after the Federal Mandate. School Years 2006–07, 2007–08 and 2008–09*, Vol. 2. Chicago, IL: Bridging the Gap Program, Health Policy Center, Institute for Health Research and Policy, University of Illinois at Chicago. Accessed October 1, 2010 at http://www .bridgingthegapresearch.org/_asset/r08bgt/WP_2010_report.pdf.

Chriqui, J. F., L. Schneider, F. H. Chaloupka et al. 2009. *Local Wellness Policies. Assessing School District Strategies for Improving Children's Health. School Years 2006–07 and 2007–08*. Chicago, IL: Bridging the Gap, Health Policy Center, Institute for Health Research and Policy, University of Illinois at Chicago.

Clark, T. 2002. *The Policy Process: A Practical Guide for Natural Resource Professionals*. New Haven, CT: Yale University Press.

Coveney, J. 2010. Analyzing public health policy: Three approaches. *Health Promot. Pract.* 11: 515–521.

Cuijpers, P., I. de Graaf, and E. Bohlmeijer. 2005. Adapting and disseminating effective public health interventions in another country: Towards a systematic approach. *Eur. J. Public Health* 15: 166–169.

Dannenberg, A. L., R. Bhatia, B. L. Cole et al. 2008. Use of health impact assessment in the U.S.: 27 case studies, 1999–2007. *Am. J. Prev. Med.* 34: 241–256.

Dodson, E. A., C. Fleming, T. K. Boehmer et al. 2009. Preventing childhood obesity through state policy: Qualitative assessment of enablers and barriers. *J. Public Health Policy* 30: S161–S176.

Dunton, G. F., M. Cousineau, and K. D. Reynolds. 2010. The intersection of public policy and health behavior theory in the physical activity arena. *J. Phys. Act. Health* 7: S91–S98.

Dye, T. 1976. *Policy Analysis*. Tuscaloosa, AL: University of Alabama.

Evenson, K. R., S. Satinsky, D. A. Rodriguez et al. 2011. Exploring a public health perspective on pedestrian planning in North Carolina. *Health Promot. Pr.*: doi:10.1177/ 1524839910381699. Epub ahead of print.

Fesperman, C., K. R. Evenson, D. A. Rodriguez et al. 2008. A comparative case study on active transport to and from school. *Prev. Chronic Dis.* 5, Available at: http://www.cdc .gov/pcd/issues/2008/apr/07_0064.htm.

Gladwin, C. P., J. Church, and R. C. Plotnikoff. 2008. Public policy processes and getting physical activity into Alberta's urban schools. *Can. J. Public Health* 99: 332–338.

Glasgow, R. E., L. M. Klesges, D. A. Dzewaltowski et al. 2006. Evaluation the overall impact of health promotion programs: Using the RE-AIM framework to form summary measures for decision making involving complex issues. *Health Educ. Res.* 21: 688–694.

Green, L. W., C. T. Orleans, J. M. Ottoson et al. 2006. Inferring strategies for disseminating physical activity policies, programs, and practices from the successes of tobacco control. *Am. J. Prev. Med.* 31: S66–S681.

Harris, E. C., A. Lindsay, J. C. Heller et al. 2009. Humboldt County general plan update health impact assessment: A case study. *Environ. Justice* 2: 127–134.

Heath, G. W., R. C. Brownson, J. Kruger et al. 2006. The effectiveness of urban design and land use and transport policies and practices to increase physical activity: A systematic review. *J. Phys. Act. Health* 3: S55–S76.

Institute of Medicine. 1997. *Linking Research to Public Health Practice. A Review of the CDC's Program of Centers for Research and Demonstration of Health Promotion and Disease Prevention.* Washington, D.C.: National Academy Press.

Jilcott, S., A. Ammerman, J. Sommers et al. 2007. Applying the RE-AIM framework to assess the public health impact of policy change *Ann. Behav. Med.* 34: 105–114.

Kahn, E. B., L. T. Ramsey, R. C. Brownson et al. 2002. The effectiveness of interventions to increase physical activity: A systematic review. *Am. J. Prev. Med.* 22: 73–107.

King, D. K., R. E. Glasgow, and B. Leeman-Castillo. 2010. Reaiming RE-AIM: Using the model to plan, implement, and evaluate the effects of environmental change approaches to enhancing population health. *Am. J. Public Health* 100: 2076–2084.

Kingdon, J. W. 2003. *Agendas, Alternatives, and Public Policies.* New York Addison-Wesley Educational Publishers.

Kramer, L., P. Schwartz, A. Cheadle et al. 2010. Promoting policy and environmental change using photovoice in the Kaiser Permanente Community Health Initiative. *Health Promot. Pract.* 11: 332–339.

Laswell, H. 1971. *A Preview of the Policy Sciences.* New York City: American Elsevier.

McGinnis, J. M. 2001. Does proof matter? Why strong evidence sometimes yields weak action. *Am. J. Health Promot.* 15: 391–396.

McLeroy, K. R., D. Bibeau, A. Steckler et al. 1988. An ecological perspective on health promotion programs. *Health Educ. Q.* 15: 351–377.

Newkirk, J. 2010. The NSPAPPH: Answering the call. *J. Phys. Act. Health* 7: S7–S8.

Pucher, J., and L. Dijkstra. 2003. Promoting safe walking and cycling to improve public health: Lessons from The Netherlands and Germany. *Am. J. Public Health* 93: 1509–1516.

Sabatier, P., and H. Jenkins-Smith. 1993. *Policy Change and Learning.* Boulder, CO: Westview Press.

Sallis, J. F., R. Cervero, W. W. Ascher et al. 2006. An ecologic approach to creating active living communities. *Annu. Rev. Public Health* 27: 1–14.

Sallis, J. F., and N. Owen. 1997. Ecological models. In: *Health Behavior and Health Education: Theory, Research, and Practice*, ed. K. Glanz, F. M. Lewis, and B. K. Rimer. San Francisco: Jossey-Bass.

Salvesen, D., K. R. Evenson, D. A. Rodriguez et al. 2008. Factors influencing implementation of local policies to promote physical activity: A case study of Montgomery County, Maryland. *J. Public Health Manag. Pract.* 14: 280–288.

Sarmiento, O., A. Torres, E. Jacoby et al. 2010. The Ciclovía–Recreativa: A mass-recreational program with public health potential. *J. Phys. Act. Health* 7: S163–S180.

Schilling, J., and L. S. Linton. 2005. The public health roots of zoning: In search of active living's legal genealogy. *Am. J. Prev. Med.* 28: 96–104.

Schmid, T. L., M. Pratt, and L. Witmer. 2006. A framework for physical activity policy research. *J. Phys. Act. Health* 3: S20–S29.

Stamatakis, K. A., T. D. McBride, and R. C. Brownson. 2010. Communicating prevention messages to policy makers: the role of stories in promoting physical activity. *J. Phys. Act. Health* 7: S99–S107.

U.S. Department of Health and Human Services. 2008. 2008 Physical Activity Guidelines for Americans. In *ODPHP Publication* No. U0036. Washington, D.C. Available at http://www.health.gov/paguidelines/ (accessed on November 1, 2008).

Yancey, A. K., M. G. Ory, and S. M. Davis. 2006. Dissemination of physical activity promotion interventions in underserved populations. *Am. J. Prev. Med.* 31: S82–S91.

APPENDIX
Glossary of Keywords Used in This Chapter

Term	Definition
Ciclovía	A temporary closing of streets to vehicle traffic to allow bicycling and walking. It also can mean a permanently designated bicycle route. It literally translates into Spanish as "bike path" and the inspiration for the idea comes from Bogotá, Colombia.
Community	The social and physical environment of neighborhoods and cities that contribute to the ecological model.
Community action model	An intervention model to influence change in communities, focused on preparation, policy, physical projects, promotions, and programs.
Ecological framework	A framework to understand health behavior choices, including whether or not to be physically active.
Health disparities	Differences in the incidence, prevalence, burden of diseases, and other adverse health conditions or outcomes between specific population groups.
Health impact assessment	A set of procedures, methods, and tools by which a policy, program, or project may be judged as to its potential effects on the health of a population and the distribution of those effects within the population.
Institutional	Organizational factors in the ecological model, such as the social and physical environment of workplaces, schools, government institutions, hospitals, and other organizations.
Interpersonal	Social factors in the ecological model, such as formal and informal social networks and support systems including family and friends.
Intervention	In this chapter, an intervention refers to an outside process to attempt to change physical activity behavior, either directly or indirectly.
Intrapersonal	Individual level factors in the ecologic model, such as genetics, physiology, motivation, and skill.
Multiple streams framework	An approach by Kingdon (2003) to understand policy change by focusing on the timing of policy actions.
Opportunity cost	The lost opportunity to do something different with that effort and money.
Outcome evaluation	A type of evaluation that assesses whether the intervention (in this case, a policy change) achieved its purpose or intent by focusing on short, intermediate, or long-term outcomes or goals.
Photovoice	This method seeks to bring about increased awareness and change of a problem through photography. In addition to photographs, the process can incorporate discussions around the photos, narratives to go with the photos, and outreach or community action.
Policy	Laws, regulations, formal and informal rules, and understandings or agreements that are adopted to guide both individual and collective behavior.
Policy analysis	The process of determining which of several policy options will be most likely to achieve a given set of goals in a particular context or setting.
Policy stream	One of the three streams in Kingdon's (2003) multiple streams framework, focused on how an issue rises or falls on the political agenda.
Political stream	One of the three streams in Kingdon's (2003) multiple streams framework, focused on the willingness of various stakeholders to place an issue on the agenda.

Problem stream	One of the three streams in Kingdon's (2003) multiple streams framework, focused on the identification of a problem to become addressed through policy.
Process evaluation	A type of evaluation that focuses on the quality and implementation of ongoing activities and interventions.
RE-AIM framework	RE-AIM stands for Reach, Effectiveness, Adoption, Implementation, and Maintenance. It is a framework that provides guidance on evaluating interventions.
Scale	Policies are considered at the local, regional or state, or national levels.
Stage approach	This functional approach to studying the policy process focuses on different stages of the policy process, rather than on their timing.

Index